ANDROGENIC DISORDERS

ANDROGENIC DISORDERS

Editor

Geoffrey P. Redmond, M.D.

President
Foundation for Developmental Endocrinology, Inc.
Beachwood, Ohio

Raven Press New York

Raven Press, Ltd., 1185 Avenue of the Americas, New York, New York 10036

Made in the United States of America

Library of Congress Cataloging-in-Publication Data

Androgenic disorders / editor, Geoffrey P. Redmond.
     p. cm.
   ISBN 0-7817-0274-7
   1. Endocrine gynecology.   2. Androgens—Pathophysiology.
3. Women—Diseases—Endocrine aspects.   I. Redmond, Geoffrey P.
   [DNLM: 1. Androgens—physiology. 2. Endocrine Diseases—
physiopathology. 3. Endocrine Diseases—therapy. 4. Skin
Appendage Diseases—physiopathology. 5. Skin Appendage Diseases—
therapy.   WJ 875 A5737 1995]
   RG163.A64   1995
   618.1—dc20
   DNLM/DLC
   for Library of Congress   94-46125
                                           CIP

9 8 7 6 5 4 3 2 1

For Ming-mei

Contents

Contributing Authors

Wilma F. Bergfeld, M.D. *Head, Clinical Research, Department of Dermatology, Cleveland Clinic Foundation, 9500 Euclid Avenue, Cleveland, Ohio 44195*

Laurence M. Demers, Ph.D. *Professor of Pathology and Medicine, Department of Pathology, The Pennsylvania State University, The Milton S. Hershey Medical Center, 500 University Drive, Hershey, Pennsylvania 17033*

Richard J. Derman, M.D., M.P.H., F.A.C.O.G. *Visiting Professor of Obstetrics and Gynecology, University of Illinois School of Medicine, Chicago, Illinois 10952*

Walter Futterweit, M.D., F.A.C.P. *Clinical Professor of Medicine, Department of Medicine, Division of Endocrinology, The Mount Sinai School of Medicine, 1 Gustave Levy Place, New York, New York 10029*

Peter A. Lee, M.D., Ph.D. *Professor of Pediatrics, Department of Pediatrics, University of Pittsburgh School of Medicine, Children's Hospital of Pittsburgh, 3705 Fifth Avenue, Pittsburgh, Pennsylvania 15213*

Shu-Yuan Liao, M.D. *Associate Clinical Professor of Medicine and Pathology, Department of Medicine, College of Medicine, University of California, Irvine, California 92717*

Sandro Loche, M.D. *Pediatric Endocrinology Service, Ospedale Regionale per le Microcitemie, USL 21, Via Jenner, Cagliari, 09121 Italy*

Maria I. New, M.D. *Professor and Chairman, Department of Pediatrics, Division of Endocrinology, The New York Hospital-Cornell Medical Center, 525 East 68th Street, Room N-236, New York, New York 10021*

Geoffrey P. Redmond, M.D. *President, Foundation for Developmental Endocrinology, Inc., Department of Endocrinology, 23200 Chagrin Boulevard, Suite 325, Building 5, Cleveland, Ohio 44122*

Karen F. Rothman, M.D. *Assistant Professor of Medicine and Pediatrics, University of Massachusetts Medical School, 210 Lincoln Street, Worcester, Massachusetts 01605*

Marty E. Sawaya, M.D., Ph.D. *Assistant Professor of Medicine and Dermatology, Department of Medicine, Division of Dermatology and Cutaneous Surgery, University of Florida College of Medicine, 1601 Southwest Archer Road, P.O. Box 100277, Gainesville, Florida 32610-0277*

Leslie R. Sheeler, M.D., F.A.C.P. *Department of Endocrinology, Innova Medical Services, 7575 North Cliff Avenue, Brooklyn, Ohio 44144*

Selma Witchel Siegel, M.D. *Assistant Professor of Pediatrics, Department of Pediatrics, Children's Hospital of Pittsburgh, University of Pittsburgh School of Medicine, 3705 Fifth Avenue, Pittsburgh, Pennsylvania 15213*

Richard F. Wagner, Jr., M.D., J.D. *Professor of Dermatology, Department of Dermatology, The University of Texas Medical Branch, 301 University Boulevard, Galveston, Texas 77555-0783*

Robert A. Wild, M.D. *Professor and Chief, Section of Research and Education in Women's Health, Adjunct Professor of Medicine (Cardiology), Department of Obstetrics and Gynecology, University of Oklahoma Health Science Center, 801 Northeast 13, CHB-215, Oklahoma City, Oklahoma 73190*

Preface

This book represents a collaboration by investigators concerned with the wide range of deleterious effects androgens can exert on women's bodies. Although there is a considerable amount of basic science in the volume, the authors are clinicians and the intent of the book is to provide the necessary knowledge base for proper care of women with androgenic disorders. This information has been difficult to find because published articles and texts, some of which are excellent, have focused on research issues. But the result of this recent intense research concern is that sufficient knowledge exists to form the basis for helping affected women in very practical ways. With current treatment methods, it is possible to reduce hirsutism, clear most cases of female acne, stabilize and sometimes improve androgenic alopecia, protect the uterus from the oncogenic effects of chronic anovulation, and make an early identification of women with important cardiovascular risk factors. Any physician who treats women needs to be informed about these matters, and this book is intended to do so.

The true incidence of androgenic disorders is unknown, in part, because general agreement on a definition is necessary for epidemiological studies to be done. A telephone survey of which I am aware suggests that about 10% of American women remove facial hair at least weekly. An unknown fraction of them have an androgenic disorder. The incidence of polycystic ovary syndrome (PCOS) is often stated to be 5% to 10%, which is of similar magnitude. A disorder that affects one out of twenty or more women is extremely common and deserves far more attention that it has so far received.

Although androgenic disorders are among the most common disorders of women and certainly the most common of all female endocrinopathies, they are little known to health professionals and to the lay public. There are several reasons for this neglect. Terminology has been confusing, so that the linguistic resources needed to develop clear concepts have been lacking. Then, the most obvious changes in androgenic disorders are those which affect appearance and the medical profession has been ambivalent about appearance as a valid reason for treatment. Because the empiric treatment of anovulation associated with androgenic disorders has advanced so greatly, there has been less pressure to understand the pathophysiology. What may be the most important aspect of androgenic disorders in public health terms—their association with insulin resistance, diabetes, and lipid abnormalities—as been slow to be recognized, so that, even now, few women with these complications are being diagnosed. Finally, the specialty structure of medicine has hindered progress because the androgenic disorders are divided among several specialties. Dermatologists generally see the skin manifestations, such as acne and androgenic alopecia; gynecologists handle the infertility; and endocrinologists treat the hirsutism. The patient being treated for polycystic ovary syndrome will most likely be seeing a gynecologist, but if adrenal involvement is suspected, an endocrinologist will be consulted. This division of labor hinders anyone from seeing the entire picture of androgenic disorders, and too often means that affected women do not obtain comprehensive care for their condition.

Fortunately, the concept of androgenic disorders as a broad category of overlapping entities is gaining currency. In the past, a variety of terms were applied including idiopathic hirsutism, cystic acne, androgenic alopecia, polycystic ovary disease, and nonclassical adrenal hyperplasia, and the use of these terms tends to be specialty-specific and inconsistent. Use of the term androgenic disorder is preferred because it is the most general and is descriptive without implying more than is known about the underlying cause. It also classifies together patients who have different manifestations of the same underlying endocrine disorder, for example, women with cystic acne and those with hirsutism.

The term that has been most misleading in actual use is polycystic ovarian disease (PCOD). Overuse of this diagnostic label has held back understanding of androgenic disorders. Polycystic ovarian disease is an anatomical term and refers to an abnormality of the structure of the ovaries. Yet patients who present with it do so because of physiological change: irregular periods, infertility, hirsutism, cystic acne, etc. Often the diagnosis is made and treatment given without ever determining if the ovaries are truly polycystic. However, the finding of presence or absence of small cysts on ultrasound does not correlate clearly with endocrine abnormalities. Often, if an ultrasound is performed, the ovaries are not, in fact, filled with small cysts. This does not mean that the ovary is not the source of the endocrine disturbance (though it sometimes is not), but it does mean that the label of polycystic ovarian disease is not factual. The opposite error also occurs. The physiology of ovulation is such that normal ovaries frequently contain small cysts and such an appearance on ultrasound often leads to a label of polycystic ovarian disease being applied to a woman in whom periods are regular, ovulation apparently normal, and there is no excess of body hair. The description of the ovaries as polycystic may be literally correct, but the endocrinopathy of the same name is not present.

My proposed solution is to abandon the term polycystic ovarian disease altogether or at least reserve it for women who have the full blown syndrome of oligoamenorrhea, annovulation, usually hirsutism or other androgen effects on the skin, and ovaries with multiple small cysts and a thickened capsule. Less complete versions can be called simply ovarian androgen excess, which is descriptively accurate and does not imply more than is there. Polycystic ovaries is also a term that is best avoided because many find it confusing and alarming. Patients imagine they have tumors in the ovary, or, if they read about the condition in medical texts, they rarely find the descriptions flattering.

The terminology for adrenal androgen excess is equally murky. Adrenal hyperplasia, like polycystic ovaries, is an anatomical term applied to what is really a physiological change. The term late-onset adrenal hyperplasia is also confusing because consistent criteria for making the diagnosis do not exist. Furthermore, late-onset adrenal hyperplasia implies a late or mild form of the classical enzyme deficiencies, but in some cases, it is not certain whether women with the late onset form have a disorder that is really related to the genetic form. The terms adrenal hyperplasia or late onset adrenal hyperplasia or partial adrenal hyperplasia should be reserved for women in whom detailed testing has in fact revealed a deficiency of an adrenal steroidogenic enzyme by measurement of levels of metabolites. Few women with excess androgen secretion have this deficiency. The most general term is adrenal androgen excess, and this term that should be used.

What about women with androgenic skin changes but normal androgen levels? This group is least well served by existing terminology because there is no common expression to describe their condition. Often they are told that nothing is wrong or that they do not have an endocrine disorder because the hormone levels measured fell into the reference range printed on the lab report. Some women in this group have rather severe androgenic changes, such as hirsutism requiring twice-a-day shaving, severe acne with progressive scarring, or oligomenorrhea and infertility. These women do have an androgenic disorder in the sense that they have abnormalities resulting from androgen action. An appropriate term would be simply increased androgen action. This does not suggest that secretion is abnormal, though sometimes it may be abnormal but difficult to document. The term puts the focus on where the problem lies: the action of, rather than the secretion of, androgenic hormones.

I believe that much of the puzzlement evoked in physicians by women with androgenic disorders can be avoided by following the suggestions made here for clarification of terms. "Androgenic disorder" is most general and refers to any situation in which a woman is experiencing unwanted effects attributable to the action of androgens. Some women in this category have increased androgen levels and therefore can be said to have androgen excess. Appropriate testing can separate these categories into subcategories of "ovarian androgen excess," "adrenal androgen excess," or "mixed androgen excess." When androgens are not elevated, the phrase increased androgen action is straightforward. In this situation, there may be some undiscovered hypersecretion or end-organ sensitivity. These terms are not mutually exclusive but refer to the three possible physiological factors in androgenic disorders: ovarian hypersecretion, adrenal hypersecretion, and end-organ hyperresponsiveness. While terms that imply knowledge of the underlying cause may seem more satisfying, they are also more vulnerable to misleading use.

The need to take appearance changes seriously is being more widely recognized as physicians listen to their patients' concerns more objectively, in part because patients have become more assertive and more insistent that their concerns be addressed. They are, quite properly, less willing to be patronized while their concerns remain unaddressed. There is also a better appreciation within the health care professions of the importance of quality-of-life issues. It needs to be pointed out that for the physician to be concerned with helping a patient's appearance does not mean an endorsement of judging people by their appearance but rather an acceptance that this practice is universal in human societies and that people should be helped to live within their society.

While specialists in androgenic disorders are now aware that patients must be evaluated for metabolic complications, there is much less recognition by health professionals at large of androgenic changes and upper-segment obesity as physical signs indicative of risk for diabetes and hyperlipidemia. This is part of a more general failure to detect and treat such abnormalities early. It is hoped that more progress will be made in this area in the next few years.

The final problem mentioned, lack of interaction between specialists of different disciplines, does seem to be improving. This book is itself evidence of the fact. The authors include medical scientists and physicians of a variety of specialties, all of whom share an interest in androgenic disorders. A recent NIH-sponsored conference on the subject attests to a similar trend. One of the editor's hopes for this volume is that it will attract others to an interest in furthering understanding of androgenic disorders.

As befits a subject with some areas of controversy, there are disagreements between different authors in this volume. As editor, I have not tried to remove these because I believe that in the present state of knowledge the reader is better served by exposure to differing viewpoints.

Geoffrey Redmond

Acknowledgments

I thank first the contributors to this volume who dived into a complex and often confusing literature and emerged with clarity. Doctor Richard Derman took a particular interest in the project and has given myself and others dedicated to improving our knowledge of androgenic disorders ideas and encouragement with his usual enthusiasm. I also benefitted from stimulating discussion about androgenic disorders with Doctors Walter Futterweit, Robert Rosenfield, Anne Lucky, Robert Wild, and others. For stimulating my nascent interest in androgenic disorders and collaboration over many years I am indebted to Doctor Wilma Bergfeld.

Mary Dettmer, Patricia Kelly, and Sandra Baskin have worked with me as nurse–practitioners in caring for women with androgenic disorders. They have made this work a pleasure and contributed greatly to research and education in this area.

I have been fortunate to have had outstanding teachers in the past who guided my efforts to learn and who gave essential encouragement. These include Doctor Gerald Cohen, in whose laboratory I did my first research on endocrinology, Doctors Akira Morishima and Jennifer Bell at Columbia University College of Physicians and Surgeons, Bruce McEwen and Lewis Krey at Rockefeller University, Lester Soyka at the University of Vermont, and O. Peter Schumacher at the Cleveland Clinic.

Several pharmaceutical companies have supported my projects in research and education regarding androgenic disorders and I wish to thank them.

Pam Alderman, Director of the Mount Sinai Medical Center Medical Library in Cleveland has given generously and cheerfully of her time and expertise; without her help and that of her staff my chapters in this book could not have been written.

Carol Siverd coordinated the project and kept contributors and myself on track and was able to remain unruffled throughout.

Kerry Willis patiently encouraged me to take on this project. Mark Placito, my editor, and others at Raven Press, were unfailingly supportive and helpful; their professionalism was exemplary.

ANDROGENIC DISORDERS

Androgenic Disorders,
edited by G. P. Redmond.
Raven Press, Ltd., New York © 1995.

1

Clinical Evaluation of the Woman with an Androgenic Disorder

Geoffrey P. Redmond

*Department of Endocrinology, Foundation for Developmental Endocrinology, Inc.,
Cleveland, Ohio 44122*

Clinical evaluation of the woman with an androgenic disorder is complex. However, despite some remaining scientific uncertainties, a diagnosis, at least in terms of which specific factors are operative, is always possible in the specific patient. However there are a number of points of confusion and this chapter will attempt to identify these areas and provide clarification. Recently, there is a greater degree of agreement among those interested in androgenic disorders as to the nature of the conditions, as evinced in recent reviews (1–4).

A careful and detailed history is essential to proper care of the woman with an androgenic disorder. Not only is it necessary to identify which manifestations she has but also which are most troubling to her. Since treatments for different manifestations may be different or even mutually incompatible, it is important to learn what the patient perceives to be her problem. There are three groups of androgenic abnormalities that may be of varying concern to different individuals or the same individual at different times in her life. Of most familiarity to the gynecologist is the associated anovulation and consequent infertility. The patient may have come for help in conceiving or she may have oligo-amenorrhea and be concerned about her prospects for future fertility. On the other hand, at many times in a woman's life fertility is not a goal and the effects on appearance may be her main concern. Finally the metabolic abnormalities—diabetes and lipid changes—may be the primary concern. It is not unusual, as in other situations, that the patient's initial complaint is not her major concern. Thus for example, a woman who has not become pregnant after years of unprotected intercourse may come for treatment of hirsutism having wrongly concluded that she is irretrievably infertile. Her goal may change when told that ovulation induction might be successful.

It must be said, however, that women have a much easier time finding help for the infertility associated with androgenic disorders than for the effects on appearance or metabolism. Until quite recently, women's health professionals primarily concerned themselves either with reproduction or with removal of the reproductive organs when this was no longer possible or desired. While not denying the central importance of childbearing to the lives of most (but not all) women, it must be pointed out that during most of a woman's life her body is not involved in being or attempting to be pregnant. Some women feel their other health concerns have been neglected and this is especially so of those with androgenic disorders.

Another point of great importance when taking a history from a woman with an androgenic disorder is to be tactful and sensitive when asking about embarrassing matters. Most of the women I see as patients have consulted with other doctors before and a high proportion have been hurt or angry with how they were treated. Androgenic changes are directly damaging to self-esteem and questions must be worded in a tactful fashion. Above all it is necessary to make it clear that you take the patient's problem seriously. A physician who considers normal concern with appearance to be a sign of vanity or neurosis will have a difficult time working with patients with androgenic disorders. I have discussed the concerns women patients have regarding androgenic and other hormonal disorders at greater length elsewhere (5).

History taking should consider the several ways in which androgenic disorders affect the body. Within each, I find it most useful to follow a developmental and continuing sequence beginning with pubertal development and continuing up to the present. Although many women with hirsutism have had hypertrichosis as little girls, few are aware of this and it is usually recalled only by their mothers. Other changes appear during the sequence of puberty and increase into adulthood.

In this discussion, I will cover what must be included in the history as completely as possible. The actual sequence may be different, based on the patient's presenting complaint. If, as is often the case, she is worried about increased hair growth, then it is best to begin with the skin manifestations. If menstrual abnormalities are the primary concern, then one can begin there.

The ways androgenic disorders affect a woman's body can be summarized into the three categories of menstruation and fertility, skin and hair, and metabolism.

CLINICAL MANIFESTATIONS

Menstruation and Fertility

Oligo-amenorrhea is one of the classical features of Stein-Leventhal syndrome. About one-third of women with androgenic disorders have abnormal menstrual patterns (6). It should be noted that the incidence seen is greatly affected by the clinical specialty of the consulting physician. A woman most concerned with menstrual abnormalities is likely to consult a gynecologist, a woman with cystic acne, a dermatologist, and so on. Each specialist therefore sees the different manifestations in different proportions.

The characteristic change of menstruation in androgenic disorders is less frequent menstruation, not dysfunctional bleeding. It is true that anovulation can *eventually* lead to excessive bleeding, but it usually does not do so initially. Because of the need to treat anovulation early with cyclic progestins to decrease the risk of endometrial cancer, it is important not to take lack of excessive bleeding as indicating the lack of potentially serious endometrial changes. Dysfunctional bleeding is not much more common in women with androgenic disorders than in others, and when present it may be due to uterine myomata or other unrelated causes (7). However there is a subgroup of women with androgenic disorders, generally markedly obese, who do have a pattern of oligomenorrhea alternating with intervals of prolonged bleeding that may last for several weeks at a time but is not usually heavy. Such women need pelvic ultrasound to examine endometrial thickness and endometrial biopsy depending on their situation, and most should have long-term progestin replacement. Dilatation and curettage (D & C) is the old remedy for such situations, but while this is sometimes necessary to obtain hemostasis with very heavy bleeding or tissue diagnosis, it does not correct the underlying hormonal abnormality and thus is not a long-term solution.

It is sometimes assumed that anovulatory women have excessive bleeding because the endometrium is not prepared for hemostasis with progesterone. However, some have menstrual periods of normal duration and amount that are infrequent. Lack of abnormally frequent or heavy bleeding does not exclude the possibility of endometrial hyperplasia or carcinoma associated with anovulation. Many women with endometrial carcinoma or precancerous lesions have had oligo-amenorrhea for many years that was not treated because either the physician or the patient thought the lack of menses to be unimportant. This is regrettable and unnecessary. All women with oligo-amenorrhea should be considered to be anovulatory and treated with progestin replacement or with other modalities as appropriate. Persistent anovulation is a disorder requiring treatment in all cases (8). In androgenic disorders, lack of menses is associated with lack of progesterone but usually not with estrogen deficiency. Adequacy of estrogen can usually be confirmed by a progestin withdrawal test, but it must be pointed out that the meaning of this test is often misunderstood. Some women who usually have normal or high estrogen levels will not bleed following progestin challenge, perhaps because at that particular time the endometrium was not stimulated. Such women still need progestin replacement.

In our experience, about a third of women with androgenic disorders have oligo- or amenorrhea. Usually this has been their menstrual pattern since adolescence. Although published studies indicate that adolescent oligo-amenorrhea is likely to be due to a persistent endocrine abnormality (9), physicians are still likely to misinterpret menstrual abnormalities in adolescent girls as a variant of normal. Often polycystic ovary syndrome (PCO) has its initial presentation as infrequent menstruation in adolescence.

A diagnostic pitfall is to attribute amenorrhea in a hirsute woman to PCO when the cause is different, such as hyperprolactinemia. When a woman presents with amenorrhea, the diagnostic procedure appropriate for amenorrhea should be carried out (10,11). Hirsutism is common and cannot be assumed to indicate PCO as the cause of amenorrhea simply because both are present. A complete workup for amenorrhea is always necessary, including assays for prolactin and follicle-stimulating hormone (FSH).

In general, oligo-amenorrhea is associated with more severe manifestations of androgenic disorders, especially marked hirsutism and android obesity (12). Most women with marked hirsutism are obese, but mild hirsutism is not unusual in slender women. Menstrual disturbances are less common in hirsute women who are not obese. Even in the presence of hirsutism or other androgenic manifestations, other causes of oligo-amenorrhea such as hyperprolactinemia must be ruled out. When oligo-amenorrhea is present it usually, but not invariably, indicates the presence of PCO rather than another form of androgenic disorder. Exceptions would be women with distinctly elevated androgens due to another cause such as late onset adrenal hyperplasia. Androgen-secreting tumors and Cushing's syndrome can also cause oligo-amenorrhea.

Infertility in association with PCO is generally due to anovulation and treatment for this is highly advanced. As it is the subject of a recent book (13), ovulation induction methods will not be discussed here. Several points need to be made, however. First, the majority of women with androgenic disorders menstruate regularly and do not have problems with fertility. Even those with oligomenorrhea may ovulate several times a year and become pregnant without treatment. I have seen many who were given an unnecessarily pessimistic prognosis about future fertility. The temptation to tell women with menstrual abnormalities that they will never be able to become pregnant should be resisted. In fact the chance of pregnancy in the face of PCO-related anovulation is relatively good and this should be communicated in order to alleviate worries which might not be verbalized.

Oligo-amenorrhea does not have to be present to make a diagnosis of an androgenic disorder, even PCO. Especially early in the course of the disease, menstruation may be normal or only an occasional period is missed. It is also true that some women with PCO have only slight or no visible androgenization, and oligo-amenorrhea may be the sole presenting abnormality (14). The degree of hirsutism, acne, or alopecia depends not only on androgen levels, but also on ethnic and individual differences. While there does seem to be a correlation between free testosterone and hirsutism scores (15,16), it seems likely that these other factors account for more of the variance between individual women with respect to terminal hair growth and other androgenic skin effects.

The syndrome described by Stein and Leventhal represents the *extreme* form of the disease, as often happens when a syndrome is first discovered. Milder androgenic disorders often lack some of the features of the extreme forms. Indeed, as stressed above, the majority of women with androgenic disorders have normal menstrual patterns.

Skin and Hair Changes

It is the skin changes that are the most characteristic and noticeable effects of androgenic disorders; they are far and away what most motivate affected women to consult doctors. While the relation of hirsutism to androgen action is generally acknowledged, the same is not true of acne and alopecia. However, the role of androgens in stimulation of the sebaceous glands and inactivation of scalp hair follicles is well established. This is discussed in Chapter 11. Acne and alopecia are as much the result of androgen action as is hirsutism.

The appearance of androgenic skin changes follows a developmental sequence. Seborrhea occurs quickly after androgen levels rise; consequently acne is usually the first skin manifestation and begins at the youngest age. Acne can begin perimenarchally but usually becomes worse after menarche. Sometimes its onset is much later for reasons which are usually unclear. Hirsutism is the result of the vellus hairs becoming thicker, darker, and stiffer terminal hairs. This requires months to years of androgen exposure and so often appears at a somewhat older age than does acne. However hirsutism too can begin around the time of menarche, though more commonly it is first noticed in the late teens and continues to increase through the early twenties. Hirsutism further increases with age, but in most women in whom it is not too severe, the later increases are relatively slight. Alopecia is uncommon before the late twenties or early thirties. When it does occur early it is an unfavorable sign in terms of future quantity of scalp hair.

This inherent ontogeny of androgenic skin changes must be kept in mind when evaluating individual patients. Because changes take time to become more severe, a given degree of hirsutism or alopecia in an adolescent or young adult is more significant than a comparable degree in an older woman. Thus a 14-year-old with oligomenorrhea due to what will eventually be severe PCO might well not yet be hirsute.

Acne

Acne is familiar to everyone, but for this reason it is often overlooked during physical examination. The acne process begins with androgen action to increase sebum production by the pilosebaceous unit. Later there is plugging in part due to abnormal stickiness of the keratin. Bacterial action chemically alters fatty acids in sebum to more irritating forms. It is important to remember however that without androgen action on the sebaceous gland acne will not occur. It is because androgens rise then that acne begins at puberty. Typically acne worsens in the late luteal phase of the cycle; this is true even in women taking nonandrogenic oral contraceptives. Why androgen effects at this time in the cycle are greater is not entirely clear.

The mildest acne lesions are termed comedones. Closed comedones are whiteheads and open comedones are blackheads. Contrary to the beliefs of mothers of teens everywhere, the dark spot of an open comedone is not dirt but melanin from broken down skin. Purely comedonal acne is not usually bothersome unless it is quite extensive. It is when inflammatory lesions appear that concern arises and the possibility of scarring exists. Papules are red raised areas; when they have fluid in them they are pustules. Inflammatory lesions greater than 5 mm in diameter are nodules and those larger than 10 mm are cysts. Cystic acne refers to acne with chronic presence of these large inflammatory lesions. Their appearance is unpleasant and often they are painful. Even without excoriation they may leave scars when they heal.

Acne is often wrongly dismissed as a trivial problem. Cystic acne should be considered a medical problem of some urgency because it is disfiguring. Over time, as more lesions appear and heal, scarring increases and becomes difficult or impossible to conceal. Pits are most visible and characteristic but there may also be small protuberances caused by destruction of elastic tissue and enlargement of pores on the facial skin. Postinflammatory hyperpigmentation may occur to a highly visible degree, especially in dark-pigmented individuals. Hyperpigmentation is especially frequent in pseudofolliculitis barbae which is caused by ingrowing of hairs removed by shaving or plucking. The distribution in hair removal areas serves to differentiate this lesion from acne. It is especially common in blacks or others with curly hair.

A common variant of acne vulgaris is acne rosacea. This is coalescent inflammation usually on the nose and malar area. It is sometimes confused with lupus but does not have the destructive effect of cutaneous lupus. The patient is distressed not only by the conspicuousness of the redness but also because it can look like the effects of alcohol excess. Chronic acne rosacea can leave permanent changes: thickening of the skin at the tip of the nose and visible capillaries on the malar area which are irreversible. It tends to occur at an older age than acne vulgaris. Although the infectious factor in rosacea may be different from acne vulgaris, it is also an androgen dependent change.

Acne is not the only skin change that can result from the excessive sebum production induced by androgens. Most women with increased androgen action have some degree of seborrheic dermatitis. This is low grade inflammation induced by sebum in the midline of the face or the scalp. Dandruff is one result of seborrhea on the scalp and there may be visible flakes of skin on the face also. Patients usually think the flaking is due to dryness but the problem is that the oiliness of the skin causes the flakes to stick and so be visible. Seborrhea of the scalp can also cause crusting and itching.

Another condition related to acne is hidradenitis supporativa. This is chronic abscess formation characteristically in apocrine sweat areas, the axillae and groin. It can occur in other intertriginous areas especially under the breasts. Obesity is also a factor in hidradenitis. Androgen action is also involved but may be less important than in acne. With time, extensive scarring can develop in affected areas. Lesions may be large and difficult to eradicate with systemic antibiotics so that incision and drainage is sometimes required.

Hirsutism

Skin areas vary greatly in their sensitivity to androgens. On the face, the most sensitive areas are the chin and neck (actually the skin under the jaw), followed by the upper lip and the cheeks. On the body the lateral aspects of the pubic region are first affected, then the linea alba, the upper thighs, and the midline of the chest followed by the lateral chest. On chest and abdomen, the more hair coverage there is lateral to the midline, the greater is the androgen effect. The face is the area which most concerns women because it is always visible. In summer or in geographical areas where clothes with little body coverage are preferred, upper leg hair or arm hair is a greater concern.

Careful inspection of the face will reveal the extent of hair growth. On the chin, dark terminal hairs are most common on the rounded area anteriorly and extending inferiorly. The midline most often has no hairs or hairs that are less stiff than the ones to the sides. The neck frequently is affected. These hairs are easier to conceal but the sensitive skin here is more easily irritated by removal methods, especially shaving. Plucking however is more injurious to the skin. The root is avulsed and injury deep in the skin occurs. There may be pseudofolliculitis initially and women who practice plucking over the long term develop an uneven, lumpy appearance to the chin which is not fully reversible. Areas which are regularly plucked may develop overall postinflammatory hyperpigmentation. Plucking is often preferred, however, because it does not have the unfeminine associations of shaving and because it produces a longer period of invisibility of the hairs.

On the upper lip, as androgen effect increases, hairs are first seen on the lateral corners and move toward the midline. Even women who shave daily rarely have as fully developed a moustache as men attain. However, the growth on the chin and neck may become heavy enough to require twice-a-day shaving for the affected woman to feel secure that it cannot be detected. The sideburn and cheek areas have the most variation in hair growth. The sideburn area is most sensitive superiorly with sideburns getting lower as androgen effect increases. Also sensitive to androgens is the skin along the mandible. Anteriorly the cheeks are least androgen sensitive but terminal hairs do appear there in some women.

Most women—and their physicians—do not have a clear idea of what constitutes a normal amount of facial and body hair for a woman. However, the misestimations are usually in opposite directions. Nearly all hirsute women do their best to conceal their extra hair, some with sufficient success to hide it from the physician as well as others. As with other subtle physical findings, hirsutism takes experience and care to recognize. When teaching endocrinology residents, I have noticed that most under- rather than over-score for hirsutism. Use of the Ferriman-Gallwey system (17) or the modified version we have developed (Fig. 1) is helpful in learning how to assess quantity of hair growth clinically. However, it is not very sensitive for detecting changes in hair growth with treatment. There have been studies of hair growth patterns in women (18), but more are needed. In our present pluricultural society, the physician should be aware of ethnic differences in quantity and distribution of hair. Considering how common hirsutism is, gynecologists or other physicians who think they see few women with hirsutism are probably failing to recognize it.

In judging their own hirsutism, women have the opposite problem: They often think they have more hair compared to other women than is actually the case. Of course, one notices changes in one's own body more readily than in others. Depic-

Grade and Definition (Enter numerical grade in box.)

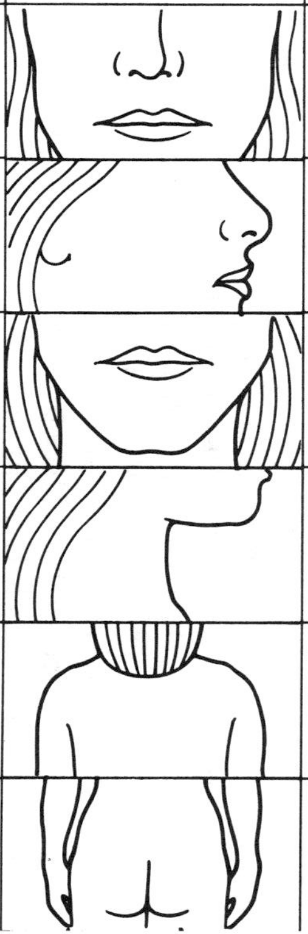

Site	1	2	3	4
Upper Lip	A few terminal hairs at outer margin or scattered over upper lip	A small moustache at outer margin or covering less than half of upper lip	A moustache extending halfway from outer margin or halfway up lip	A moustache extending to mid-line and covering most of upper lip
Sideburn Area	A few scattered terminal hairs	Scattered terminal hairs with small concentrations	Light coverage of entire area	Dense coverage of entire area
Chin	A few scattered terminal hairs	Scattered terminal hairs with small concentrations	Complete but light coverage	Complete and heavy coverage
Lower Jaw and Upper Neck	A few scattered hairs	Scattered hairs with small concentrations	Light coverage of entire area	Complete and dense coverage of entire area
Upper Back	A few scattered terminal hairs	More terminal hairs, but still scattered	Complete but light coverage	Complete and dense coverage
Lower Back	Some sacral hair (area of coverage less than 4 cm wide)	With greater lateral extension	Three-quarter coverage	Complete coverage

FIG. 1. Hirsutism rating scale (*continued on p. 9*). (Modified from ref. 17.)

Region		Grade 1	Grade 2	Grade 3	Grade 4
Upper Arm		☐ Sparse growth affecting not more than a quarter of the limb surface	☐ More than this; coverage still incomplete	☐ Complete but light coverage	☐ Complete and dense coverage
Thigh		☐ Sparse growth affecting not more than a quarter of the limb surface	☐ More than this; coverage still incomplete	☐ Complete but light coverage	☐ Complete and dense coverage
Chest		☐ Terminal circumareolar hairs or midline hairs	☐ Both terminal circumareolar hairs and midline hairs	☐ Three-quarter coverage	☐ Complete coverage
Upper Abdomen		☐ A few midline terminal hairs	☐ More terminal hairs, still midline	☐ Half coverage	☐ Full coverage
Lower Abdomen		☐ A few midline terminal hairs along linea alba	☐ A midline streak of terminal hair	☐ A midline band of terminal hair not more than 1/2 width of pubic hair at base	☐ An inverted V-shaped growth 1/2 width of pubic hair at base
Perineum		☐ Perianal terminal hair	☐ Lateral extension of terminal hair to edge of gluteal cleft	☐ Three-quarter coverage of buttocks	☐ Complete coverage of buttocks
Column Subtotals					

Total Score

tion of women's skin in the media contributes to this. When women are photographed in fashion magazines or even in men's magazines, what might seem defects are concealed. Hair can be concealed by lighting, by soft focus or by prior removal with waxing. This leads to the impression that normal women have only pubic and axillary hair but none on other locations. Even axillary hair is removed by most American women as is leg hair. Some visible terminal hairs are also normal around the areolae and along the linea alba but as these are not visible under clothes, many women think they are the only ones who have hair there. Although hair is normal in these locations, many do not know that it is normal. Hair on the breast may be particularly of concern since this appears to be a masculinizing change on what is thought of as one of the most feminine parts of a woman's body.

Alopecia

Of all the androgenic skin changes, alopecia is the most distressing to women affected by it. Yet it is scarcely mentioned in endocrinology or gynecology texts or training programs. Dermatologists are aware of it but less familiar with the underlying endocrine etiology. Yet it is a major cause of distress in otherwise healthy women. For this reason, it is important to learn to recognize androgenic alopecia as the result of an abnormality of hormone action (19).

"Alopecia" simply means loss of scalp hair. It has many causes including infection and autoimmunity. However, by far the most common causes are endocrine. Endocrine alopecia is usually referred to as androgenic alopecia or sometimes as androgenetic alopecia, the latter to emphasize a genetic factor. I prefer the former term; it is not a coinage and does not misleadingly imply a genetic element that, though probable, cannot be demonstrated by the physical finding of alopecia in the androgenic distribution.

Androgenic alopecia has a characteristic distribution which is almost always sufficient to indicate the diagnosis of endocrine alopecia. However, the term is somewhat misleading since alopecia that occurs at menopause, often in women with very low androgen levels, has an identical distribution. The etiology of excess androgen action or inadequate estrogenic action is indicated not by the pattern of loss but by the related circumstances such as age of onset and progression.

The most sensitive area for androgenic alopecia is the vertex, followed by the crown. Indeed the vertex is the part of the scalp on which everyone's hair is thinnest. Thinning around it is not unusual even when there is no diminution elsewhere. Some women have progression to the point of having a bald spot on the vertex. Vertex hair thinning is easily concealed by bringing back the hair on the top of the head or sides; women who choose such styles may make their alopecia inapparent to others including physicians. Thinning on the top of the head is harder to conceal. The mildest degree is simply a widened part but in more marked cases the shiny skin of the scalp becomes visible.

Textbooks typically list one of the signs of virilization in women as anterior hair line recession. This does indeed occur in severe androgen excess. However in androgenic alopecia, one of the striking features is that the anterior hair line is preserved. This is in contrast to the situation in men in whom some anterior hairline recession is usual, even in those with little or no balding. In women, a normal anterior hair line does not rule out androgenic alopecia. Thinning over the temples behind the anterior hairline is common. Some women are unaware or unbothered by this, but others find it disturbing.

I use a grading system of minimal–mild–moderate–severe. Minimal means that there may be some widening of the part or thinning at the vertex, but it is barely noticeable. With mild alopecia, thinning is definite but scalp is not readily visible from the top or back. In moderate alopecia, the scalp is still covered by hair but is visible through it. Marked alopecia is frank baldness with areas of scalp completely visible.

It is important to differentiate androgenic alopecia from other forms. The most dramatic form of alopecia is areata which has three degrees of severity. Alopecia areata refers to loss of hair from discrete areas with other areas being completely unaffected. It is most commonly noticed on the scalp but can affect other regions such as the eyelashes or the pubic, leg, or axillary regions. In alopecia areata totalis, all hair is lost from the scalp but other areas still have hair. In alopecia areata universalis, all body hair is lost. Androgenic alopecia never affects hair other than on the scalp, so when there is loss of hair on these other areas, the underlying process is usually areata. However, occasionally women with androgenic alopecia will notice some thinning of eyebrow or eyelash hair, and it is not unusual to have some thinning of pubic hair after menopause. The cause of these changes is unknown although they might be minute areas of alopecia areata in some affected people. A useful point of differentiation is that androgenic alopecia is more marked on top and spares the sides, while alopecia areata, although it can affect the crown, is usually more pronounced on the sides.

Alopecia can result from trauma to the hair from several causes. It is important to recognize these when they are present but equally important not to attribute androgenic or alopecia areata to mishandling. Androgenic alopecia is far more common than the traumatic forms. Trichotillomania is the elegant name for the habit of hair pulling. Some women with this habit are not aware of it or may deny it is the cause of their thin hair. Stopping the practice is difficult. Far more common is traction alopecia in which the hair is pulled out at the root during styling. This is common in African-American women who often use pomade to style their hair which increases the force transmitted during traction. Cornrows and similar styles also involve strong traction being placed on the hair and alopecia around each braid is common. Ponytails and other styles which involve pulling or brushing the hair back can also cause traction alopecia. Sometimes, wearing of a hair band can cause breakage of the hair underneath and a resulting area of thinning.

Cure of these forms of alopecia is simple, at least in principle: Avoid placing traction on the hair. A brush should be used instead of a comb (the idea that repeated brushing of hair is beneficial is the opposite of the truth since it subjects the hair to greater traction than combing), any curling should be done loosely, and combing with hot air from the blow dryer should be avoided. A blow dryer can be used but the heat should be turned off.

Other hair-care or styling practices rarely are a factor in alopecia. Modern perms, dyes, etc. in these days of product liability are generally safe. The only common practice which tends to injure hair is bleaching, either by itself or as the first step in dying with a lighter color. Bleaching should be avoided by women concerned about alopecia. African-American women should avoid hair treatments which utilize dye. Shampoos are frequently asked about but do not seem to be a factor in alopecia.

Acanthosis Nigricans

This exotic-sounding lesion was once thought to be rare (20,21) but is now known to be present in as many as 10% of markedly obese women. Dunaif suggests that about 50% of obese women with PCO have acanthosis nigricans (ACN) (22). It is important because it is often a marker of insulin resistance and diabetes. In Dunaif's study, PCO women with ACN had higher insulin responses to glucose than those without it. While the incidence of diabetes in women with ACN is less than originally reported, it is high. It is likely that women with ACN who have normal glucose tolerance when tested are at greatly increased risk of developing diabetes, but this has not been demonstrated in prospective studies. A distinct syndrome comprising ACN, PCO, and insulin resistant diabetes has been suggested. While it is true that these three entities are often found in the same woman, it is unclear that it represents a distinct syndrome. Rather, there is a close association between ACN and androgenic disorders, particularly PCO. ACN can also be a marker for occult malignancy, especially of the gastrointestinal tract but also elsewhere. This possibility should be considered in those over 40.

It is likely that ACN was presumed rare is because it is distributed on areas rarely inspected in the physical examination: the back of the neck, which in women is nearly always hidden by hair, and the axillae. It can also appear on other intertriginous regions such as the lower edge of the breast, within abdominal fat folds and anywhere else that skin rubs against skin. ACN, except in certain very rare conditions, is invariably seen in people who are very obese.

ACN consists of hyperpigmentation, hypertrophy of skin markings, and a velvety appearance of the affected area. In marked cases there are dark brown skin tags in the affected areas. The most distinguishing of these features is the hypertrophy of skin markings, because many people, especially if they are obese, have some hyperpigmentation in intertriginous areas.

ACN is most difficult to detect in those with very light or very dark complexions. Darkly pigmented blacks often are darkest in the areas on which ACN characteristically appears. This should not be misinterpreted as ACN. Very fair Caucasians may have minimal hyperpigmentation, but ACN can be found if the typical skin areas are inspected carefully. Some patients with ACN, or their mothers if the patient is a teenager, think ACN is dirt. It does not wash off, however.

ACN can be found with mild obesity but seems especially associated with more severe obesity. In particular individuals, ACN tends to correlate with the degree of obesity, increasing when weight is gained and decreasing or even disappearing if weight is lost. As ACN gets more severe, hyperpigmentation increases, the skin-marking hypertrophy is greater, and skin tags appear or become larger and more numerous. It is probably true that more severe ACN is more likely to be associated with diabetes, but this has not been demonstrated. Some patients with marked ACN, especially adolescents, have glucose levels after oral glucose that are not at all elevated, though insulin levels may be.

ACN seems to be a marker for diabetes, but it is not itself the result of diabetes. It is possible that insulin resistant diabetes and ACN are independent complications of the obese state. Treatment of diabetes or of the androgenic disorder does not decrease ACN; the only known effective treatment is weight loss. When achieved, this invariably results in lightening or disappearance of the lesion.

While ACN is important as a marker for PCO and diabetes, there is not an invariable relationship between these entities. ACN may occasionally occur without clinically evident endocrine or metabolic abnormalities, and both PCO and diabetes can occur without ACN. ACN tends to be associated with more severe manifestations of androgenic disorders, but it is not clear that PCO in which ACN is present is a distinct form of the disease. Nonetheless ACN is extremely important as a marker.

Presentation of Polycystic Ovary Syndrome in Adolescence

The oligo-amenorrhea of PCO usually begins, as do the other abnormalities, in adolescence. Although it is widely believed that oligomenorrhea is normal in the first years after menarche, this is not in fact the case. With infrequent exceptions, normal teenagers have regular cycles. This unfortunate misconception frequently leads to delay in diagnosis because the amenorrhea of PCO is mistakenly thought to be normal for the patient's stage of development. If fact, about half of adolescent girls with amenorrhea continue to have amenorrhea in the ensuing years. Other features of PCO may take more time to establish themselves. Hypertrichosis may be present prepubertally, although it is often unnoticed, but sexual hair does not begin normally until the beginning of puberty. Increase in facial and body hair is a slow process and usually is not complete until the end of the teens or later. Similarly, the thickened capsule and multiple cysts of PCO are the result of anovulatory cycles and may not be apparent in the first years after menarche, although many girls with PCO do show multiple cysts on ultrasound. Some normal girls show very small cysts in their ovaries also, because the normally developing ovary passes through a stage in which it appears to contain multiple small cysts. This may be an incidental finding on a pelvic ultrasound done for another reason such as pelvic pain. Parents should not be told their daughter has "polycystic ovaries" because of such a finding. PCO is a physiological disturbance with an inconsistent relationship to ovarian anatomy.

Thus both false-negative and false-positive diagnoses of PCO occur with adolescents. Both can be avoided by recognizing the points made here. Oligo-amenorrhea should be considered as presumably abnormal in teenagers. Hirsutism, when present, will be milder in the young teenager than in older women. Ovarian morphology by ultrasound can be misleading. Awareness of these pitfalls and consideration of all the clinical data usually makes it possible to determine whether a teenager has PCO or not.

Physicians should restrain themselves from giving unfavorable prognoses regarding fertility to adolescent girls in whom they have diagnosed PCO. In the first place, most women with androgenic disorders are able to become pregnant; only a minority ever consult an infertility specialist. Secondly, the prognosis for successful ovulation induction is good. One can accurately say in most cases that the likelihood ofpregnancy either spontaneously or with the help of hormonal medication is high.

Obesity and Androgenic Disorders

That there is an association between androgenic disorders and obesity in women cannot be doubted; it is less easy to account for the specifics of the relationship. Obesity was part of the original syndrome of Stein and Leventhal (23) and in most physicians' minds is characteristic of women with androgenic disorders. However, there are many mildly and some quite hirsute women who are slender or only slightly obese. Certainly obesity does not in itself cause androgen excess because most obese women do not have androgen excess. It has been reported, however, that mean free testosterone levels are higher in obese women with normal ovulatory cycles (24). However, the subjects were not characterized as to pattern of obesity or waist–hip ratio. It is possible that only a subgroup of obese women have elevated androgen levels, but that this subgroup is large enough to raise the mean in studies of obese women when fat distribution is not characterized. Not all forms of obesity are alike. Nonetheless most women with severe hirsutism, for example those who shave daily, are obese. It is not clear that onset of obesity after adolescence can cause new development of an androgenic disorder in a woman without previous androgenization, although it may make existing hirsutism worse. Alternatively, it is possible that hyperandrogenism can cause obesity, but how it would do so is unclear although hyperinsulinism is a possible etiologic factor. It has not been established how effectively weight reduction can ameliorate hyperandrogenism, in part because significant weight reduction in this group of women is so rarely achieved. There is, however, one study (24a) which did show a decrease of testosterone and androstenedione into the normal range and resumption of ovulation in PCO women who lost a significant amount of weight. Several were then able to achieve pregnancy despite being infertile before. This confirms the empirical observation that weight reduction does restore ovulation in many obese infertile women. However, the androgenic hair changes seem to be less readily reversible, perhaps because the action of androgen on the hair follicle may not be fully reversible, at least at the modestly lower androgen levels that may result from weight reduction. However weight reduction is worthwhile because it is the most effective means of improving the metabolic abnormalities discussed below.

There is an important distinction between two quite different patterns of body fat distribution in obesity. In gynecoid obesity, there is an exaggeration of the normal female fat distribution with large hips, buttocks and thighs. The breasts may or may not be large, and the upper body is less affected that the lower body. Alternative terms are lower segment or pear-shape obesity. With android obesity in contrast, the hips, buttocks and thighs are relatively thin and the extra fat is mainly on the upper body and abdomen. People with android obesity tend to have much larger intraabdominal fat deposits as shown by computed tomography (CT) scan. They have a pot- or beer-belly appearance. The two types of obesity can be distinguished also in men. They are further discussed and illustrated in Chapter 13.

Lower segment obesity is more likely to be of childhood onset, but the form obesity takes cannot be accounted for simply by age of onset. While it seems plausible that sex steroid levels determine the form of obesity, with estrogen tending to promote distribution in the hips, buttocks, and thighs, while androgens promote deposit in the abdomen, this has not been proven. Women seem to have one or the other fat distribution after puberty, which then persists for life. Weight loss reduces the degree of obesity but, unfortunately, not its pattern.

The most objective criterion for distinguishing android from gynecoid obesity is that of the waist–hip ratio. In the android form, body circumference is greater at the waist than the hips; in the gynecoid form the hips are wider than the waist as is normal for a woman. It appears to be intraabdominal fat which increases health risk because of its direct portal drainage into the liver. This can be quantitated by abdominal CT scan. It is likely that increased waist–hip ratio appears as a risk factor because it is associated with increased intraabdominal fat.

The health implications of the different fat distributions are considerable (25). Android obesity is associated with increased risks of androgenization, diabetes, dyslipidemia, heart disease, breast cancer and endometrial cancer. While gynecoid obesity is not innocuous, it is far less a risk factor for cardiovascular disease.

Metabolic Abnormalities Associated with Androgenic Disorders

Glucose Intolerance and Non–Insulin Dependent Diabetes Mellitus

The relationship of androgenic disorders, obesity, and glucose intolerance is discussed in detail in Chapter 13. These associations are of major importance for women's health (26). While it is not known exactly what proportion of women with premenopausal onset of non–insulin dependent diabetes mellitus (NIDDM) are android or androgenized, it is likely that many or most of them are. This has obvious implications for screening. In women with these appearance changes, the likelihood of clinical diabetes is high. A three-hour glucose tolerance test (GTT) and hemoglobin A_{1c} should be obtained as the necessary and sufficient work-up. The fasting blood glucose is the most commonly ordered test, but is the *least* sensitive because fasting glucose is the last parameter to become abnormal in the progression toward diabetes. A three-hour formal GTT is necessary. To diagnose diabetes, two or more values above 200 mg/dL is a criterion sometimes recommended but overly stringent. Diabetes is present when blood glucose levels are high enough to cause complications. The exact threshold is not known, but it seems almost certain that these can occur with abnormal glucose tolerance in which fasting and two-hour postprandial glucose values are above the strict normals of 110 and 140 mg/dL respectively. Most of the literature on this subject is old and derived from screening programs that are no longer considered to be useful. However, stricter criteria apply to someone who is identified not in mass screening, but whose GTT was done because of physical changes—android obesity, oligomenorrhea, or ACN—that are known to be associated with diabetes.

If the GTT is done with simultaneous insulin levels, a much higher proportion of women with these risk factors will be found to be abnormal. This is usually not necessary in a clinical setting because specific treatment is not available for insulin resistance in the absence of elevated glucose values.

The hemoglobin A_{1c} is related to the integrated blood glucose concentration over the preceding two- to three-month interval. It is not sensitive enough for diagnosis but gives helpful information about the severity of blood glucose abnormality and is the most useful index of treatment success.

NIDDM shows a strong familial tendency but seems to require obesity for the tendency to be expressed. However, obesity itself is often familial. A family history of NIDDM is another reason to test a patient with an androgenic disorder for diabetes.

Most of the women I see with androgenic disorder–associated diabetes did not know they had diabetes. It was identified when testing was performed because of the associated physical changes. This is disturbing because it suggests that NIDDM is usually diagnosed late after symptoms or even complications have appeared. The classical symptoms of polyuria, polydipsia, and weight loss with increased food intake are those of Type I, or insulin dependent, diabetes which is a quite different disorder. By the time such symptoms appear in a patient with NIDDM, the condition has been present for many years and complications may be present.

Dyslipidemia

Despite the national publicity about the value of detecting and treating lipid abnormalities, most women who need treatment are not receiving it. The relationship of lipid abnormalities to androgen action in women is discussed in Chapter 13. A low HDL-cholesterol value seems to be associated with high free testosterone values, although it is not clear that this effect is distinct from the effect of obesity (27,28).

The clinical signs which suggest the presence of diabetes also can be associated with dyslipidemia. Direct physical changes such as xanthomas are rare in lipid disorders, but android obesity, ACN, and elevated free testosterone levels seem to be associated with unfavorable lipid profiles as they are with glucose intolerance and NIDDM. In general, a lipid profile should be done in the same women for whom there is an indication for diabetes testing. An additional factor of importance is a family history of premature coronary heart disease (CHD).

Psychological Concerns

Studies of the effects of androgenic manifestations on women's psychological well-being are generally lacking. Those that have been published are often in conflict, especially those concerning the effects of hyperandrogenism on women's sexuality (29). This is quite surprising in view of all the interest in both the biology and the cultural aspects of gender in the past thirty years. While the more extreme gender problems such as ambiguous genitalia and transsexualism have been much studied, the far more common problems of hirsutism and alopecia have not. This might be because these latter matters are not considered serious enough to merit attention or, alternatively, it may be that mild gender ambiguity is more disturbing than extreme forms which are more easily distanced from. Whatever the cause, women with androgenic changes rarely find sympathy or understanding for their plight. However, anyone who listens sympathetically to the concerns of women with noticeable signs of androgen excess cannot fail to note how distressing these are to the affected woman.

Our society is hypocritical about matters of appearance. On the one hand, a concern with how one looks is considered vain. Women are frequently embarrassed to speak to a physician about appearance concerns for fear of being thought vain or superficial. The women's movement has criticized social concern with female beauty as yet another form of oppression of women. Yet this also encloses a criticism. If a woman is concerned with how she looks, she is simply going along with her oppressors. No philosophical position validates concern with appearance. Stereotyping is not frequent; women who think too much about how they look are not only vain but superficial, selfish, or frivolous.

The contrary ideal is never articulated because in fact there is none. If being vain is a fault, what is the alternative? Certainly not being sloppy. Several points need to be made here at the risk of saying what is not popular. First, people are judged all the time on their appearance and all know this. Those who do not dress or groom properly are penalized socially and professionally. Those physicians (often, but by no means always, male) who counsel women not to be concerned with their appearance are unlikely to give this counsel to their spouses or daughters.

It is useful to rethink one's attitudes toward appearance. First, the issue is not beauty but being able to look normally appealing to others. This means looking neat, clean, youthful (very important in our culture), lively, vital, and energetic. Looking old, tired, or depressed is not acceptable in America. Nor is looking dirty and ill-kempt, which is how some women with hirsutism fear they look.

While gender roles are now changing, gender ambiguity is no less a source of discomfort. This may not be true for rock stars, but it is true in business and ordinary socializing. Women with hair loss feel they have lost an important sign of femininity and youth. Their anxiety is rarely about their own sexuality but about how they will seem to others. Occasionally a woman with hirsutism will make a remark like, "I sometimes think I should have been a man." Expressed here is not doubt about her being biologically and psychologically female, but a fear that how she looks is not what is expected for her social gender role. Sense of self is involved also. To be told that no one else will notice hirsutism or alopecia is rarely reassuring when a woman feels that her outer appearance does not accord with her inner sense of who she is.

I have not found in my observation of women with androgenic changes that there is any correlation between concern about these and other aspects of personality. Some probably do fit to some degree the stereotype of the vain woman, spending great amounts of time in front of mirrors and having as primary concerns that her makeup and hair remain intact. They may be selfish in their dealings with others. But every other sort of character trait is also found among this group of women. Some take great care over their appearance and others do not. There are housewives, physicians, nurses, attorneys, factory workers, construction crew members, police officers, secretaries, teachers, etc. It is normal to be bothered by androgenic changes and no particular personality type is associated with this concern. The physician working with women with androgenic disorders needs to recognize this and avoid prejudicial judgements.

Hair loss is especially disturbing because hair is the one part of one's body that can be easily modified and so styling it is an expression of individuality. Some women who are greatly bothered by even mild alopecia have had unusually abundant and attractive hair which attracted favorable notice their entire lives. When alopecia occurs, what has seemed a personal asset is lost. If this is kept in mind when working with women in this situation, the distress their alopecia evokes will seem less excessive. Indeed, in my opinion, it is for the patient rather than the physician to decide how bothersome is an appearance change. We cannot really judge what something like this means to another. There are certainly some women with mild or moderate alopecia who do not notice or do not care. Obviously they will rarely come to a doctor for hair loss. The same is true of hirsutism. However, that some women are not bothered by a mild degree of alopecia or hirsutism does not mean that other women with a comparable change are neurotic to be distressed by it or to seek treatment.

Having said all this I must admit that some of the women I have seen for alopecia or androgenic complaints do have psychological problems. However the same is true of patients I or any other physician sees for any other complaint. The presenting complaint of an androgenic disorder does not suggest the likelihood of psychological abnormality. However I do suspect that many women who come to a specialist for these problems are relatively assertive as a group. This is because they are self-selected for having the determination to keep on seeking an answer for their problem in the face of repeated discouragement. Some of the women I have seen have sought help unsuccessfully for more than a decade. One I remember from a rural area told me she had been to 16 physicians before coming to me. Some are told, obviously incorrectly, that nothing can be done about their problem. Others are advised that loss of scalp hair or excessive and visible facial hair are not important enough to justify the cost of testing or medication. Some are the victims of even less sensitive attitudes. An appropriate reaction on the part of a patient to such a dismissal is anger.

Many women who initially may seem to be overreacting to their alopecia or hirsutism—for example, by withdrawing from social activities—improve when treatment has been successful. I particularly remember one young woman who would not go out except to work because she was convinced that people were staring at the back of her head where her hair was thin. It seemed that she had some degree of paranoia or agoraphobia. When her hair came back after about 2 years of treatment, however, she started going out and eventually married. She *was* overreacting, but correction of the physical change which so distressed her resulted in her resuming a normal life.

Androgenic disorders in themselves do not generally require intervention by a psychiatrist or psychologist. They do, however, require a sympathetic attitude on the part of physician and nurse and other health care professionals. Many patients are afraid of criticism or derisive remarks and one should phrase matters carefully to avoid increasing anxiety about appearance being gender inappropriate or that the patient is vain or wasting the doctor's time. It is best to avoid talking about "too many male hormones" or commenting that the hirsute patient does have a lot of hair. One women I saw was told by her previous endocrinologist that she "certainly had a hairy bottom," a remark she never forgot. It is best to reinforce normality by explaining that many women have facial and body hair and that the media give an unrealistic idea of how much hair is normal for a woman. Similar reassurances can be given for other androgenic changes.

When they receive sympathetic attention, women with androgenic disorders can be among the most appreciative of patients.

REFERENCES

1. Sperling LC, Heimer WL. Androgen biology as a basis for the diagnosis and treatment of androgenic disorders in women. I, II. *J Am Acad Dermatol* 1993;28:669–683, 901–916.
2. Kvedar JC, Gibson M, Krusinski PA. Hirsutism: evaluation and treatment. *J Am Acad Dermatol* 1985;12:215–225.
3. Redmond GP, Bergfeld WF. Diagnostic approach to androgenic disorders in women: acne, hirsutism and alopecia. *Cleve Clin J Med* 1990;57:424–427.

4. Redmond GP, Bergfeld WF. Treatment of androgenic disorders in women: acne, hirsutism and alopecia. *Cleve Clin J Med* 1990;57:428–432.
5. Redmond G. *The good news about women's hormones*. New York: Warner Books; 1995.
6. Redmond GP, Gidwani G, Gupta M, Bedocs N, Skibinski C. Menstrual patterns in women with androgenic disorders. *Fertil Steril (Program Suppl)* 1989;S126.
7. Long CA, Gast MJ. Menorrhagia. *Obstet Gynecol Clin North Am* 1990;17:343–359.
8. Speroff L, Glass RH, Kase NG. *Clinical gynecological endocrinology and infertility*. 4th ed. Baltimore: Williams and Wilkins; 1989;165–231.
9. Southam AL, Richart RM. The prognosis for adolescents with menstrual abnormalities. *Am J Obstet Gynecol* 1966;94:637–645.
10. Redmond GP. Solving the mystery of menstrual dysfunction. *Postgrad Med* 1989;85:127–132.
11. Doody KM, Carr BR. Amenorrhea. *Obstet Gynecol Clin North Am* 1990;17:361–387.
12. Redmond GP, Bergfeld WF, Gupta M, Bedocs NM, Skibinski C, Gidwani G. Menstrual dysfunction in hirsute women. *J Am Acad Dermatol* 1990;22:76–78.
13. Collins R, ed. *Ovulation induction*. New York: Springer-Verlag; 1991.
14. McKenna TJ, Moore A, Magee F. Amenorrhea with cryptic hyperandrogenemia. *J Clin Endocrinol Metab* 1983;56:893–896.
15. Redmond GP, Bergfeld W, Gupta M, Bedocs C, Skibinski C, Gidwani G. Clinical and biochemical findings in 500 women with androgenic disorders. *The Endocrine Society Program Abstracts*; Seattle, WA. June 1989;330.
16. Redmond GP, Bergfeld W, Gupta M, Parker R, Subichin S, Bedocs N, Gidwani G. Comparison of hormonal abnormalities in women with different manifestations of androgen excess. In: Genazzani AR, Volpe A, Facchinetti F, eds. *Research in gynecological endocrinology*. London: Parthenon; 1986;187–190.
17. Ferriman D, Gallwey JD. Clinical assessment of body hair growth in women. *J Clin Endocrinol Metab* 1961;21:1440–1447.
18. Thomas PK, Ferriman DG. Variation in facial and pubic hair growth in white women. *Am J Phys Anthropol* 1957;5:171–180.
19. Bergfeld WF, Redmond GP. Androgenic Alopecia. *Dermatol Clin* 1986;5:491–500.
20. Kahn CR, Flier FS, Bar RS, et al. The syndromes of insulin resistance and acanthosis nigricans. *N Engl J Med* 1976;295:739–745.
21. Flier JS, Kahn CR, Roth J. Receptors, antireceptor antibodies and mechanisms of insulin resistance. *N Engl J Med* 1979;300:413–419.
22. Dunaif A. Diabetes mellitus and polycystic ovary syndrome. In: Dunaif A, Givens JR, Haseltine FP, Merriam GR, eds. *Polycystic ovary syndrome*. Boston: Blackwell Scientific; 1992;347–358.
23. Stein IF, Leventhal ML. Amenorrhea associated with bilateral polycystic ovaries. *Am J Obstet Gynecol* 1935;6:189–205.
24. Wajchenberg BL, Achando SS, Marconides JAM, Germak OA, Mathor MB, Kirschner MA. Free testosterone levels during the menstrual cycle in obese versus normal women. *Fertil Steril* 1989;51:535–537.
24a. Bates GW, Whitwoorth NS. Effects of body weight reduction on plasma androgens in obese, infertile women. *Fertil Seril* 1982;38:406–409.
25. Redmond GP. Obesity in women. In: Redmond GP, ed. *Lipids and women's health*. New York: Springer-Verlag; 1991;119–131.
26. Redmond GP. In: Redmond GP, ed. *Lipids and women's health.* Androgens in women: Their effects on lipid and carbohydrate metabolism. New York: Springer-Verlag; 1991;81–105.
27. Wild RA, Bartholomew MJ. The influence of body weight on lipoprotein lipids in patients with polycystic ovary syndrome. *Am J Obstet Gynecol* 1988;159:423–427.
28. Redmond GP, Skibinski CI, Bedocs NM, Van Lente F, Beck GJ. Hirsutism and elevated testosterone levels in women are associated with lower values of HDL-cholesterol. *The Endocrine Society Annual Meeting Abstracts*; San Antonio TX 1992, p.277.
29. Ehrhardt AA. Psychological consequences of androgen effects. In: Dunaif A, Givens JR, Haseltine FP, Merriam GR, eds.: *Polycystic ovary syndrome*. Boston: Blackwell Scientific; 1992;341–346.

Androgenic Disorders,
edited by G. P. Redmond.
Raven Press, Ltd., New York © 1995.

2

Biochemistry and Laboratory Measurement of Androgens in Women

Laurence M. Demers

Department of Pathology, The Milton S. Hershey Medical Center, The Pennsylvania State University, Hershey, Pennsylvania 17033

The synthesis and release of androgenic steroids in women are a normal part of adrenal and ovarian steroidogenesis and contribute to the physiologic expression of the female reproductive system (1). Excessive production of androgens occurs, however, in a number of endocrine disease states and produces undesirable symptoms characteristic of androgen excess, such as hirsutism and the virilizing manifestations of testosterone (2). Androstenedione, dehydroepiandrosterone (DHA) and testosterone are considered to be the principal androgenic steroids responsible for these effects in women (3). The synthesis and release of androgenic steroids in women can be linked to two major steroid secreting organs, the ovary and the adrenal. During the reproductive years of a woman's life, the ovary releases androgenic steroids primarily in the form of androstenedione. This steroid is produced by the ovary in a cyclical fashion under the timed regulatory control of the hypothalamic–pituitary axis during the course of the normal menstrual cycle. Secretion of androstenedione by the ovary during the follicular phase of the menstrual cycle is approximately half that secreted during the luteal phase of the cycle. Under normal circumstances, only small amounts of the other androgenic steroids, DHA and testosterone, are directly released from the ovary. With the onset of menopause, the quiescent ovary continues to secrete small amounts of androstenedione.

The adrenal, in contrast to the ovary, is a major source of androgenic steroids in women (4). DHA is the dominant androgenic steroid released from the adrenal; it occurs primarily in the sulfate form as DHA-S. The amount of DHA-S produced by the adrenal is substantial and the amount released is second in concentration only to that of cortisol. The adrenal also produces androstenedione; however, the amount synthesized and released is considerably less than that of DHA-S. Approximately 50% of the circulating androstenedione level in the reproductive age woman is derived from the adrenal.

Testosterone itself is the most potent androgen in terms of biologic efficacy, and yet it is the least concentrated of the androgenic steroids found in the circulation of women. Testosterone is not usually synthesized or released directly either by the ovary or the adrenal gland but is formed primarily by extraglandular conversion of either androstenedione from the ovary and adrenal or DHA-S from the adrenal (5). Much of the extraglandular conversion of testosterone takes place in the liver and skin. During the reproductive years, a woman produces approximately 300 μg of testosterone per day, primarily through the extraglandular conversion of androstenedione and DHA-S to testosterone.

As mentioned previously, ovarian androstenedione secretion falls under pituitary gonadotropin regulatory control and thus plasma levels fluctuate depending on the phase of the menstrual cycle. Luteinizing hormone is the principle gonadotropin that stimulates ovarian production of androstenedione (6). Adrenal secretion of DHA-S and androstenedione, in contrast to ovarian secretion, is not influenced by menstrual cyclicity but is affected by nonmenstrual factors such as stress and those factors that influence the 24-hr circadian rhythm of adrenal steroid release through higher-center neuroendocrine mechanisms. The 24-hr biologic rhythm of corticotropin-releasing factor (CRF) and adrenocorticotropin (ACTH) release stimulates the secretion of adrenal androgens in a manner similar to that of cortisol release, with a higher output in the A.M. and a diminished secretion in the late P.M.

Recently, a pituitary factor that is not ACTH has been implicated in the specific control of adrenal androgen output (7). Although it is still controversial, a few laboratories have reported on the isolation of a glycopeptide from human pituitary extracts that shows sequence homology to an 18–amino acid n-terminal region of the propiomelanocorticotropin (POMC) pituitary peptide, the precursor peptide of ACTH and melanocyte-stimulating hormone (MSH). The term CASH (cortical androgen stimulating hormone) has been used to describe this peptide (7). From a biologic perspective, there is ample clinical evidence to support the suggestion that the adrenal androgen pathway may fall under pituitary control separate from ACTH (8). The observed divergence in cortisol and DHA-S secretion found at adrenarche and the divergent pattern of adrenal androgen hypersecretion found in different disease states associated with altered adrenal androgen release tend to support the notion that the adrenal androgen pathway does fall under separate control by a pituitary factor that is not ACTH.

Androgen Biosynthesis (1)

All androgens are formed from the steroid substrate pregnenolone, which is derived from cholesterol originating primarily from low-density lipoproteins (LDL cholesterol) found in the circulation. The biochemical pathways of steroidogenesis leading from pregnenolone to androstenedione and testosterone in the ovary can differ somewhat depending on the phase of the menstrual cycle and whether steroidogenesis is taking place in the follicle or corpus luteum. In contrast, in the adrenal, a single pathway to adrenal androgen biosynthesis exists.

Pregnenolone is first synthesized from cholesterol by the removal of a six-carbon fragment under the catalytic action of a cytochrome P450 side-chain cleavage enzyme. (Fig. 1) This enzymatic step is believed to be the major rate limiting step in the steroid biosynthetic pathway. In the ovary, this step is influenced by the pituitary gonadotropin luteinizing hormone (LH), while in the adrenal, ACTH activates this important enzymatic step. Pregnenolone once formed is then converted either to progesterone when steroidogenesis is taking place in the corpus luteum or to 17α-

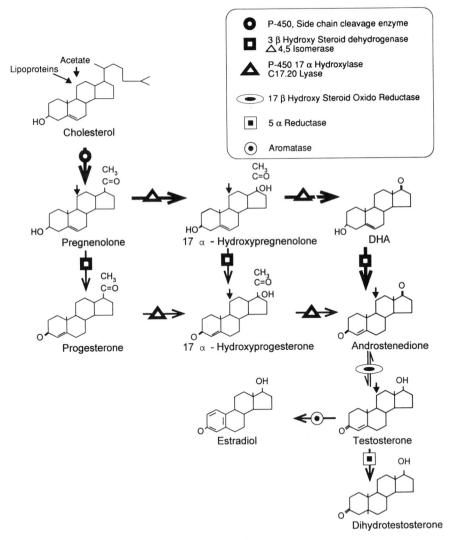

FIG. 1. The biosynthetic pathway of androgens in the ovary and adrenal cortex. The dominant pathway is indicated by the heavy arrows. Each step in the biosynthetic pathway is mediated by a specific enzyme as noted in the figure.

hydroxypregnenolone when synthesis is taking place in the ovarian follicle. Pregnenolone transformation to 17α-hydroxypregnenolone, in contrast, predominates in the adrenal. Formation of progesterone from pregnenolone requires the dual action of the enzymes 3β-hydroxysteroid dehydrogenase and Δ4,5-ketosteroid isomerase. This reaction shifts the double bond from the Δ5 B ring to the Δ4 A ring of the basic steroid molecule.

Both pregnenolone and progesterone are substrates for a P-450 17α-hydroxylase enzyme which catalyzes the formation of 17α-hydroxypregnenolone and 17α-hydroxyprogesterone. 17α-hydroxyprogesterone predominates in the corpus luteum while 17α-hydroxypregnenolone is the dominant 17-hydroxy steroid intermediate in the ovarian follicle as well as in the adrenal. Following the 17-hydroxylation step, the two-carbon side chain, C20 and C21, is then cleaved by the same P-450 17α-hydroxylase enzyme, which has inherent C17,20 lyase enzyme activity. The net result is a 17-keto androgenic steroid.

In the case of 17α-hydroxypregnenolone, the product of the 17,20 lyase enzyme is DHA, a Δ5 steroid. Androstenedione, a Δ4 steroid, can be synthesized from 17α-hydroxyprogesterone; however, this is not considered to be the major pathway for the synthesis of androstenedione. Investigators in the field of steroid metabolism suggest that formation of androstenedione from DHA is the predominant pathway in both the ovary and adrenal.

Most of the DHA made on the adrenal undergoes sulfation at the 3-hydroxyl position before secretion. This renders DHA more polar and water soluble for independent and noncarrier protein transport through the circulation. The result is that DHA-S is the predominant form of DHA found in the circulation.

Androstenedione is produced from DHA through the dual action of the enzymes 3β-hydroxysteroid dehydrogenase and Δ4,5 isomerase. Androstenedione is then available for conversion to testosterone primarily at sites outside of the adrenal and ovary. Synthesis of testosterone from androstenedione is a reversible reaction step that is catalyzed by the enzyme 17β-hydroxysteroid oxidoreductase. This enzyme produces the reversible reduction of the 17-keto group of androstenedione. Approximately 75% of the circulating testosterone in women is derived from peripheral conversion of androstenedione. Only small amounts of testosterone are released directly from either the ovary or adrenal. Testosterone once formed is then available for conversion to estradiol through aromatization of the A ring by the enzyme aromatase, or it is metabolized to its active product dihydrotestosterone (DHT) by the enzyme 5α reductase. This enzyme is found in androgen-sensitive tissues like the liver and certain skin areas that are prone to androgen-targeted hair growth.

Androgen Secretion

The secretory activity of ovarian and adrenal steroid secreting cells is coupled closely to hormone biosynthesis since little hormone is stored in either organ sys-

TABLE 1. *Production, plasma levels, and metabolic clearance rates of androgens in women*

Steroid	MCR (L/day)	Serum level (ug/dl)	Production rate (mg/day)
Androstenedione	2,070	0.04–0.240	2–3 (follicular phase) 4–5 (luteal phase)
DHA	1,640	0.02–2.0	7.0–8.0
DHA-S		100–360	8.0–16.0
Testosterone	690	0.02–0.08	0.20–0.30

DHA, dehydroepiandrosterone; DHA-S, dehydroepiandrosterone sulfate; MCR, metabolic clearance rate.

tem. Once formed, steroids are secreted or metabolized almost immediately. Over the years, the measurement of metabolic clearance rate (MCR) has become an important tool to assess hormone secretion. The determination of the MCR couples both hormone glandular release and blood flow through the gland as a function of hormone production. The administration of a radiolabeled form of the steroid has been the basis for an isotope dilution technique that allows for the calculation of the metabolic clearance rate for each steroid (9). Multiplying the MCR by the concentration of hormone in the blood provides the rate of total hormone production. These calculations have been used to determine androgen production rates in women as shown in Table 1. The adrenal glands in women secrete on a daily basis approximately 4 mg DHA, 10 mg DHA-S, 1.5 mg androstenedione, and 75 μg of testosterone. The ovaries, in contrast, secrete approximately 1.5 mg androstenedione during the follicular phase and 3 mg androstenedione per day during the luteal phase of the menstrual cycle. Approximately 2 mg DHA and 50 μg of testosterone are secreted by the ovaries on a daily basis.

Androgen Transport and Bioavailability

Both androstenedione and DHA lack specific protein carriers like cortisol-binding globulin or sex hormone–binding globulin that facilitate transport of cortisol, testosterone, and estradiol through the aqueous environment of the blood circulation. When released into the blood stream, androstenedione is primarily transported weakly bound to albumin. DHA in contrast undergoes the addition of a sulfate group at the 3-hydroxyl position. This facilitates its transport thought the circulation as the more polar DHA-S without the need for a carrier protein. Free DHA, like androstenedione, is also transported weakly bound to albumin.

Testosterone, in contrast to DHA and androstenedione, shares with estradiol the same carrier protein, sex hormone–binding globulin (SHBG), for about three-quarters of its transport needs (10). About 25% of testosterone is carried weakly bound to albumin and less than 2% circulates as absolute free testosterone (Fig. 2). This distribution of testosterone to the different protein carriers has led to the concept of expressing testosterone levels as either total testosterone or free and weakly bound testosterone with the weakly bound form reflective of albumin-bound testosterone

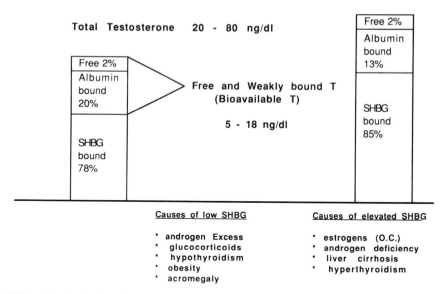

FIG. 2. The distribution of total testosterone to its plasma-binding proteins in women. Free and weakly (albumin-) bound testosterone (bioavailable T) is approximately 22% of the total testosterone level. Alterations in circulating levels of the sex hormone binding globulin (SHBG) can be caused by hormonal and disease factors as listed.

(11). Most steroid biochemists consider the free and weakly bound testosterone to be the bioavailable form of testosterone that responds to testosterone receptor uptake when blood perfuses androgen receptor target tissues. Changes in the availability of SHBG levels with disease or drug therapy can influence the interpretation of total testosterone levels. Thus measurement of the free and albumin-bound form of testosterone is important for the proper interpretation of elevated total serum testosterone levels. As will be discussed under the section on the laboratory measurement of androgens, the measurement of free and weakly bound testosterone has largely replaced the measurement of absolute free testosterone for providing an estimate of bioavailable testosterone in the circulation.

Androgen Metabolism

Androgenic steroids undergo a variety of metabolic transformations resulting in a class of largely biologically inactive 17-ketosteroids (Fig. 3) (12). DHA-S is converted to free DHA by a sulfatase enzyme. DHA in turn can be metabolized to several ketosteroids including 11-hydroxy (11-OH) DHA, 16-OH DHA, and androstenedione through the catalytic activity of 11-hydroxylase, 16-hydroxylase, and the 3β-hydroxysteroid dehydrogenase, Δ4,5 isomerase complex respectively. Androstenedione in turn can be metabolized to 6-OH androstenedione, 11-OH androstenedione, androsterone, etiocholanolone, and epiandrosterone through a series

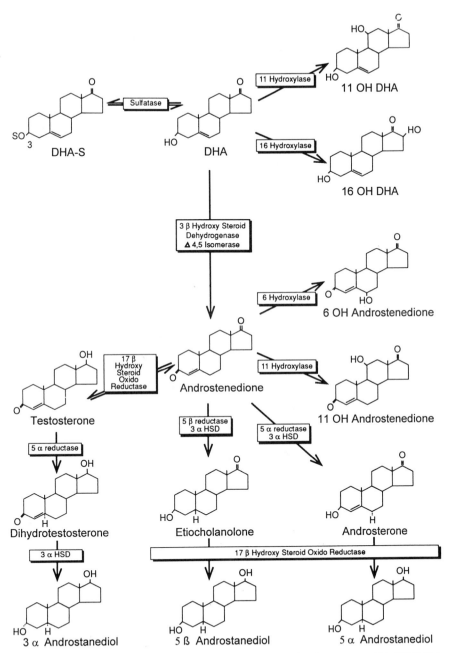

FIG. 3. The metabolism of androgenic steroids from dehydroepiandrosterone sulfate (DHA-S) in vivo to active and inactive metabolites. Testosterone and its active product, dihydrotestosterone, are the most potent androgens formed. Enzymes mediating each metabolite are noted for each reaction.

of hydroxylase- and reductase-mediated reactions in addition to its conversion to testosterone through the action of a 17β-hydroxysteroid oxidoreductase enzyme. This latter enzyme also catalyzes the formation of etiocholanolone and androsterone to 5β- and 5α-androstanediol, respectively. Testosterone itself is further metabolized to its active product, DHT in androgen target tissues under the influence of a 5α-reductase enzyme located in the cytosol of these tissues. DHT can be further metabolized to 3α-androstanediol, which becomes conjugated to glucuronide for excretion by the kidneys as 3α-androstanediol glucuronide (3α-diol G). This latter reaction takes place in the liver and skin. 3α-Diol G has been proposed as a useful marker for androgen metabolism in the skin when the cause of hirsutism is not associated with overt adrenal or ovarian androgenic steroid overproduction. This form of hirsutism is believed to be a consequence of overexpression of the 5α-reductase enzyme within the pilosebaceous unit of the skin.

Androgens and Adrenarche

Before the age of 8 years, the circulating blood levels of the androgenic steroids in prepubertal children are very low. The production of androgens by the prepubertal ovary and the adrenal is extremely minimal during the period of early childhood. For yet unexplained reasons, sometime around the age of 8 or 9 and before the onset of puberty, the adrenal androgen pathway becomes active and the process termed adrenarche begins (13). DHA-S levels begin to rise in the circulation and continue to increase throughout the adolescent period. Peak blood levels of DHA-S are reached in the mid twenties and are then maintained throughout a woman's reproductive life and well into menopause. The blood levels of DHA-S then begin to decline about the seventh decade of life and continue a downward trend thereafter. The consequences of this decline in terms of an expression of abnormal physiology or an association with the pathology of aging has not been elucidated. It is interesting to note, however, the striking parallel between DHA-S blood levels and bone density changes with age. The process of bone mass accrual in children begins about the same time during the early prepubertal period as the appearance of significant levels of DHA-S (14). Maximum bone density is usually achieved in the early twenties. In contrast, at the other end of the age spectrum, the increase in bone resorption and subsequent decline in bone mass in the seventh and eighth decades of life occur in the exact time period when a noticeable decline in circulating DHA-S levels occurs. This period has been described as the adrenopause, a time when the adrenal androgen pathway ceases to be functional. There is, however, still no direct clinical or biochemical evidence to support the notion that DHA-S is an obligatory participant in the process of bone mass accrual or maintenance.

Although androstenedione production from the adrenal is also increased in young children at the time of adrenarche, the principal source of this androgenic steroid in the circulation of girls comes with puberty and maturation of the ovary. Androstenedione levels are maintained throughout reproductive life and decline slightly with the onset of menopause. As mentioned previously, the senescent ovary does continue to secrete low levels of androstenedione well into menopause in spite of the lack of cyclical ovarian activity.

Laboratory Diagnosis of Androgen Excess

Excessive androgen excretion in women occurs in a variety of ovarian and adrenal disease states with clinical manifestations occurring in the form of increased hair growth in androgen-sensitive areas, acne, male pattern baldness, clitoral hypertrophy, and deepening of the voice (12). The relative contributions of the adrenal and ovary to excessive androgen production are thus important to know, and they are usually determined by the measurement of androgenic steroids in the circulation. The laboratory diagnosis of androgen overproduction is usually made after the clinical symptoms are manifest and the need to identify the source of androgen hypersecretion becomes important. The ovary is the more common source of androgen excess in women with moderate or severe hypersecretion. This is due to the prevalence of polycystic ovarian disease (PCOD), a disorder associated with increased androgen production by the ovaries. Measurement of androstenedione and total testosterone in concert with gonadotropins in women with suspected PCOD sets the stage for eliciting ovarian hypersecretion in a screening sense. In women with mild to moderate hirsutism who have ovulatory menstrual cycles, the clinical suspicion then switches to the adrenal, and the measurement of DHA-S and total testosterone is then considered in a screening sense.

In the presence of mild to moderate increases in total testosterone, the need to determine free and weakly bound testosterone becomes important because SHBG levels are reduced and free testosterone is disproportionately elevated in conditions of true androgen excess as well as other non–androgen-related disorders.

In some women, mild to moderate hirsutism can occur in the absence of overt elevations in either adrenal or ovarian androgens. The explanation usually given is that these patients may have increased androgen sensitivity of androgen-sensitive skin with elevated pilosebaceous unit levels of 5α-reductase and excessive hair growth in spite of apparently normal circulating androgen levels. Blood levels of 3α-diol G, the conjugated metabolite of DHT has been shown to be elevated in the blood of these women.

Androstenedione

Androstenedione, the major androgenic steroid secreted by the ovary, is routinely measured by radioimmunoassay. Highly specific antibodies that show little or no cross-reactivity with related steroids allow for the direct measurement of this steroid in serum or plasma without the need for extraction and chromatography. The circulating level of androstenedione ranges from 0.4 to 2.4 ng/ml (1.4 to 8.4 nmol/L) in premenopausal women and 0.3 to 1.3 ng/ml (1.0 to 4.6 nmol/L) in postmenopausal women.

Androstenedione levels as reported previously reflect both ovarian and adrenal secretion, with approximately 50% coming from each gland. Elevations are observed in diseases of ovarian and adrenal androgen excess such as PCOD, ovarian carcinoma, adrenogenital syndromes encompassing C-21 and C-11 hydroxylase deficiency, Cushings syndrome, and adrenal carcinoma.

Dehydroepiandrosterone Sulfate

DHA-S is the major androgen precursor secretory product released by the adrenal. Over 90% of DHA is sulfated before secretion from the adrenal. Ninety percent of DHA-S in the circulation of women is derived from the adrenal. DHA-S is determined directly in serum or plasma by radioimmunoassay with the use of highly specific antibodies. Free DHA can also be determined directly with highly specific radioimmunoassays, although DHA-S is the preferred analyte in most cases when a hirsute workup becomes necessary. The concentration of DHA-S ranges from 1,000 to 3,600 ng/ml (2.7 to 9.8 μmol/L) in adult, premenopausal women and 300 to 2,000 ng/ml (0.8 to 5.4 μmol/L) in women over the age of 70.

DHA-S secretion normally reflects the circadian rhythm of the CRF–ACTH axis with slightly higher output levels in the A.M. and reduced secretion in the P.M. The differences in A.M./P.M. levels, however, are not as pronounced as one sees for cortisol, since DHA-S has a much longer half-life in the circulation. The circulatory levels of DHA-S, as mentioned previously, are age related, with reduced levels found in young children, increased levels observed with adrenarche and puberty, and maximal levels achieved during the second decade of life with a decline occurring in the elderly, particularly in patients over the age of 70 (15).

DHA-S levels are increased with Cushing's syndrome as well as with the adrenogenital syndromes where deficiencies of pivotal hydroxylase enzymes such as 21- and 11-hydroxylase lead to reduced cortisol biosynthesis and steroid substrate overflow through the 17-keto adrenal androgen pathway as a consequence of compensatory ACTH secretion to the point of the enzyme block. The highest circulatory levels of DHA-S are found in patients with adrenal carcinoma.

Total and Free Testosterone

Over 75% of the circulating testosterone found in women is derived from the peripheral conversion of androstenedione to testosterone by the liver and by androgen-sensitive tissues like the skin (1). Total testosterone levels range from 20 to 80 ng/dl (0.7 to 2.8 nmol/L) in reproductive age women. Total testosterone levels are routinely determined by a direct radioimmunoassay using highly specific antibodies that obviate the need for organic solvent extraction and chromatographic purification. Because of the influence of SHBG levels (the binding protein that transports approximately three-quarters of testosterone in the circulation of women) and with alterations in circulating albumin with disease, there is frequently a need to determine the level of free and weakly (albumin-) bound hormone, in order to properly interpret true androgen excess. Any disease condition that compromises liver protein synthesis or enhances protein excretion can have a direct effect on the total level of hormone. Testosterone itself can cause a decrease in the level of SHBG through direct effects on the synthesis of this protein by the liver. Conversely, increases in SHBG brought about by estrogenic steroids and birth control pills can artifactually elevate the total testosterone level and present a biochemical picture of testosterone excess. Thus, the assessment of free and weakly (albumin-) bound testosterone is a useful indicator to identify the true level of free and bioavailable hormone to make an accurate diagnosis of testosterone overproduction. In normal women, the free and weakly bound testosterone is approximately 20% of the total testosterone level.

Most clinical endocrine laboratories now offer the determination of free and weakly bound testosterone to accurately assess the bioavailability of testosterone to androgen-sensitive tissues. The most common method for determining free and weakly bound testosterone employs ammonium sulfate precipitation to separate SHBG-bound testosterone from free and albumin-bound testosterone. The basis of the method is to preincubate the patient serum sample with a small amount of tritium-labeled testosterone, equilibrate the labeled steroid with the binding proteins in the sample, and then precipitate the SHBG-bound steroid with ammonium sulfate. The amount of ammonium sulfate used is important to selectively precipitate SHBG-bound testosterone. The supernate reflects free and weakly bound testosterone and is counted and expressed as percent free and weakly bound. The mass of free and weakly bound testosterone is then calculated by multiplying the total testosterone level by the percent free and weakly bound.

Only two-thirds of women with hirsutism have elevated total testosterone levels, while approximately 90% of patients with hirsutism have elevated free and weakly bound testosterone. Consequently, the measurement of free and weakly bound testosterone can be of use in interpreting mild to moderate elevations in total testosterone. The highest levels of testosterone occur in women who have ovarian carcinoma.

In the overall scheme of assessing patients with hirsutism and virilization, the laboratory determination of circulating androgens can be of immediate help in eliciting the presence and source of the androgen overproduction. Although hirsutism by itself is a relatively benign condition and is most commonly associated with PCOD, the need to rule out a potentially more serious underlying disorder such as an ovarian or adrenal malignancy is paramount. When androstenedione or testosterone levels are markedly elevated, the problem points to the ovary. When DHA-S is markedly raised, the concern shifts to the adrenal. Androgen excess arising from adrenogenital syndromes is frequently associated with DHA-S excess but not to the extent observed when DHA-S overproduction is a result of an adrenal carcinoma. The laboratory workup of patients presenting with signs and symptoms of androgen

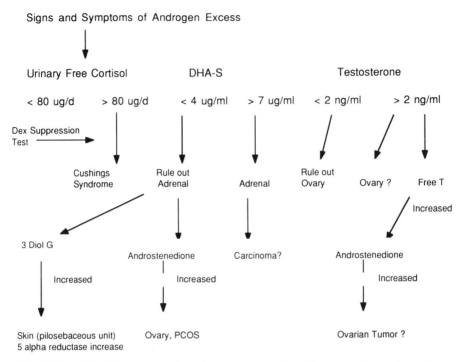

FIG. 4. The clinical laboratory workup of patients presenting with signs and symptoms of androgen excess. Urinary free cortisol is used to rule out Cushing's syndrome. DHA-S is used to rule out adrenal androgen overproduction while testosterone and androstenedione are used to rule out an ovarian source of androgen excess. 3 α androstanediol glucuronide (3 α diol G) is determined in cases of hirsutism that present without DHA-S excess.

excess is presented in Fig. 4. Interpretation of serum androgen levels is further discussed in Chapter 5.

Since hirsutism is a commonly presenting symptom that suggests androgen excess, a serum androgen profile is usually obtained in patients who present with this clinical anomaly. After obtaining a urinary free cortisol to rule out the probability of Cushing's syndrome, the serum androgen profile usually consists of measuring DHA-S and testosterone by radioimmunoassay. Androstenedione is added when the clinical picture is accompanied by menstrual cycle irregularities and there is a high degree of suspicion that the ovary may be involved.

When DHA-S and androstenedione are either normal or only minimally elevated and the testosterone is raised, the determination of free and weakly bound testosterone may be of use in determining whether the elevation is simply a consequence of a binding-protein abnormality or true androgen excess. Patients with a true androgen excess will have an elevated free and weakly bound testosterone when expressed either as a percentage or as mass testosterone. The expected pattern of elevation of the androgenic steroids in different forms of hirsutism is shown in Fig. 5.

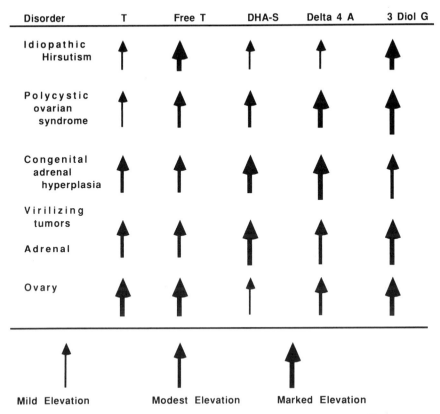

Disorder	T	Free T	DHA-S	Delta 4 A	3 Diol G

Idiopathic Hirsutism

Polycystic ovarian syndrome

Congenital adrenal hyperplasia

Virilizing tumors

Adrenal

Ovary

Mild Elevation   Modest Elevation   Marked Elevation

FIG. 5. The pattern of serum androgen elevations in various forms of hirsutism. T, testosterone; Free T, free and weakly (albumin-) bound testosterone; DHA-S, dehydroepiandrosterone sulfate; Delta 4 A, androstenedione; 3 Diol G, 3 alpha androstanediol glucuronide.

The use of gonadal or adrenal steroid administration can sometimes be used to distinguish the source of androgen excess. Gonadal steroids in the form of an oral contraceptive will induce a suppression of androgen secretion when excess androgens are a result of ovarian hypersecretion. By the same token, cortisol administration will produce negative feedback to the CRF–ACTH axis, reducing adrenal steroidogenesis and DHA-S output if the adrenal axis is implicated as a result of overstimulation from a central or ectopic source. These approaches are detailed in Chapter 5.

REFERENCES

1. Degroot LJ. *Endocrinology*. 3rd ed. Philadelphia: W.B. Saunders; 1995.
2. Ehrmann DA, Barnes RB, Rosenfield RL. Hyperandrogenism, hirsutism and the polycystic ovary syndrome. In: Degroot LJ, ed. *Endocrinology*. Philadelphia: W.B. Saunders; 1995.
3. Rosenfield RL, Lucky AW. Acne, hirsuitism and alopecia in adolescent girls: clinical expression of androgen excess. *Clin Endocrinol Metab* 1993;22:507.

4. Kirchner MA, Bardin CW. Androgen production and metabolism in normal and virilized women. *Metabolism* 1972;21:667–688.
5. Abraham GE. Ovarian and adrenal contributions to peripheral androgens during the menstrual cycle. *J Clin Endocrinol Metab* 1974;39:340–346.
6. Erickson GF, Magoffin DA, Dyer CA, Hofeditz C. The ovarian androgen producing cells: a review of structure/function relationships. *Endocr Reviews* 1985;6:371–399.
7. Parker LN. Andremarche. *Endocrinol Metab Clin North Am* 1991;20:71–83.
8. Cutler GB, Davis ES, Johnsonbaugh RE, Loriaux DL. Dissociation of cortisol and adrenal androgen secretion in patients with secondary adrenal insufficiency. *J Clin Endocrinol Metab* 1979;49:604–609.
9. Tait JF. The use of isotopic steroids for the measurement of production rates in vivo. *J Clin Endocrinol Metab* 1963;23:1285–1297.
10. Handelsman DJ. Testosterone and other androgens: physiology, pharmacology and therapeutic use. In: DeGroot LJ, ed. *Endocrinology*. Philadelphia: W.B. Saunders; 1995.
11. Pardridge WM, Demers LM. Bioavailable testosterone in salivary glands. *Clin Chem* 1991;37(2): 139–140.
12. Wilson JD, Foster DW. *Williams textbook of endocrinology*. 8th ed. Philadelphia: W.B. Saunders; 1992.
13. Parker LW. Adrenal androgens. In: Degroot LJ, ed. *Endocrinology*. Philadelphia: W.B. Saunders; 1995.
14. Parker LN, Sack J, Fisher D, Odell W. The andremarche: prolactin, gonodotropins, adrenal androgens and cortisol. *J Clin Endocrinol Metab* 1978;46:396–403.
15. Orentreich N, Brind J, Rizer R, Vogelman J. Age changes and sex differences in serum DHAS concentrations throughout adulthood. *J Clin Endocrinol Metab* 1984;59:551–560.

Androgenic Disorders,
edited by G. P. Redmond.
Raven Press, Ltd., New York © 1995.

3

Androgen Action at the Cellular Level

Marty E. Sawaya

Department of Medicine, Division of Dermatology and Cutaneous Surgery, University of Florida College of Medicine, Gainesville, Florida 32610

Androgen hormones exert a variety of effects upon mammalian tissues, including modification of gene expression and control of cellular growth and differentiation. Historically, the effects of androgens have been classed as either androgenic or anabolic (1).

The androgenic effects are those associated with differentiation of the male phenotype which occur primarily in the reproductive tract tissues, as well as skin. The anabolic effects occur within nonreproductive tissues such as liver, kidney, and muscle.

The primary mechanisms of androgen action may not differ significantly from tissue to tissue, even though the consequences of androgen action may vary. For example, an important consequence of androgen action is the stimulation of cellular growth, which may include increases in cell size (hypertrophy), in cell number (hyperplasia), or both, depending on the tissue. An example of this is the submaxillary gland where testosterone stimulates DNA synthesis, with cellular proliferation within the tissue (2), whereas in the mouse kidney, the primary growth effect of androgens is hypertrophy, with little or no DNA synthesis (3). These tissue-specific growth effects from androgens probably reflect the particular genes that respond to the hormone, rather than the fundamental differences in the mechanisms of hormone action.

Current research is now understanding and unraveling the detailed biochemical and molecular events that are initiated by androgens, leading to cellular growth. Several gene products produced by different androgen-responsive tissues are now major models of study for establishing the mechanisms of "Androgen action at the cellular level."

INTRACELLULAR MECHANISMS OF ANDROGEN HORMONE ACTION

Enzymes/Cofactors

The last few years have revealed an explosion of information on the molecular mechanisms of androgen hormone action (4,5). Androgens, like other steroids such as estrogens, progestins, and glucocorticoids, stimulate the production of growth factors, cytokines and proteases, which have an effect on cellular metabolic functions (6,7). Several organs in the body are target tissues for androgen hormone action, such as testes, ovary, adrenal, brain, and skin.

Steroids passively diffuse through the cell membrane where further metabolic transformations can take place. Androgens such as dehydroepiandrosterone (DHEA) and androstenedione, weak precursors, can be metabolically transformed to potent androgens, testosterone (T) and dihydrotestosterone (DHT) (Fig. 1). Specific enzymes are needed for these transformations to take place, either locally within the organs or at other target tissue sites, thus affecting another organ. For example, the testes or ovary can transform DHEA to T, which can then circulate to the skin, and we now know that structures within the skin, namely the hair follicle and sebaceous gland, have the potential to form potent androgens locally, instead of relying on circulating levels of hormones (6,8,9).

Local versus systemic production of androgens is an important aspect to consider when evaluating specific diseases/disorders. In the past, it was thought that androgen-related skin disorders, such as acne, androgenetic alopecia, and hirsutism, were due to an elevated systemic production of T and DHT from gonadal sources such as ovary, testes, or prostate. We now know that the enzymes for transforming DHEA to DHT are located in sebaceous glands and hair follicles of skin, and that the amounts of these enzymes will vary with body site location: higher levels of enzymes are found on scalp and facial and genital skin than on leg, abdomen, and back (6,8,9).

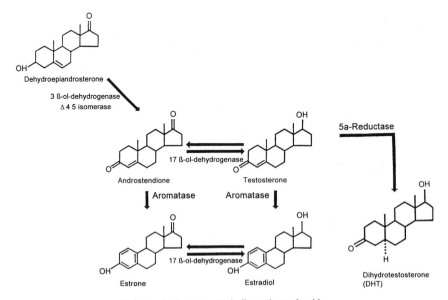

FIG. 1. Androgen metabolic pathway in skin.

In skin, the enzymes in the androgen metabolic pathway are shown in Fig. 1, where DHEA is converted to DHT via Δ5, 3β-hydroxysteroid dehydrogenase, 17β-hydroxysteroid dehydrogenase, and 5α-reductase. The cytochrome P-450 aromatase enzyme (Aromatase) converts T and androstenedione to estradiol and estrone, respectively. The conversion of androgens by these enzymes is dependent on oxidized and reduced pyridine cofactors, NAD, NADH, and NADPH.

It has been found that women have higher levels of the aromatase enzyme in scalp hair follicles than their male counterparts (9,10). Thus while the same enzymes may be present the level of enzymes produced can vary between men and women, effecting skin conditions such as hair loss, commonly known as androgenic alopecia (8,9).

The oxidized/reduced pyridine cofactors are important since these cofactors are required for the enzymic conversions to take place, and they can determine the direction of synthesis for reversible reactions, such as those involving the 17β-hydroxysteroid dehydrogenase enzyme (9). The cofactors are synthesized in other metabolic pathways such as the TCA (Krebs) cycle, the pentose phosphate pathway, etc. It has been suggested (8,11,12) that the levels of reduced or oxidized cofactors are influenced by androgens themselves in a negative feedback inhibition fashion as was shown for the glucose-6-phosphate dehydrogenase enzyme in the pentose phosphate pathway limiting the production of NADPH.

Fig. 1 describes the general pathway for steroid metabolism in skin. It should be emphasized that there are many more steps in the cascade that for simplicity's sake were not listed. Most, if not all, of the enzymes shown have been identified and characterized in whole human skin from face to genital areas. Differences in biochemical characteristics have been described for the 5α-reductase enzyme from skin versus that of prostatic origin, suggesting that there are two separate 5α-reductase enzymes, I and II (8,13,14) respectively, and that substrates for one enzyme may not work as well for the other enzyme. Hence, antiandrogens found to be effective for prostate diseases may have different or altered effects when used to treat skin disorders (8).

FORMING AN ACTIVATED ANDROGEN RECEPTOR COMPLEX

Phosphorylation

From Fig. 2, once DHT or T is formed systemically or locally, it binds to a specific intracellular receptor, the androgen receptor (AR), which forms an activated hormone–receptor complex (HRC). The AR is dependent on other cellular factors to activate it to form the HRC. Steroid receptors are phosphoproteins, phosphorylated by specific kinases, usually either a serine or a tyrosine residue (15–18). In several reports (15–18) there has been evidence to suggest that steroid receptors are inactivated and kept in an "unoccupied" state when they are dephosphorylated, indicating that ligand binding is dependent on the phosphorylation of the receptor. It

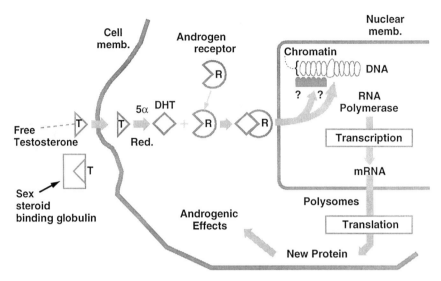

FIG. 2. Cellular mechanism of androgens.

is also thought that the AR must be in a sulfhydryl-reduced state for optimum hormone binding to occur at the ligandbinding site of the AR (19). Thus, the phosphorylating and sulfhydryl reducing enzymes are necessary for AR activation to form the HRC, which can then bind to specific gene sites to alter protein synthesis.

Sulfhydryl Reduction by the Thioredoxin Enzyme System

The sulfhydryl reducing factor in skin is believed to be a thioredoxin enzyme system (TR) that influences intramolecular disulfide bonding of the AR, which affects hormone binding to its specific site (6,8,9). The TR is found in many tissues of the body and has many functions: an electron transfer protein common to all living cells, a reducer of free radicals at the surface of skin, an antioxidant in reduction of methionine residues, a reducer of disulfide links in proteins, and an electron donor in ribonucleotide reductases for RNA synthesis (20). The TR enzyme also utilizes reduced pyridine cofactors NADPH.

Previous investigators have shown that TR and other sulhydryl oxidative–reductive enzymes, such as protein disulfide isomerase (21), glutathione transhydrogenase, sulfhydryl oxidase, and the disulfide interchange enzyme (22), are important for activating other classes of steroid receptors. Investigations have shown that these sulfhydryl oxidating–reducing enzymes are important for activation of the glucocorticoid receptor in skin (23). Elevated or suppressed TR levels have been found in certain skin diseases; for example, elevated TR levels were found in psoriasis and keloids, hyperproliferating disorders (24,25), whereas levels were found to be suppressed in alopecia areata (26).

Inhibitor Protein

An endogenous cellular factor found in skin called inhibitor protein, an 18-kDa protein, was found in human hair follicles (6,8,9) and shown to be important in regulating T or DHT hormone binding to the AR binding site. Other inhibitor-type substances have been found for rat uterus, ventral prostate, liver, etc. and are thought to interact with steroid receptors at various levels. For example, low molecular weight inhibitors extracted from cytosol have been found for the glucocorticoid receptor (27) and thought to inhibit one or more of the following: hormone binding to the receptor, transformation of the receptor, and translocation to the nucleus (28). Another inhibitor type substance (or more than one) has been found for reproductive tissues, the ovary and uterus, which works in a similar fashion for the estrogen receptor and progesterone receptors (29,30).

The inhibitor protein in skin may be binding near the hormone binding site of the AR to alter the conformational shape of the receptor, discouraging or blocking steroid binding to its ligand binding site, hence giving an overall effect of limiting or regulating hormone binding (31).

INTRANUCLEAR MECHANISMS OF ANDROGEN ACTION

AR Gene and Functional Domains

The binding of the HRC to chromatin initiates the sequence of events that culminates in the observed biologic response, Fig. 2. The direction and magnitude of the reaction and its effect on the expression of specific genes are, however, dictated by the metabolic and differentiation states of the cell (32). Since it is also accepted that steroids function through modulation of gene transcription, we now know that there is direct binding of the HRC to a cis-acting DNA sequence, termed the hormone response element (HRE), which is within or flanking the gene under androgen control. AR, in its activated state as the HRC, binds to the HRE, which stimulates transcription, and in most cases the HRE behaves as a classical enhancer element, since it functions independently of orientation and position and can confer hormone regulation on a heterologous promotor. Studies of sequence analysis of a variety of HREs has identified a short palindromic consensus sequence that defines the binding site for the AR (32). It has been found that a small 15-base pair of oligonucleotides contain these HRE sequences, which confers androgen regulation upon nearby promotors (33,34). The HRE sequences that are spatially close for various steroids may explain the multiple control of single genes by several steroid hormones.

The hypothesis that the cis-acting DNA element, the HRE, binds the AR complex to stimulate transcription is also consistent with data showing that the AR must undergo dimerization for binding to DNA. Many transcriptional factors, including members of the steroid receptor family, undergo dimer formation in acquiring high affinity DNA binding (35). Dimerization of the AR, and of other steroid receptors such as the progesterone, glucocorticoid, and estrogen receptors (35), was demonstrated with the mobility shift assay using wild-type and truncated forms of the receptors.

Recent studies (35) have demonstrated AR expressed in baculovirus which displays high affinity AR binding, androgen-dependent nuclear translocation, and phosphorylation. AR dimerization required ligand binding to the receptor when the amino-terminus domain of the AR was present. It was concluded that intramolecular interactions between the amino-terminus and steroid binding domains are regulated by the specificity of hormone binding which modulates receptor dimerization and DNA binding.

The AR protein is encoded by a single gene containing eight exons and located on the x chromosome (36) . Analysis of the cloned AR sequences shows that they correspond to various other receptors in the steroid family. Cloning the AR gene has contributed to our understanding of the molecular basis of disease (37,38).

Like other members of the steroid receptor family, the AR gene comprises four functional domains (Fig. 3). Domain I is composed of parts of the N-terminal end, encoded by exon 1 of the gene, that promote transactivation of certain target genes. Domain II is a DNA-binding domain, located near the center of the polypeptide, which facilitates binding of the AR protein onto specific target genes. The DNA-binding domain is characteristic of a conserved cysteine-rich sequence that forms finger-like structures that are metal ion–stabilized polypeptide configurations found in DNA-binding proteins (32).

Domain III is the hinge domain, which is thought to be responsible for binding other proteins and may have some negative control of transcription. A protein associated with this area is a nuclear matrix–associated acceptor protein (NAP), a small molecular weight protein, less than 20 kDa, that has been found in various tissues (6,9,32).

NAPs have been found in animal (39) and human (40) models and are important

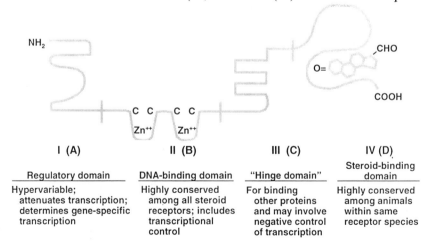

I (A)	II (B)	III (C)	IV (D)
			Steroid-binding domain
Regulatory domain	DNA-binding domain	"Hinge domain"	
Hypervariable; attenuates transcription; determines gene-specific transcription	Highly conserved among all steroid receptors; includes transcriptional control	For binding other proteins and may involve negative control of transcription	Highly conserved among animals within same receptor species

FIG. 3. Domains of steroid receptors.

in mediating high affinity binding of the AR–HRCs to DNA. It may be that the AR binds directly to NAP, using either the hinge region or the zinc fingers of domain II, the DNA-binding domain.

The NAPs that have been isolated and extracted from pools of other nonhistone nuclear proteins have been found to be tissue specific and unique in specificity for mediating high, saturable binding of HRCs to DNA. Studies have shown that removing NAP from nuclear chromatin using detergents revealed loss of high affinity binding (39,40).

The NAP has been found to be a 12-kDa protein for AR in skin (40), a 10-kDa protein for progesterone receptors in avian oviduct (39), a 20-kDa protein for the AR in rat ventral prostate (41), and several other weights for the estrogen receptor (39). Researchers are engaged in characterizing the DNA fragments associated with these NAPs with the intent of finding specific DNA sequences necessary for HRC binding, as well as the specific androgen-regulated genes signaling synthesis of cellular proteins altering growth and differentiation.

Domain IV is the hormone-binding domain, located near the C-terminus of the protein, which is responsible for the specificity and affinity of ligand binding (32). It is the hormone-binding domain that determines the specificity for the steroid. Studies with mutated receptor molecules indicate that in the absence of androgen, this domain inhibits AR binding to DNA, an effect that is attenuated in the presence of hormone (42).

Mutated AR/Gene Defects

Many studies of AR gene expression are primarily in animals with the testicular feminization mutation (Tfm), which has an X-linked mutation where there are diminished ARs in tissues of the body (43). The androgen resistance syndromes in general have been studied in subjects with affected families where analysis of the patterns of inheritance has provided insight into the pathogenesis and has made it possible to define distinct subgroups of the disorders. The molecular processes by which androgens act within cells have been identified (43), and techniques are now within our reach to assess these processes in biopsy material from affected subjects and in fibroblasts cultured from skin biopsies, or by use of the polymerase chain reaction. As a consequence we now have greater insight into the roles of the various genes involved in normal androgen action.

The molecular defects responsible for androgen resistance seen in the androgen insensitivity syndrome (AIS) disorders (Table 1) occur mainly at three sites in the pathway for androgen action (Fig. 2): at the enzyme 5α-reductase and at the androgen receptor, and receptor-positive resistance occurs where subsequent phases of gene site activation/stimulation abnormalities have been detected. It is now known that several mutations in the 5α-reductase enzyme have been found, along with a variety of defects in the AR, rendering considerable genetic heterogeneity in these syndromes.

Studies by Nakao et al. (44) have shown that a single amino acid substitution in

TABLE 1. *Mutations that cause AIS disorders*

Syndrome	Level of mutation		
	5α-R	AR	Postreceptor effect
Familial pseudoherm aphroditism	+ +[a]		
Incomplete AIS		+ +	
Idiopathic male infertility		+[b]	
Reifenstein syndrome		+	
Complete AIS		+	+/?

[a]Severe.
[b]Mild.
AIS, androgen insensitivity syndrome; 5α-R, 5α-reductase; AR, androgen receptors.

AIS, androgen insensitivity syndrome; 5α-R, 5α-reductase; AR, androgen receptor. the steroid-binding domain of the human AR leads to the androgen insensitivity syndrome, Reifenstein syndrome. From this point mutation in the steroid-binding domain, these patients exhibit phenotypic variation ranging from azospermia and gynecomastia, to more severe defects such as hypospadias or even the presence of a pseudovagina. Elucidating the molecular basis of these variant AISs has provided new insights into the molecular mechanisms of androgen action. To date, studies of the molecular basis of AIS have revealed complete and partial deletions of the AR gene (43,44), as well as mutations in the 5α-reductase enzyme (Table 1). In one patient (45), two structural alterations in the AR gene were reported, both of which contributed to AR dysfunction. Others (43,44) have found single base substitutions within the DNA- and hormone-binding regions of exons 2–8 that appear to underlie the disorder in the majority of cases to date where a gene defect has been found.

ANDROGEN GENE EXPRESSION AT OTHER LEVELS

Androgens affect gene expression at levels other than transcription. Alterations in mRNA stability (46,47), protein processing (48), and protein turnover (49,50) have all been documented. It still remains to be determined whether these are primary effects of androgens or secondary effects resulting from androgen action at other sites. The distinction between primary and secondary effects should also be made for transcriptional regulation by steroids in general, not to mention androgens alone, for in some cases, hormonal induction of transcription has been shown to be indirect (51,52).

At the molecular level, androgens can exert their effects at several levels. From nuclear assays, it has been shown that urinary proteins can be hormonally induced in mouse liver (53), and that ovalbumin and ovomucoid can be induced in chick oviduct (54) by increases in transcription of the corresponding genes. On the other hand, androgen induction of rat prostatic steroid-binding proteins (55) and mRNAs of the mouse kidney (56) may involve posttranscriptional mechanisms. Induction of ornithine decarboxylase in mouse kidney involves protein stabilization (49,57).

Other study models have dissected the molecular mechanisms of androgen action, including the steroid-binding protein in rat prostate (55,58), the sex-limited protein gene in mouse liver (59,60), and the mouse mammary tumor virus (58,61, 62). Transfection experiments with cloned sequences indicate that the AR regulation of these genes is conferred by nearby DNA elements. Overlap in gene expression is seen in the case of the mammary tumor virus, where the glucocorticoid response HRE within the long terminal repeat of the viral genome is responsible for progestin and androgen effects (61,58).

RECEPTOR RECYCLING

Very little is known about the specific mechanisms involved in receptor recycling. However, after their action in the nucleus, the HRC state becomes deactivated and the AR reenters the cytoplasm of the cell where it is thought that the sequence of events is repeated (18,28).

Recycling aside, the amount of AR in the cytoplasm or nucleus is regulated. The androgens themselves are most likely involved in the regulation of their own receptors and the enzymes that mediate their conversion to more or less potent derivatives for excretion (28).

ANDROGENS IN THE AGING PROCESS

Cellular changes that occur during the aging process affect reproduction, fertility, tumorigenic processes, and even alter hair growth in skin (6,7,9,28,39). Age-related molecular proteins have been found to affect gene expression by masking specific positive or negative HRE sites important for growth and differentiation of normal cells (39,40). These age-related nucleoacidic, nonhistone proteins are thought to mask and occlude certain gene sites that can alter cell growth, as seen in the aging process.

ANDROGENS AND ONCOGENES

The viral oncogenes encode proteins that are associated with the transformation of normal cells to cancer cells. The cellular oncogenes, called proto-oncogenes, from which the viral oncogenes were derived have important roles in growth and differentiation of normal cells. Androgens, directly or in conjunction with altered oncogenic products, appear to be important in the growth and differentiation of cancer cells (7). The amino acid sequence of many of the steroid receptors, including AR, is similar to the *erb*-A (Avian erythroblastosis virus) oncogene product, which indicate that a superfamily of transcription factors may exist which regulate normal and malignant growth and differentiation. Results imply that these two classes of proteins have important interrelationships.

The *erb*-A oncogene is a retrovirus which induces erythroblastosis and sarcomas in birds and transforms erythroblasts and fibroblasts in vitro (7). Some investigators

(7,28,39) believe that these viral oncogenes regulate gene transcription by acting through cellular receptors similar to those seen for the steroid receptors, including AR, estrogen, progesterone, and glucocorticoid receptors. The *erb*-A gene exhibits significant similarity to the steroid receptor's DNA-binding domain, region C of the receptor, but it is most variable in region E, the hormone-binding domain, the area most varied between the different classes of receptors. It may be that the gene products from these viral oncogenes have different functions depending on the tissue in which they appear. It has been found that the human c-*erb*-A genes are located in close proximity to the chromosomal breakpoints in two leukemias, indicating an association with these cancerous states (7).

Androgens and glucocorticoids can affect oncogene mRNA and AR expression in certain cells. Two cell lines, the DDT-MF-2 and R3327H-G8–A1 (7), are derived from tumors of the male reproductive tissues, and have been used to study the relationship of steroids and oncogene c-*sis* with cell growth and receptor concentration. Both cell lines contain AR and glucocorticoid receptors, and are sensitive to platelet derived growth factor (PDGF), which is a product of the c-*sis* oncogene. Androgens stimulate growth and increase the concentration of AR in both cell lines, whereas glucocorticoids inhibit both of these events and arrest the cells in the G_1 phase of the cell cycle. Androgens administered at the same time as the glucocorticoids do not prevent this block. Usually these cells synthesize and secrete PDGF which regulates progression through the cell cycle in an autocrine fashion. The glucocorticoids inhibit the expression of the c-*sis* gene, resulting in cell cycle arrest. Adding PDGF to these arrested cells allows them to progress through the cell cycle and overcome the effects of the glucocorticoids. Even so, the AR concentration is still suppressed, indicating that the effects of glucocorticoids on the AR level and cell cycle progression are mediated by two independent processes (7).

Direct correlations of androgen hormonal status and oncogene expression have been performed. In experiments using four prostatic cancer cell lines, large amounts of Ha-ras and myc mRNA were detected in all of the lines tested, with lower amounts of N-ras, Ki-ras, myb, fms, fos, and sis observed in some of the cell lines, with no transcripts for fes, int-1, or abl. An androgen-dependent line, PC 92, has shown higher levels of fos mRNA in addition to the myc and Ha-ras mRNAs. When the androgens were withdrawn, subsequent inhibition of growth occurred, fos mRNA levels decreased to minimal levels and Ha-ras mRNA levels dropped by more than 50%; however, myc levels were unchanged (7). It may be that the fos expression is reduced due to inhibition of cell growth, or that decreased expression is a cause of the inhibition, but overall the studies suggest that there is a direct correlation of androgen status and oncogene expression.

CONCLUSIONS

While a great deal of knowledge on the mechanisms of androgen-regulated gene expression now exists, information relating to specific androgen associated diseases is lacking. A number of experimental systems have been developed and show promise as models for molecular studies of androgen regulation. Further development of these models may show greater insight into androgen related disease processes, as well as shape more effective treatment options to prevent or treat diseases in the future.

REFERENCES

1. Bardin CW, Catterall JF. Testosterone: a major determinant of extragenital sexual development. *Science* 1981;24:1285–1294.
2. Gresik EW. Postnatal developmental changes in submandibular glands of rats and mice. *J Histochem Cytochem* 1980;28:860–870.
3. Mills NC, Mills TM, Yurkiewicz WJ, Bardin CW. Actions of androgens on the kidney of female mice: strain differences in the DNA and β-glucuronidase responses. *Int J Androl* 1979;2:371–384.
4. Ringold G. Steroid hormone regulation of gene expression. *Ann Rev Pharmacol Toxicol* 1985; 25:529–566.
5. Yamamoto KR. Steroid receptor regulated transcription of specific genes and gene networks. *Ann Rev Genet* 1985;19:209–252.
6. Sawaya ME, Hordinsky MK. Advances in alopecia and androgenetic alopecia. *Adv Dermatol* 1992;7:211–227.
7. Shepel L, Gorski J. Steroid hormone receptors and oncogenes. *Biofactors* 1988;1:71–83.
8. Sawaya ME, Hordinsky MK. The antiandrogens, when and how they should be used. *Dermatol Clin* 1993;11:65–72.
9. Sawaya ME. Steroid chemistry and hormone controls during the hair follicle cycle. *Ann NY Acad Sci* 1991;642:376–385.
10. Sawaya ME, Penneys NS. Immunohistochemical distribution of aromatase and 3β-hydroxysteroid dehydrogenase in human hair and sebaceous gland. *J Cutan Pathol* 1991;19:309–314.
11. Schweikart HU, Wilson JD. Regulation of human hair growth by steroid hormones. II: Androstenedione metabolism in isolated hairs. *J Clin Endocrinol Metab* 1874;39:1012–1019.
12. Sawaya ME, Honig LS, Garland LD, Hsia SL. 3β-hydroxysteroid dehydrogenase activity in sebaceous glands of scalp in male-pattern baldness. *J Invest Dermatol* 1988;91:101–105.
13. Andersson S, Bishop RW, Russell DW. Expression, cloning and regulation of steroid 5α-reductase, an enzyme essential for male sexual differentiation. *J Biol Chem* 1989;264:16249–16255.
14. Itami S, Kurata S, Sonoda T, Takayasu S. Characterization of 5α-reductase in cultured human dermal papilla cells from beard and occipital hair. *J Invest Dermatol* 1991;96:57–61.
15. Migliaccio A, Rotondi A, Auricchio F. Calmodulin stimulated phosphorylation of 17β-estradiol receptor on tyrosine. *Proc Natl Acad Sci USA* 1984;81:5921–5925.
16. Woo DL, Fay SP, Griest R, Coty W, Goldfine I, Fox CF. Differential phosphorylation of the progesterone receptor by insulin, epidermal growth factor, and platelet-derived growth factor receptor tyrosine protein kinases. *J Biol Chem* 1986;261:460–467.
17. Housley PR, Pratt WB. Direct demonstration of glucocorticoid receptor phosphorylation by intact L-cells. *J Biol Chem* 1983;258:4630–4635.
18. Nielsen CJ, Sando JJ, Pratt WB. Evidence that dephosphorylation inactivates glucocorticoid receptors. *Proc Natl Acad Sci USA* 1977;74:1398–1402.
19. Peleg S, Schrader WT, O'Malley BW. Sulfhydryl group content of chicken progesterone receptor: effect of oxidation on DNA binding activity. *Biochemistry* 1988;27:358–367.
20. Schallreuter KU, Wood JM. The role of thioredoxin reductase in the reduction of free radicals at the surface of the epidermis. *Biochem Biophys Res Commun* 1986;136:630–637.
21. Edman JC, Ellis L, Blacher RW, Roth RA, Rutter WJ. Sequence of protein disulfide isomerase and implications of its relationship to thioredoxin. *Nature* 1985;317:267–270.
22. Lambert N, Freedman RB. Kinetics and specificity of homogeneous protein disulfide-isomerase in protein disulfide isomerization and in thiol protein-disulfide oxidoreduction. *Biochem J* 1983;213: 235–243.
23. Sawaya ME, Lewis LA, Hsia SL. Presence of a converting factor for androgen receptor proteins in isolated human hair follicles and sebaceous glands. *FASEB J* 1989;2:4765.

24. Sawaya ME, Cohen RJ, Taylor JR. Type I and II glucocorticoid receptor analysis in patients with psoriasis. *J Invest Dermatol* 1991;96:618.
25. Sawaya ME, Kirsner RS, Nemeth AJ, Weiss DS, Hsia SL. Elevated type II glucocorticoid receptor binding in keloids and hypertrophic scars. *J Invest Dermatol* 1990;94:575.
26. Sawaya ME, Hordinsky MK, Schmieder GJ. Calcium-calmodulin dependent activation of glucocorticoid receptors in alopecia areata. *J Invest Dermatol* 1991;96:595.
27. Bailly A, Salias N, Milgrom E. A low molecular weight inhibitor of steroid receptor activation. *J Biol Chem* 1977;252:858–862.
28. Grody WW, Schrader, WT, O'Malley BW. Activation, transformation, and subunit structure of steroid hormone receptors. *Endocr Rev* 1982;3:141–163.
29. Jensen EV, Suzuki T, Kawashima T, Stumpf WE, Jungblut PW, DeSombre ER. A two step mechanism for the interaction of estradiol with rat uterus. *Proc Natl Acad Sci USA* 1968;59:632–640.
30. Shen G, Thrower S, Lin L. Uterine estrogen receptor binding of oligo(dT)-cellulose: an inhibitor from hypothalamic cytosol. *Biochem J* 1979;182:241–246.
31. Sawaya ME, Mendez AJ, Hsia SL. Presence of an inhibitor to androgen binding to receptor protein in human sebaceous gland and hair follicle. *J Invest Dermatol* 1988;90:605.
32. Berger FG, Watson G. Androgen regulated gene expression. *Annu Rev Physiol* 1989;51:51–65.
33. Klock G, Strahle U, Schutz G. Oestrogen and glucocorticoid responsive elements are closely related but distinct. *Nature* 1987;329:734–736.
34. Strahle U, Klock G, Schutz G. A DNA sequence of 15 base pairs is sufficient to mediate glucocorticoid and progesterone induction of gene expression. *Proc Natl Acad Sci USA* 1987;84:7871–7875.
35. Wong C, Zhou Z, Sar M, Wilson EM. Steroid requirement for androgen receptor dimerization and DNA binding. *J Biol Chem* 1993;268:19004–19012.
36. Lubahn DB, Brown TR, Simental JA, et al. Sequence of the intro/exon junctions of the coding region of the human androgen receptor gene and identification of a point mutation in a family with complete androgen insensitivity. *Proc Natl Acad Sci USA* 1989;86:9534–9538.
37. Lubahn DB, Joseph DR, Sullivan PM, Willard HF, French FS, Wilson EM. Cloning of human androgen receptor complementary DNA and localization to the X chromosome. *Science* 1988;240: 327–330.
38. Chang CS, Kokontis J, Liao ST. Molecular cloning of human and rat complementary DNA encoding androgen receptors. *Science* 1988;240:324–326.
39. Spelsberg TC, Rories C, Rejman JJ, Goldberger A, Fink K, Lau CK, Colvard DS, Wiseman G. Steroid action on gene expression: possible roles of regulatory genes and nuclear acceptor sites. *Biol Reprod* 1989;40:54–69.
40. Sawaya ME, Kraffert CA, Hsia SL. A nuclear matrix associated receptor protein involved in the chromatin binding of the androgen receptor regulating human hair follicle growth in androgenetic alopecia. *J Invest Dermatol* 1991;96:595.
41. Ho K, Snoek R, Quarmby V, Viskochil DH, et al. Primary structure and androgen regulation of a 20 kilodalton protein specific to rat ventral prostate. *Biochemistry* 1989;28:6367–6373.
42. Godowski PJ, Rusconi S, Miesfield R, Yamamoto K. Glucocorticoid receptor mutants that are constitutive activators of transcriptional enhancement. *Nature* 1987;325:365–368.
43. Hiort 0, Huang Q, Sinnecker G, Sadeghi Nejad AB, et al. Single strand conformation polymorphism analysis of androgen receptor gene mutations in patients with androgen insensitivity syndromes: applications for diagnosis, genetic counseling, and therapy. *J Clin Endocrinol Metab* 1993;77:262–266.
44. Nakao R, Yanase T, Sakai Y, Haji M, Nawata H. A single amino acid substitution in the steroid binding domain of the human androgen receptor leads to Reifenstein syndrome. *J Clin Endocrinol Metab* 1993;77:103–107.
45. McPhaul MJ, Marcelli M, Tilley WD, et al. Molecular basis of androgen resistance in a family with a qualitative abnormality of the androgen receptor and responsive to high dose androgen therapy. *J Clin Invest* 1991;87:1413–1421.
46. Brock ML, Shapiro DJ. Estrogen stabilizes vitellogenin mRNA against cytoplasmic turnover. *Cell* 1983;34;207–214.
47. Paek I, Axel R. Glucocorticoids enhance stability of human growth hormone mRNA. *Mol Cell Biol* 1987;7:1496–1507.
48. Rabindran SK, Danielson M, Firestone GL, Stallcup MR. Glucocorticoid dependent maturation of viral proteins in mouse lymphoma cells isolation of defective and hormone independent cell variants. *Somat Cell Mol Genet* 1987;13:131–143.

49. Isomaa VV, Pajunen AE, Bardin CW, Janne OA. Ornithine decarboxylase in mouse kidney. Purification, characterization and radioimmunological determination of the enzyme protein. *J Biol Chem* 1983;258:6735–6740.

50. Seely JE, Poso H, Pegg AE. Effect of androgens on turnover of ornithine decarboxylase activity are brought about by changes in the amount of enzyme protein as measured by radioimmunoassay. *J Biol Chem* 1982;257:7549–7553.

51. Chen CLC, Feigelson P. Hormonal control of alpha-globulin synthesis and its mRNA in isolated hepatocytes. *Ann NY Acad Sci* 1979;349:28–45.

52. Widman LE, Chasin LA. Multihormonal induction of alpha globulin in an established rat hepatoma cell line. *J Cell Physiol* 1982;112:316–326.

53. Derman E. Isolation of cDNA clone for mouse major urinary proteins: age and sex related expression of mouse urinary protein genes is transcriptionally controlled. *Proc Natl Acad Sci USA* 1981;78:5425–5429.

54. Compere SJ, McKnight GS, Palmiter RD. Androgens regulate ovomucoid and ovalbumin gene expression independently of estrogen. *J Biol Chem* 1981;256:6341–6347.

55. Page MJ, Parker MG. Effect of androgen on the transcription of rat prostatic binding protein genes. *Mol Cell Endocrinol* 1982;27:343–355.

56. Berger FG, Loose DS, Meisner H, Watson G. Androgen induction of messenger RNA concentrations in mouse kidney is post transcriptional. *Biochemistry* 1986;25:1170–1175.

57. Seely JE, Poso H, Pegg AE. Effect of androgens on turnover of ornithine decarboxylase in mouse kidney: studies using labeling of the enzyme by reaction with difuoromethylornithine. *J Biol Chem* 1982;257:7549–7553.

58. Parker MG, Webb P, Needham M, White R, Hain J. Identification of androgen response elements in mouse mammary tumor virus and the rat prostate C3 gene. *J Cell Biochem* 1987;35:285–292.

59. Schreffler DC. The S region of the mouse major histocompatibility complex (H-2): genetic variation and functional role in complement system. *Transplant Rev* 1976;32:140–167.

60. Stavenhagen J, Loreni F, Hemenway C, Kalff M, Robins DM. Molecular genetics of androgen dependent and independent expression of mouse sex limited protein. *Mol Cell Biol* 1987;7:1716–1724.

61. Cato ACB, Henderson D, Ponta H. The hormone response element of the mouse mammary tumor virus DNA mediates the progestin and androgen induction of transcription in the proviral long terminal repeat region. *EMBO J* 1987;6:363–368.

62. Darbre P, Page M, King RJB. Androgen regulation by the long terminal repeat of mouse mammary tumor virus. *Mol Cell Biol* 1986;6:2847–2854.

Androgenic Disorders,
edited by G. P. Redmond.
Raven Press, Ltd., New York © 1995.

4

Interpretation of Androgen Levels in Women

Geoffrey P. Redmond

*Department of Endocrinology, Foundation for Developmental Endocrinology, Inc.,
Cleveland, Ohio 44122*

Androgenic disorders are conditions characterized by excessive androgen action in women. Given this quite simple definition it would be expected that measurement and interpretation of serum levels of androgens in these conditions would be straightforward. That this is not the case is testified to by the enormous volume of medical literature on the subject. There is probably no area of endocrinology about which there is as much confusion as the interpretation of laboratory results in androgenic disorders. Areas of controversy are: what proportion of androgenized women have elevated blood levels of androgens, which circulating androgens are biologically important, what is the glandular origin of the circulating androgens, and what other biochemical abnormalities are associated. This chapter will address these issues to show that adequate information exists to make clinical decisions regarding treatment even though not all theoretical issues have been resolved.

ANDROGENS IN WOMEN

It should not be a surprise that women have biologically active levels of androgens. Normal men, conversely, have biologically significant levels of estrogens, often as high as those in women during the menstrual phase of the cycle. It is an artificial distinction to regard male and female hormones as appropriate for only one gender each. Nonetheless, androgen levels and action are of course much less in women than in men. Normal laboratory ranges vary, but a typical range for testosterone in an adult woman would be 20 to 50 ng/dL. Men have levels 10 to 15 times higher, though there can be overlap in certain situations. In midpuberty, a boy can have levels scarcely above the range of the adult woman. However, it is in later puberty that the most distinctive male gender traits—facial hair and increased muscle bulk—occur when testosterone levels rise above those in women. In adulthood there is generally no overlap. For a woman to have a testosterone level as high as 150 to 200 ng/dL is rare and suggestive of a tumor or severe endocrine disturbance. When levels below 150 ng/dL occur in men, decreased libido and erectile dysfunction are common. Thus, while testosterone is present in adults of both sexes, the levels differ considerably, and when those of one sex approach those of the other, alterations of function are frequent. Women with elevated androgens almost never have testosterone levels in the normal range of men.

The most striking feature of androgen levels in women presenting with an androgen related complaint is their variation with age. All major androgens, total testosterone, free testosterone, androstenedione, dehydroepiandrosterone (DHEA), and DHEA-A, show a similar pattern (1,2). Values are unmeasurably low before puberty, then rise, peaking in the late teens or early twenties, and then gradually decline. In normal women, DHEA and DHEA-S levels decrease with age (3). Testosterone and androstenedione have been less thoroughly studied. Most studies have been cross-sectional so the developmental pattern in individual women may be different. However, there is at least one report that women with high androgen levels during puberty continue to have high levels into adulthood (4).

What controls this developmental pattern is not known, nor is it clear whether it is due to changes in the function of the ovary or adrenal or both. Most likely, both are involved because there is a mutual influence between ovarian and adrenal androgen secretion. It is clearly not due to senescence since secretion declines at an age when ovarian function and ovulation are still unimpaired.

Testosterone secretion in women has some diurnal variation, with higher levels late in the day. This may be one reason why values obtained during an office visit may be normal in obviously androgenized women: the values measured at that moment are not representative of overall integrated secretion. There is no practical solution to this because repeated androgen determinations are expensive as well as inconvenient. A better solution is to recognize that a single androgen level, however precise, is only a means to approximate overall secretion. Thus a high normal value may represent oversecretion if levels are that high most of the 24-hour day. It is essential to be aware of the indistinctness of the zone between normal and abnormal in interpreting androgen levels. This may seem an obvious point but it is one often ignored in practice. Certainly if a women is experiencing excessive androgen action, a single normal testosterone level does not exclude the possibility of a subtle hypersecretory state. Admittedly this may not be provable in the clinical setting, but the physician will deal with more such borderline states than clear-cut ones when working with androgenic disorders, and it is useful to be aware of possible explanations.

In the perimenopause and after, androgen levels in women are lower than they were during the menstrual years. A testosterone level in the high-normal level for a menstrual age woman would be considered elevated if obtained after menopause. There is a common misimpression that androgen levels rise after menopause. While a small subset go on to have hyperthecosis, the great majority of postmenopausal women have quite low levels—even those who develop androgenic changes. This is commonly attributed to the lower levels of sex steroid–binding globulin, which result from low estrogen levels. However, androgen action in postmenopausal women has rarely been studied, and the reason for the slight virilization that sometimes occurs in women's sixth decade or later is unclear. Most women with gradual and subtle androgenic changes after menopause have low, rather than elevated, androgen levels. Their free testosterone is also low because it depends not only on levels of sex hormone–binding globulin (SHBG) but also on levels of total testosterone. Whether the same amounts of free testosterone somehow diffuse more freely into the tissues, or whether the lack of estrogen somehow potentiates androgen effects (commonly assumed but unproven), or whether it is simply accumulation of slow androgen action over the decades is unclear. Perhaps all three mechanisms are involved.

While it is clear that testosterone, especially in its free form, is the most active circulating androgen, the relative importance of androstenedione and DHEA and its sulfate are less so. These are inactive as androgens but may be converted to testosterone and so presumably form a pool of testosterone precursor. There is good evidence that many young women with marked acne have increased DHEA-S levels (5). However, determination that DHEA-S is involved in a particular young woman may be difficult because mean values in the late teens and early twenties are considerably about the usual reference range of up to 300 or 350 μg/dL. Treatment with small doses of dexamethasone to suppress DHEA-S to normal is discussed in Chapter 14. DHEA-S appears to be controlled by mechanisms different from those that control secretion of testosterone, so blood levels of these two androgens are often dissociated.

Androstenedione levels are more usually, but not invariably, correlated with testosterone levels. Elevation of androstenedione without elevation of testosterone is almost never seen, although the converse is not necessarily so. Some women with elevation of testosterone do not have increased androstenedione levels. This means that measurement of androstenedione is less important than either testosterone or DHEA-S but it is still useful in forming an estimate of the total androgen burden. There is probably an additive effect of the different circulating androgens but no formula to combine them has been devised. The usual upper normal limit for androstenedione is 250 ng/dL, but values over 200 may be indicative of a subtle state of androgen overproduction, especially if testosterone is also elevated.

Tumor Levels

A common concern in the evaluation of the androgenized woman is the possibility of an adrenal or ovarian tumor. These are in fact extremely rare; my experience suggests that the incidence is considerably less than 1% in women presenting because of an androgenic disorder. The most serious cause is adrenal carcinoma. While hirsutism may indeed be a presenting feature, there are usually other signs present. The usual empirical rule is that a testosterone level over 200 ng/dL, an androstenedione level over 400 ng/dL, and a DHEA-S level over 600 μg/dL should prompt expeditious ruling out of tumor. It may be better to set the level a little lower, at 150 ng/dL, for testosterone.

Few androgenized women have levels as high as these, and as a result, adrenal and ovarian imaging studies are only occasionally necessary for androgenic disorders. Pelvic exam or ultrasound will rule out large ovarian tumors but cannot exclude the possibility of a small, benign thecal cell tumor deep in the ovary. In the current state of technology, CT scan of the adrenals without contrast is the appropriate study to look for an adrenal tumor. Carcinoma will be unmistakable. However, many normal women have "incidentalomas" of a few millimeters in the adrenal, hence a small abnormal area cannot be assumed to be the source of androgen hypersecretion.

Venous sampling studies are nowadays rarely performed. There is difficulty of being certain of the exact placement of the catheter. Additionally, during the luteal phase and perhaps before it, one ovary predominates over the other in sex steroid secretion, and therefore much higher androgen secretion from one ovary does not necessarily establish a tumor in that ovary. A similar situation may obtain in thecal cell hyperplasia. Even though both ovaries appear to be involved, based on their histopathological appearance after removal, androgen secretion may be much higher from one ovary at the time of sampling. In such cases, removal of one ovary might seem a tempting therapeutic option, but it would not be curative. Similarly, with a small adrenal lesion of unclear significance, detection of only slightly increased secretion from that adrenal does not necessarily establish that a functioning tumor is present. However, there is still a place for venous sampling studies (6), for example to establish that a mass seen on imaging studies is actually the source of elevated androgens, provided caution is exercised in their interpretation. When androgen levels are suppressible, however, venous sampling is generally inappropriate.

The levels found in late-onset 21–hydroxylase deficiency can be as high as those found with functioning tumors so that adrenocorticotropic hormone (ACTH) stimulation testing is essential when evaluating the woman with a marked elevation of testosterone. Since a tumor may behave as if it has an enzyme block, however, imaging studies are sometimes still necessary.

Androgen secreting tumors and Cushing's disease and syndrome are discussed in detail in Chapters 8 and 10.

OVARIAN AND ADRENAL CONTRIBUTIONS

One of the classic issues concerning androgenic disorders concerns the source of circulating androgens. Until recently, the relative roles of adrenal and ovary were frequently debated. Now it is recognized that both can be involved (6) and that individual women with androgenic disorders vary greatly in the contributions of ovary and adrenal (7). Ovarian hyperandrogenism tends to present at a younger age and is more likely to be associated with obesity (frequently but not invariably android), oligomenorrhea, and infertility. However there are many exceptions to these generalizations; the relative ovarian and adrenal contributions cannot be determined without formal suppression testing. Clinical application of these tests is further discussed in Chapter 14.

It does seem that androgen hypersecretion by either gland can somehow produce hypersecretion by the other. Clearly, adrenal hypersecretion can be a factor in women who have been assigned the diagnosis of polycystic ovary disease (PCOD) (8). This is another reason why the distinction between ovarian and adrenal disorders is not absolute. Nor has it been proven that ovarian and adrenal components do not vary over time in the same woman.

Testosterone and androstenedione can be of either adrenal or ovarian origin, but DHEA-S is almost exclusively ovarian. An elevated DHEA-S thus does indicate an adrenal source but only for itself, not for testosterone or androstenedione. While it is probably true that when elevations of either of these androgens are accompanied by a high DHEA-S, their source is somewhat more likely to be adrenal, but there are too many exceptions for this to be relied on in diagnosis.

STIMULATION AND SUPPRESSION TESTING

Dynamic testing is necessary to determine the nature of androgen hypersecretion. In most cases, the question is the relative adrenal versus ovarian origin of the androgen or androgens whose levels are elevated. For this, dexamethasone suppression testing is most helpful. Our protocol employs a dose of 0.375 mg orally q.i.d. for about 8 days. It is essential to administer the dexamethasone for several days in order to have adequate suppression of adrenal androgen secretion. While a single bedtime dose of dexamethasone is often used to test suppressibility of cortisol secretion, several days of administration are required to suppress adrenal biosynthesis and secretion of androgens. Failure to recognize this fact has frequently led to underestimation of the adrenal contribution to circulating androgens.

A convenient way to administer the dose is to use one and one-half of a 0.25 mg tablet four times daily. The patient is told to continue to take the medication until blood has been drawn at the end of the test. A very few patients complain of mild stimulation or insomnia during the test, but we have not seen serious side effects in several hundred tests carried out over the last few years. Facial rounding, weight gain, or striae have not occurred. Dexamethasone does sometimes restore ovulation, however, so patients should be informed of the need for contraception.

At the end of the test, whatever androgens were initially elevated are measured again, together with a serum cortisol. If the latter is not suppressed, it suggests that the patient has not been compliant with the regimen. In our experience, this is infrequent, but is important to discover because otherwise the test will be interpreted to show ovarian hyperandrogenism. If a particular androgen was not elevated initially, there is no need to repeat the level at the end of the dexamethasone course. If DHEA-S is the only androgen elevated, formal suppression testing as described here is not usually necessary because DHEA-S is always mainly adrenal in origin. However, if extremely high levels are present, suppression testing may be warranted as part of the evaluation of a possible adrenal tumor.

The postdexamethasone androgen levels represent the ovarian contribution. By dividing the final androgen level by the initial one, an estimate of the fraction originating from the ovary is determined. A rise in level at the end of the test simply indicates that nearly all the androgen is ovarian; dexamethasone does not stimulate androgen release.

It should be realized that the interpretation of the test is a clinical approximation and not strictly anatomical. There is some evidence of ovarian cells which respond to ACTH stimulation. It is more accurate to state that what is tested is the fraction of the androgen that is under ACTH control, but even this may not be definitive because of the possibility of some suppression of luteinizing hormone (LH) by dexamethasone. Finally, the lowering of testosterone may be due to suppression of precursor androstenedione secretion resulting in less substrate for peripheral conversion, rather than to release of testosterone itself. These theoretical limitations are not problematic in clinical practice, because for therapeutic decisions it is the ACTH dependence of the androgen rather than its exact anatomical origin which is most important. Partial dexamethasone suppressibility by itself may not be sufficient to rule out a tumor, however, if androgen levels are extremely high.

Stimulation testing is mainly performed to rule out one of the forms of adrenal hyperplasia. This subject is discussed in detail in Chapter 11. Generally, between 250 and 1,000 µg of synthetic 1–24 ACTH subunit (Cortrosyn [r], Organon) is administered intravenously, and blood samples are obtained at 0, 30, and 60 min. Steroid metabolites that are measured are 17-hydroxyprogesterone, 17-hydroxypregnenolone, and ll-desoxycortisol (compound S) to look for 21-hydroxylase deficiency, 3β hydroxysteroid dehydrogenase deficiency, and 11-hydroxylase deficiency respectively. Cortisol is measured as well to confirm that adrenal stimulation has in fact occurred. An alternative diagnostic method is to measure urinary metabolites by gas chromatography/mass spectroscopy, but this technology is not generally available in clinical laboratories.

It is not clear which patients need stimulation testing to look for adrenal hyperplasia. In children, the presence of genital ambiguity at birth or early appearance of androgen-mediated pubertal changes in boys or girls (if severe) indicate the need for such testing. When the late onset or nonclassical form is being sought, the situation is less certain. We employ such testing when androgen elevation is severe. It should be noted that the group of women whose androgens are suppressed with dexamethasone will include those with classical or nonclassical adrenal hyperplasia. However, it is impractical as well as costly to test all women with androgenic disorders for enzyme defects.

MEASURES OF 5α-REDUCTASE ACTIVITY

A few years ago there was considerable interest in tests that would measure dihydrotestosterone (DHT) metabolites produced in the skin (9,10). The idea was that those with idiopathic hirsutism, that is, pronounced hirsutism with normal androgen levels, might have increased conversion of testosterone to its more active metabolite DHT by the 5α-reductase enzyme in the target organ (11). The metabolite most often measured is 3α-androstanediol glucuronide (3α diol G). Once thought to be specific for skin conversion of testosterone to DHT, this is now known to reflect metabolism in other sites as well. Its clinical utility is questionable (12). At best it simply confirms that the patient's hair follicles are especially sensitive to testosterone, something that is apparent from the clinical finding of hirsutism.

OTHER USEFUL TESTS

Prolactin

Although some reports indicate that prolactin is increased in women with PCOD in comparison to normals, the levels are still within the normal range. There is sometimes confusion on this point. Androgenic disorders and mild hyperprolactinemia are common endocrinopathies in otherwise healthy women and, as a result, they not infrequently coexist. These are almost always separate conditions needing separate evaluations and, when necessary, separate treatments. It is especially important not to misinterpret definite hyperprolactinemia (values over 30 to 35 pg/ml) as due to an androgenic disorder. MRI of the pituitary is necessary in such cases to rule out the possibility of a prolactinoma. Treatment of hyperprolactinemia with bromocryptine will not correct any coexisting androgen excess. Indeed hyperprolactinemia may be associated with low androgens because of the suppression of ovarian activity.

LH and FSH

Somehow the idea that the LH-to-FSH (follicle-stimulating hormone) ratio is the definitive test for PCOD has become widespread (13). (Elevated is usually defined as greater than 2.5 or 3.0.) The popularity of this ratio is unfortunate because this determination is of very limited utility in diagnostic evaluation of androgenic disorders. While it is an important observation that LH secretion by the pituitary is increased in PCOD (14), it does not follow that its ratio to LH will be elevated on a given occasion. Indeed we have seen many women who would otherwise meet criteria for PCOD who do not have an elevated LH/FS ratio. Similarly, it is possible that a woman without PCOD might have LH levels above those of FSH just by random fluctuation. Another fallacy in relying on LH/FSH is not recognizing that the ratio is not of direct pathophysiological significance. The cause of androgenic skin and hair changes in PCOD and other forms of androgenic disorder is the action of testosterone and other androgens. Hence direct measurements of these steroids are most closely tied to the severity of the disturbance and, when used with stimulation or suppression tests as indicated, show the origin of the hypersecretion. LH/FSH is less useful in deciding therapy than the levels of the androgenic steroids whose action is actually causing the skin and hair changes.

This is not to say that the disordered secretion of gonadotropins in androgenic disorders is not of considerable interest in trying to unravel the nature of the abnormal control mechanisms. However as a clinical test it is of limited value. Certainly dexamethasone suppression testing is a more direct means of quantitating the ovarian contribution to hypersecretion of androgens.

Thyroid Hormones

Thyroid dysfunction does not seem to be a feature of androgenic disorders. However, questions about the normality of thyroid function commonly arise because of the suspicion of thyroid enlargement, because of concerns, most often on the part of the patient, that obesity may have a metabolic cause, or because thyroid abnormalities can occasionally be the cause of menstrual dysfunction. Thyroid-stimulating hormone (TSH) is most sensitive and, if normal, makes an abnormality of thyroid function improbable.

CONCLUSIONS

Skillful use of the laboratory is essential for proper diagnosis and treatment of women with androgenic disorders. However, test results are sometimes ambiguous and have meaning only within the context of the individual's clinical findings. Nowhere is this more true than with androgenic disorders. The preceding chapter has attempted to outline the use of the major tests and point out possible pitfalls in their interpretation.

REFERENCES

1. Redmond GP, Bergfeld W, Gupta M, Parker R, Subichin S, Bedocs N, Gidwani G. Comparison of hormonal abnormalities in women with different manifestations of androgen excess. In: Genazzani AR, Volpe A, Facchinetti F, ed. *Research in gynecological endocrinology.* London: Parthenon; 1986;187–190.
2. Redmond GP, Bergfeld W, Gupta M, Bedocs C, Skibinski C, Gidwani G. Clinical and biochemical findings in 500 women with androgenic disorders. In: *The Endocrine Society Program Abstracts*; Seattle, WA, June 1989; 330.
3. Orentreich N, Brind JL, Rizer RL, Vogelman JH. Age changes and sex differences in serum dehydroepiandrosterone and dehydroepiandrosterone sulfate throughout adulthood. *J Clin Endocrinol Metab* 1984;59:551.
4. Apter D, Vihko R. Endocrine determinants of fertility: serum androgen concentrations during follow-up of adolescents into the third decade of life. *J Clin Endocrinol Metab* 1990;71:970–974.
5. Marynick SP, Chakmakjian ZH, McCaffree DL, Herdon JH, Jr. Androgen excess in cystic acne. *N Engl J Med* 1983;308:981–986.
6. Moltz L, Schwartz U. Gonadal and adrenal androgen secretion in hirsute females. *Clinics Endocrinol Metab* 1986;15:229–245.
7. Redmond GP, Gidwani G, Bergfeld W, Skibinksi C, Gupta M, Parker R, Bedocs N. Regulation of excessive androgen secretion in women: role of ACTH responsive endocrine tissue. *Fertil Steril Program Suppl* 1987;83.

8. McKenna TJ, Cunningham SK. Adrenal abnormalities in polycystic ovarian syndrome and the impact of their correction. In: Dunaif A, Givens JR, Haseltine F, Merriam GR, eds.: *Polycystic ovarian syndrome*. Boston: Blackwell Scientific; 1992;183–193.

9. Horton R, Hawks D, Lobo R. 3 alpha-androstanediol glucuronide in plasma: a marker of androgen action in idiopathic hirsutism. *J Clin Invest* 1982;69:1203–1206.

10. Lookingbill DP, Horton R, Demers LM, et al. Tissue production of androgens in women with acne. *J Am Acad Dermatol* 1985;12:481–487.

11. Horton R, Lobo R. Peripheral androgens and the role of androstanediol glucuronide. *Clin Endocrinol Metab* 1986;15:293–306.

12. Salman K, Spielvogel RL, Shulman LH, et al. Serum androstanediol glucuronide in women with facial hirsutism. *J Am Acad Dermatol* 1992;26:411–414.

13. Yen SSC, Vela P, Rankin J. Inappropriate secretion of follicle-stimulating hormone and luteinizing hormone in polycystic ovarian disease. *J Clin Endocrinol Metab* 1970; 30:435.

14. Kazar RR, Kessel B, Yen SSC. Circulating luteinizing hormone pulse frequency in women with polycystic ovary syndrome (PCO). *J Clin Endocrinol Metab* 1987;65:233.

Androgenic Disorders,
edited by G. P. Redmond.
Raven Press, Ltd., New York © 1995.

5

Androgens in Infancy, Childhood, and Adolescence

Peter A. Lee and Selma Witchel Siegel

Department of Pediatrics, University of Pittsburgh School of Medicine, Children's Hospital of Pittsburgh, Pittsburgh, Pennsylvania 15213

Beginning early in fetal life, the adrenal cortex and the testes secrete androgens. During the neonatal period, significant testicular testosterone secretion occurs in male infants. Subsequently, there is minimal androgen secretion in both sexes until adrenarche. Androgens are C19 steroids (Fig. 1) with primarily anabolic and virilizing effects. Androgens, similar to other adrenal and gonadal steroids, contain the basic structure of steroid molecules consisting of 17 carbon atoms organized as three hexane (6-carbon) and one pentane (5-carbon) rings. The methyl groups at C-10 and C-17 are the 18th and 19th carbon atoms. Typically, in most commercial laboratories, plasma androgen levels are measured by specific radioimmunoassays. Other methods include colorimetric assays, high performance liquid chromatography, or gas-liquid chromatography.

The biosyntheses of adrenal and gonadal steroids utilize similar enzymatic pathways (Fig. 2). Tissue specificity of particular enzymes and enzyme activity account for the precise pattern of steroid secretion. Cholesterol, either derived from receptor-mediated endocytosis of low-density lipid (LDL) particles or synthesized within the cell, is the starting material for steroidogenesis. The rate limiting step in steroidogenesis is the conversion of cholesterol to pregnenolone by the side chain cleavage enzyme, P450scc. Enzymes common to the adrenal glands and the gonads are P450scc, 3β-hydroxysteroid dehydrogenase, and 17α-hydroxylase/17,20-lyase (CYP17). Enzymes specific to the adrenal gland are 21-hydroxylase (CYP21), 11 β-hydroxylase (CYP11B1), and aldosterone synthetase (CYP11B2) (1). Enzymes located within the gonads are 17β-hydroxysteroid dehydrogenase and aromatase.

Three protein components compose the functional unit for the mitochondrial steroid hydroxylases: P450scc, CYP11B1, and CYP11B2. These components are a cytochrome P450-type hemoprotein, a flavoprotein electron transport system (adrenodoxin reductase), and an iron–sulfur protein (adrenodoxin). The microsomal steroid hydroxylases are CYP21 and CYP17. The protein encoded for by CYP17 has both 17α-hydroxylase and 17,20-lyase activities (2).

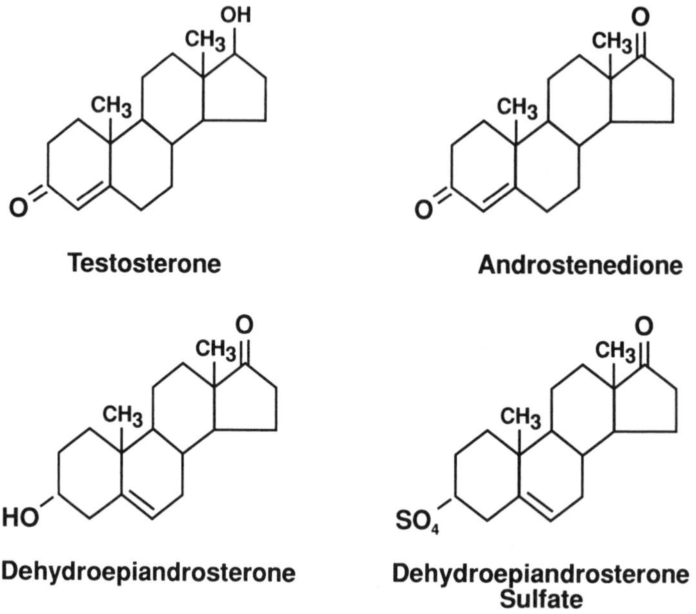

FIG. 1. Structure of common androgens (methyl groups at carbon 18 and 19).

Hence, both the adrenal and the gonads can synthesize dehydroepiandrosterone (DHEA) and androstenedione. The relative androgenic potency of DHEA is approximately 5% and that of androstenedione approximately 10% compared to testosterone. DHEA alone has little virilizing effect and does not promote growth or skeletal maturation during childhood (3). In adults, circulating DHEA is derived from the adrenal cortex (approximately 70%) and the gonads (approximately 30%). Also, in adult men, approximately 70% of the circulating androstenedione is secreted by the adrenal cortex and the remainder is secreted by the testes. In the adult women, the proportion of androstenedione derived from the adrenal cortex varies from 50% to 70% depending on the phase of the menstrual cycle.

Testosterone is the most potent circulating androgen. Within the cells of androgen target tissues, testosterone may be converted to dihydrotestosterone through the action of 5α-reductase (4). Both testosterone and dihydrotestosterone bind to the androgen receptor which acts as a ligand dependent transcription factor (5). The androgen receptor binds to an androgen response element within the regulatory portion of a target gene to affect gene transcription (6). The greater affinity of the androgen receptor for dihydrotestosterone contributes to its androgenic potency. Testosterone can be converted to estradiol, which affects gonadotropin secretion through the estradiol receptor in the hypothalamus and pituitary and may influence androgen dependent sexual dimorphism of fetal brain development. Conversion of testosterone to estradiol can occur within the ovary, testes, or peripheral tissues such as the liver and adipose tissue. In the adult woman, 50% of the plasma testosterone is secreted and 50% is derived from peripheral conversion (7).

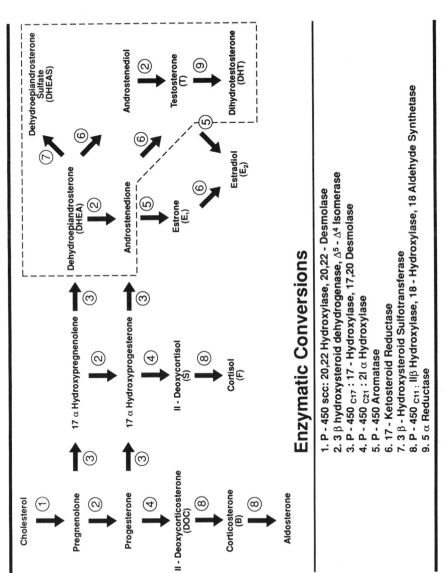

Enzymatic Conversions

1. P - 450 scc: 20,22 Hydroxylase, 20,22 - Desmolase
2. 3 β hydroxysteroid dehydrogenase, Δ^5 - Δ^4 Isomerase
3. P - 450 c_{17} : 17 - Hydroxylase, 17,20 Desmolase
4. P - 450 c_{21} : 21 α Hydroxylase
5. P - 450 Aromatase
6. 17 - Ketosteroid Reductase
7. 3 β - Hydroxysteroid Sulfotransferase
8. P - 450 c_{11} : 11β Hydroxylase, 18 - Hydroxylase, 18 Aldehyde Synthetase
9. 5 α Reductase

FIG. 2. Metabolic pathways for the synthesis of steroids (androgens within dashed lines). Numbers in circles indicate the enzymes mediating the conversions.

61

Peripheral metabolism of testosterone leads not only to active metabolites (estradiol and dihydrotestosterone) but also to inactive metabolites. These latter are largely excreted in the urine as 17-ketosteroids and polar compounds. For adrenal androgens, metabolites are conjugated prior to excretion as 17-ketosteroids by the kidney. Complete 24-hour urinary measurements for 17-ketosteroids can provide an integrated assessment of androgen secretion.

Similar to many hormones, androgens circulate in association with binding proteins. Circulating androgens are bound to sex hormone–binding globulin (SHBG) (8), loosely bound to albumin, or free (dialyzable). Levels of SHBG, a beta globulin synthesized in the liver, are increased by estrogens and thyroid hormone. Since the bound hormone is less available for biologic activity, degradation, and excretion, the bound fraction constitutes a reservoir. Testosterone levels can be measured and expressed as total testosterone, bioavailable or non–SHBG-bound testosterone, or free (dialyzable) testosterone. During childhood, the low SHBG levels have minimal effects upon the very low free hormone levels. In contrast, after sexual maturity, the quantity of SHBG affects free hormone levels. From infancy through late childhood (9), there is a decrease in serum SHBG levels and an increase in free sex steroid levels. In boys, there is a relative increase in bioavailable testosterone (10). Among girls, a progressive increase in bioavailable testosterone and estradiol occurs (11). In women with hyperandrogenism, the elevated androgen levels are associated with decreased SHBG levels, which results in greater free testosterone levels.

Androgen actions in boys include male sexual differentiation during fetal life, male sexual maturation during puberty, initiation and maintenance of spermatogenesis, and feedback regulation of gonadotropin secretion at the hypothalamus and pituitary. In girls, androgens are responsible for the development of sexual hair and serve as precursors for estrogen biosynthesis.

FETAL ANDROGEN PRODUCTION

Blood levels of androgens during fetal life, neonatal life, and childhood are listed in Table 1 (9,12–19). Amniotic fluid (20,21) and cord blood levels (19) reflect fetal androgen secretion from both adrenal and gonadal sources, while cord blood values reflect placental contributions as well.

Adrenal Androgen Production

By 8 weeks of gestation, the adrenal gland contains a large, centrally located fetal zone and a thin outer layer of neocortex. This outer cortex differentiates into the three zones of the adult cortex, zona glomerulosa, zona fasciculata, and zona reticularis. These three zones are recognizable at birth. Early during the first year of life, the fetal zone involutes and disappears.

The fetal adrenal gland begins secreting steroids by the second month after con-

TABLE 1. *Androgen levels in fetal and neonatal life [Mean (Range)]*

	Testosterone (T) (ng/dL)		Androstenedione (A) (ng/dL)		DHEAS (µg/dL for fetal values) (ng/dL for birth, age)
	Male	Female	Male	Female	
Fetal					
2nd Trimester	87	10			132
	(55–115)	(5–16)			(70–236)
3rd Trimester		11			144
		(4–19)			(55–254)
Birth					
Cord	50	29	87	93	648
	(15–120)	(10–62)	(26–147)	(17–163)	(120–1490)
Peripheral blood	228	46	197	174	
	(10–485)	(18–74)	(34–381)	(23–325)	
Age					
Day 1	208	66	178	174	919
	(75–487)	(24–115)	(65–310)	(80–410)	(160–3570)
Week 1	49	13	46	42	220
	(17–117)	(7–37)	(17–68)	(14–91)	(60–450)
Week 2–Month 4	174	9	38	25	90
	(39–362)	(6–19)	(8–62)	(6–10)	(40–400)
Month 5–24	14	10	13	8	38
	(4–122)	(4–16)	(5–50)	(3–56)	(20–200)

Conversions to SI units: T: ng/dL × 34.67 = pmol/L, A: × 34.91, DHEAS: × 34.67; DHEAS: µg/dL × 27.21 = nmol/L DHEAS, dehydroepiandrosterone sulfate.

ception. While the fetal zone is capable of producing all steroids secreted by the adult adrenal cortex, the production of mineralocorticoids and glucocorticoids (C21 steroids) is relatively low due to decreased 3β-hydroxysteroid dehydrogenase activity. High steroid levels, similar to those occurring in the fetus because of placental steroids, have been shown to inhibit 3β-hydroxysteroid dehydrogenase activity (22). The fetal adrenal primarily secretes dehydroepiandrosterone sulfate (DHEAS) and pregnenolone sulfate. DHEAS, formed from DHEA by the enzyme steroid sulfotransferase, serves as a substrate for placental estrogen synthesis. Fetal plasma DHEAS levels rise progressively until the last 8 weeks of gestation (16). After birth, DHEAS levels decline concomitantly with regression of the fetal zone of the adrenal cortex. DHEAS production then remains low until puberty.

Gonadal Androgen Production

Normal Male Development

At 6 to 7 weeks of fetal life, in the presence of the *sry* gene, testicular differentiation of the bipotential gonad has begun. By 8 weeks of gestation, Leydig cells have begun to secrete testosterone. Fetal testosterone levels peak (200–600 ng/dL) at about 15 weeks of gestation and decline thereafter (23). This early testosterone secretion is critical for male sexual differentiation. Testosterone acts locally to stabilize the development of the Wolffian ducts into the epididymis, vas deferens, seminal vesicles, and ejaculatory ducts. Dihydrotestosterone induces male differentiation of the external genitalia.

Although gonadotropin-releasing hormone (GnRH) is present within the hypothalamus and luteinizing hormone (LH) and follicle-stimulating hormone (FSH) are detectable in the pituitary gland by 10 weeks of gestation, the hypophysial portal system does not mature until later in fetal life. It appears that human chorionic gonadotropin (hCG) is responsible for this early testosterone secretion because hCG levels and concentrations of hCG receptors in the fetal testis correlate with fetal testosterone levels (24). During the second half of gestation, pituitary gonadotropins appear to play a role in complete Leydig cell differentiation, testicular descent, and normal development of the external genitalia. In hypogonadotropic hypogonadism or anencephaly, inadequate male development may occur.

Normal Female Development

While there is evidence of aromatization of androgens to estrogens in the fetal ovary in early gestation, the ovaries are relatively quiescent with minimal steroidogenesis during fetal life. The role of gonadotropins or ovarian steroids in fetal ovarian development is unclear. Early fetal ovarian differentiation is normal in individuals with 45,X Turner syndrome. In the absence of androgens, female-external genital differentiation occurs.

Abnormal Androgen Levels in the Male Fetus

In the absence of adequate testosterone levels during fetal life, the genitalia of male fetuses may be underdeveloped. Typically, ambiguous genitalia with palpable inguinal gonads are found at physical examination. Traditionally, these disorders have been classified as causes of male pseudohermaphroditism (Table 2). Impaired testosterone biosynthesis can be due to decreased side chain cleavage activity, decreased 3β-hydroxysteroid dehydrogenase activity, decreased 17α-hydroxylase/17, 20-lyase activity, decreased 5α-reductase activity, and decreased 17β-hydroxysteroid dehydrogenase activity. Cortisol biosynthesis is also impaired in patients with decreased side chain cleavage activity, decreased 3β-hydroxysteroid dehydrogenase activity, or decreased 17α-hydroxylase/17,20-lyase activity. Since müllerian inhibiting hormone levels are normal, müllerian duct derivatives are absent.

Target organ resistance to androgen action characterizes the androgen insensitivity disorders. In the complete androgen insensitivity syndrome, differentiation of the external genitalia is female. Genital ambiguity and pubertal virilization occur in the partial forms. On the basis of genital skin androgen receptor analysis, this group of disorders can be classified as receptor positive or receptor negative. Deletions and point mutations in the androgen receptor gene on the X chromosome have been identified (6).

TABLE 2. *Causes of androgen deficiency in the male fetus*

I. Biosynthetic defects in testosterone synthesis
  A. Affecting adrenal cortical and testicular steroid synthesis
    1. P450 scc: 20,22-desmolase deficiency
    2. 3β-hydroxysteroid dehydrogenase deficiency
    3. $P450_{C17}$: 17-hydroxylase, 17,20-lyase deficiency
  B. Affecting testicular steroid biosynthesis
    1. 17-hydroxysteroid dehydrogenase
II. Defects in androgen responsiveness
  A. Androgen insensitivity syndromes
    1. Complete—female phenotype with inguinal testes
    2. Partial—partially virilized, including micropenis
  B. 5α-reductase deficiency
III. Dysgenetic testes
  A. Gonadal dysgenesis (absent portions of Y chromosome)
  B. 46XY gonadal dysgenesis (unrecognized Y deletions)
IV. Excessive maternal ingestion of progestins or estrogens

Dysgenetic testes with Leydig cell aplasia or hypoplasia results in fetal androgen deficiency. Physical findings include ambiguous or female external genitalia. Asymmetric differentiation of the external genitalia suggests gonadal dysgenesis secondary to chromosomal anomalies.

Abnormal Androgen Levels in the Female Fetus

Exposure of a female fetus to excessive androgen levels induces virilization of the external genitalia (Table 3). Traditionally, this condition has been labeled female pseudohermaphroditism. Inborn errors of cortisol biosynthesis, the virilizing congenital adrenal hyperplasias, are the most common cause of prenatal virilization. Decreased conversion of steroid precursors into cortisol results in increased adrenal

TABLE 3. *Causes of androgen excess in the female fetus*

I. Fetal source
  A. Virilizing adrenal hyperplasias
    1. P450c21 (21-hydroxylase deficiency)
    2. P450c11 (11-hydroxylase deficiency)
    3. 3β-hydroxysteroid dehydrogenase deficiency
  B. Disorders of sexual differentiation
    1. Gonadal dysgenesis
    2. Hermaphroditism
II. Placental source
  A. P450 aromatase deficiency
III. Maternal source
  A. Virilizing adrenal hyperplasia
  B. Virilizing tumors
    1. Ovarian
    2. Adrenal
  C. Exogenous virilizing hormones
    1. Testosterone and other androgens
    2. Certain synthetic progestins

androgen production. Once the hypothalamic–pituitary–adrenal axis has matured, the decreased adrenal cortisol secretion leads to increased adrenocorticotropic hormone (ACTH) secretion and, hence, continued excessive adrenal androgen production. The virilizing congenital adrenal hyperplasias are 21-hydroxylase deficiency, 11β-hydroxylase deficiency, and 3β-hydroxysteroid dehydrogenase deficiency. In 21-hydroxylase deficiency and 11β-hydroxylase deficiency, excessive quantities of androstenedione are secreted. In 3β-hydroxysteroid dehydrogenase deficiency, increased levels of DHEA are found. The adrenal androgens undergo peripheral conversion to testosterone and dihydrotestosterone.

Additional causes of excessive androgen levels in the female fetus include placental aromatase deficiency (25). Any maternal source of elevated androgens can induce virilization of the female fetus. Maternal sources include exogenous steroids (androgens and synthetic progestins with androgenic properties) administered during the pregnancy and endogenous hyperandrogenism secondary to undertreated maternal virilizing congenital adrenal hyperplasia, virilizing adrenal or ovarian tumors, and luteomas of pregnancy. Genital defects unrelated to prenatal androgen levels may occur. Such defects often occur in association with other congenital anomalies.

NEONATAL ANDROGEN PRODUCTION

Normal Male Androgen Production

Assuming that androgen metabolism is relatively constant in children, circulating androgen levels reflect androgen production. In girls, androgen levels decline rapidly after birth reflecting decreased adrenal secretion and ovarian quiescence (15,17). In contrast, in boys, active testicular steroidogenesis occurs during the first few months of life (9,12,14). The involution of the fetal zone of the adrenal cortex leads to a rapid decline in DHEAS levels. Adrenal androgen secretion remains minimal until the onset of adrenal pubertal maturation, adrenarche. After birth, gonadotropin and sex steroid levels rapidly decline.

However, sex differences occur, with higher testosterone levels in boys (12–15). During the first week of life, gonadotropin levels rise. For the first several months of life, the hypothalamic–pituitary–testicular axis is active. The episodic gonadotropin secretion leads to testicular testosterone secretion. During this neonatal period, the functioning of negative feedback mechanisms of the hypothalamic–pituitary–testicular axis can be assessed.

Abnormal Androgen Production

Taking advantage of the increased activity and functioning negative feedback, LH, FSH, and testosterone can be measured in a child with ambiguous genitalia (26), micropenis (27), or undescended testes (28). With testicular failure, gonadotropins are elevated and testosterone is low. Gonadotropins and testosterone are low in hypogonadotropic hypogonadism. Elevated gonadotropins with elevated testosterone levels indicate androgen insensitivity (29). Appropriate LH, FSH, and testosterone levels for age suggest normal function of the hypothalamic–pituitary–testicular axis. Once the hypothalamic–pituitary axis becomes quiescent (down-regulated), such testing cannot be performed until puberty.

Excessive adrenal androgen secretion in the virilizing congenital adrenal hyper-plasias may lead to clitoromegaly or premature pubarche. Affected males have nor-mal male genitalia but may develop phallic enlargement or premature sexual hair. In 21-hydroxylase and 11β-hydroxylase deficiencies, androstenedione and 17-hydrox-yprogesterone are elevated (Fig. 2). In 11β-hydroxylase deficiency, 11-deoxycor-tisol levels are elevated. In 3β-hydroxysteroid dehydrogenase deficiency, DHEA and 17-hydroxypregnenolone are elevated and increased ratios of 17-hydroxypreg-nenolone to 17-hydroxyprogesterone and DHEA to androstenedione occur. Periph-eral conversion of these weak androgens to testosterone occurs.

ANDROGEN PRODUCTION DURING CHILDHOOD

Normal Androgen Production

Circulating androgen levels are low due to the quiescence of the hypothalamic–pituitary–gonadal axis and low adrenal androgen production (Tables 4,5) (30–39). Mean testosterone levels in boys and girls are undetectable in many assays. Indeed, the levels are so low that it is unclear if sex differences occur.

Abnormal Androgen Production

In premature adrenal pubertal maturation or premature adrenarche, circulating androgen levels are sufficient to induce development of pubic and axillary hair

TABLE 4. *Androgen levels in males childhood and puberty [Mean (Range)]*

	Testosterone (ng/dL)	Androstenedione (ng/dL)	DHEA (ng/dL)	DHEAS (μg/dL)
Age 2–6 years	8 (3–17)	24 (8–50)	40 (<10–100)	11 (<5–65)
Adrenarche	12 (6–50)	40 (15–68)	153 (36–378)	51 (17–107)
Tanner 2 (gonadarche)	80 (29–215)	53 (26–85)	280 (100–525)	107 (44–196)
Tanner 3	258 (96–600)	75 (43–124)	360 (150–600)	122 (52–292)
Tanner 4	425 (213–725)	99 (52–176)	415 (177–670)	199 (88–365)
Adult	601 (350–941)	122 (72–218)	489 (205–860)	240 (112–420)

TABLE 5. *Androgen levels in female childhood and puberty[a] [Mean (Range)]*

	Testosterone (ng/dL)	Androstenedione (ng/dL)	DHEA (ng/dL)	DHEAS (μg/dL)
Age 2–6 years	<10	25 (8–50)	28 (15–130)	11 (<5–65)
Adrenarche > 7 years	7 (3–19)	57 (18–92)	150 (65–230)	68 (20–190)
Tanner 2 (gonadarche)	18 (6–29)	77 (29–112)	283 (130–540)	92 (35–195)
Tanner 3	27 (8–53)	126 (45–190)	348 (160–610)	115 (50–235)
Tanner 4	38 (13–62)	150 (50–250)	394 (190–794)	150 (70–290)
Adult	40 (20–70)	165 (55–280)	490 (170–850)	180 (70–290)

[a]Values for general reference purposes only and represent calculations from references in which various assays were used. Mean values and ranges are expected to vary for various assays.

(pubarche), acne, and increased body odor. Typically, skeletal maturation is appropriate for chronologic age. Gonadarche occurs at an appropriate age without compromising adult height. Observation over time is often the only treatment necessary for this apparently benign condition. A retrospective analysis has shown that the incidence of polycystic ovary disease was higher in girls who sought medical attention for premature pubarche (40). This finding suggests that disorders which may not become clinically apparent until adult life may present as pubarche and can be difficult to differentiate from premature adrenarche.

During childhood, premature adrenarche should be differentiated from more pathologic causes of hyperandrogenism (41). Phallic enlargement, clitoromegaly, increased growth velocity, and accelerated skeletal maturation often suggest a less benign source of the excessive androgen secretion such as virilizing congenital adrenal hyperplasia. While random adrenal androgen and steroid precursors may be elevated in the virilizing congenital adrenal hyperplasias, ACTH stimulation tests are often necessary to differentiate mild forms of congenital adrenal hyperplasia from premature adrenarche (42). In some instances, it may be difficult to distinguish a mildly affected individual from a manifesting heterozygotic carrier especially with the high frequency of heterozygotic carriers for this common autosomal recessive disorder in the population. Molecular genetic analysis can also be helpful in such patients (43). For patients with mild forms of congenital adrenal hyperplasia and appropriate skeletal maturation, longitudinal re-evaluation may be helpful to determine whether glucocorticoid replacement therapy would be beneficial. Prepubertal patients who present with premature pubarche and have borderline elevation of basal and ACTH-stimulated adrenal steroids (17-hydroxyprogesterone incremental response >200 ng/dL) merit close observation until regular menstrual cycling develops. There is no clear indication for glucocorticoid suppressive ther-

TABLE 6. *Etiology of androgen excess during childhood*

Boys
  Central precocious puberty
    Associated with CNS dysfunction
      Congenital anomalies
      Hypothalamic hamartomas
      Optic gliomas
        Neurofibromatosis
      Postinflammatory lesions
      Postradiation lesions
      Posttraumatic lesions
      Septo-optic dysplasia
      Tuberous sclerosis
      Tumors
        Astrocytomas
    Secondary to chronic exposure to sex steroids
      Congenital adrenal hyperplasia
      Untreated androgen-secreting tumor
  Peripheral precocious puberty
    Adrenal androgen-secreting adenomas and carcinomas
    Chronic primary hypothyroidism
    Congenital virilizing adrenal hyperplasia
    Exogenous sex steroids or hCG
    Gonadotropin-independent precocious puberty
    hCG secreting tumors
      Chorioepitheliomas
      Choriocarcinomas
      Germinomas
      Hepatoblastomas
      Teratomas
    Hydrocephalus
    Leydig cell tumors
    LH secreting pituitary adenomas
Girls
  Adrenal adenomas and carcinomas
  Congenital virilizing adrenal hyperplasia
  Cushing's disease
  Exogenous androgen
  Ovarian tumors
    Arrhenoblastoma
    Teratoma

apy unless virilization is excessive (i.e., clitoromegaly) or skeletal maturation is significantly advanced.

Other uncommon causes of hyperandrogenism in boys (Table 6) include gonadotropin-dependent and gonadotropin-independent etiologies of sexual precocity such as familial gonaodtropin-independent precocious puberty and androgen-secreting tumors. One dramatic example of the effects of autonomous androgen secretion during childhood is the Leydig cell tumor (44). Primary cortisol resistance is a rare cause of sexual precocity. For girls, additional sources of excessive androgen production (Table 6) are androgen-secreting tumors (adrenal adenomas, adrenal carcinomas, ovarian arrhenoblastomas, or teratomas) and exogenous androgens.

ADRENAL ANDROGEN PRODUCTION AT PUBERTY

Adrenarche

Adrenarche is the onset of increased adrenal androgen secretion which begins in late childhood (ages 6–8 years). Increased plasma DHEAS levels herald the onset of the first significant hormone change of puberty. Subsequently, DHEA and androstenedione levels increase (Tables 4,5). This augmentation of adrenal androgen production precedes the physical manifestations of pubarche, that is, sexual hair, increased body odor, and acne. There is an increased prominence of the zona reticularis. It is unclear if adrenarche is due to endogenous adrenal factors or is secondary to the effects of a currently unidentified hormone. In terms of enzyme activity, a relative decrease in 3β-hydroxysteroid dehydrogenase activity and a relative increase in CYP17 activity seem to occur. Before adrenarche, DHEAS levels are not suppressible by glucocorticoids before adrenarche, suggesting a mechanism of control during prepubertal years that is independent of ACTH (37).

Adrenarche occurs independently of gonadarche (45–48). Early adrenarche is not associated with a pubertal response to GnRH stimulation (49) or increased gonadotropin secretion (50). Adrenarche occurs at the appropriate age in the absence of gonadarche in patients with hypergonadotropic hypogonadism such as Turner syndrome or with hypogonadotropic hypogonadism such as Kallmann syndrome. Precocious puberty due to gonadarche may occur in the absence of adrenarche. Further, gonadarche occurs in the absence of adrenarche as illustrated by patients with Addison's disease who are taking replacement glucocorticoid therapy (51).

GONADAL ANDROGEN PRODUCTION AT PUBERTY

Normal Testicular Androgen Production

With the onset of increased nocturnal gonadotropin secretion, testosterone is secreted during sleep. An increase in an early morning plasma testosterone indicates that pubertal development is imminent (52). Salivary testosterone levels can also be used as a laboratory marker of testosterone secretion in pubertal males (53). The production of testosterone and other androgens progressively increases such that adult male levels are achieved by mid-puberty (Table 4). Free or dialyzable testosterone levels also increase (54).

The somatic features that indicate maturation of the male reproductive system are androgen dependent. Androgen-mediated effects include sexual hair in the pubic area and the axillae, acne (55), development of apocrine glands, increased bone and muscle mass (56), and maturation of the external genitalia. Seminiferous tubule development occurs secondary to gonadotropin, primarily FSH, and androgen stimulation. Pubertal gynecomastia commonly occurs in mid puberty due to a relatively greater estradiol/testosterone ratio.

Normal Ovarian Androgen Production

Since androgens are necessary precursors for estradiol synthesis within the ovary, ovarian androgen production increases during puberty. Adrenal androgen production also increases. Circulating levels (Table 5) reflect both sources. Androgen effects in normal female puberty include development of sexual hair, maturation of the labia majora, acne, and apocrine gland secretion.

Among healthy adolescent girls followed prospectively, androgen levels appear to be predictive of androgen levels during their reproductive years (57). In other words, those with lower androgen levels continued to have lower levels, while those with higher androgen levels continued to have higher levels. Further, those girls with higher androgen levels had lower fertility rates.

Inadequate Androgen Production in Boys

Every boy with delayed puberty suffers from inadequate androgen production. Delayed puberty can be due to constitutional delay, gonadotropin deficiency. or testicular failure. Undervirilization may occur in phenotypic male patients with partial androgen insensitivity.

Normal adolescent boys may become concerned about what they perceive as a lack of adequate virilization or masculinization in comparison with their peers. In these situations, it is important to determine whether androgen levels are appropriate for age and stage of pubertal development (Table 4). Boys and their parents may benefit from discussion that the extent of pubic, chest, facial, and general body hair development varies among normal men and is dependent on genetic factors. If their concern is related to penile size, they can be counseled that this is a common worry and that actual penis size is difficult to judge during a quick glance in the locker room. After an examination to verify normal development, they should be reassured that they have a normal sized penis.

Inadequate Testosterone Production in Girls

Inadequate androgen effects are rare in girls. Phenotypically female patients with complete androgen insensitivity have scant or absent sexual hair. Female patients with panhypopituitarism may also lack sexual hair and other androgen-mediated secondary sexual characteristics. Generally, girls with Addison's disease have normal sexual hair. In girls with Turner's syndrome, adrenal androgen production is appropriate for age.

Excessive Androgen Production in Boys

No clear entity of excessive androgen production occurs in pubertal boys. Even among boys with untreated congenital adrenal hyperplasia with excessive adrenal androgen production, adjustments in the hypothalamic–pituitary–testicular axis maintain circulating testosterone levels within the normal adult range (58) for men.

Exogenous androgens may cause excessively elevated circulating androgen levels. The immediate effect may seem to provide the desired increase in body bulk, especially in the actively training individual. However, down-regulation of the hypothalamic–pituitary–testicular axis results, with subsequent decreased spermatogenesis and reduced testicular volume. Other long-term consequences may include untoward effects on muscles including the heart, and premature aging.

Excessive Androgen Production in Girls

Hirsutism and irregular menses are common clinical manifestations of hyperandrogenism in pubertal and postpubertal women. Elevated androgen (testosterone, DHEA, androstenedione, or free testosterone) levels should be documented to confirm the hyperandrogenism because not all patients who complain of hirsutism or amenorrhea have hyperandrogenism. Idiopathic hirsutism is the term used when hyperandrogenism, increased circulating levels of androgens, is not present.

Hyperandrogenism indicates excessive androgen production from the ovaries, the adrenal glands, or both sources. The etiology of hyperandrogenism may be difficult to ascertain in pubertal and postpubertal women (59). Regardless of the primary source of the excessive androgens, prolonged hyperandrogenism can induce polycystic changes in the ovaries. Polycystic ovary disease encompasses a heterogeneous group of disorders which result in excessive ovarian androgen production (60).

Mild or attenuated forms of 21-hydroxylase congenital adrenal hyperplasia are the most common causes of adrenal hyperandrogenism (60–63). The criteria to diagnose mild forms of 21-hydroxylase deficiency, 3β-hydroxysteroid dehydrogenase deficiency, and 11β-hydroxylase deficiency are poorly defined because of the overlap of stimulated hormone levels between heterozygotic carriers and mildly affected individuals. Information may be gained by assessing the ratios of steroid hormone precursor substrates and products such as the increased ratios of 17-hydroxypregnenolone to 17-hydroxyprogesterone and DHEA to androstenedione in 3β-hydroxysteroid dehydrogenase deficiency. Patients with hyperandrogenism and elevated incremental 17-hydroxyprogesterone elevations following ACTH administration may meet diagnostic criteria for nonclassical congenital adrenal hyperplasia. Yet, the decision to initiate glucocorticoid suppressive therapy should primarily depend on the extent of the clinical symptoms resulting from hyperandrogenism rather than focus on an incremental elevation greater than 2.5 standard deviations above the mean for normal women (64). Some patients appear to have adrenal hyperandrogenism without achieving the diagnostic criteria for congenital adrenal hyperplasia (65). Additional molecular genetic evaluation of patients may improve diagnostic classification.

ANDROGENS IN NONENDOCRINE ILLNESS

Adaptive alterations in endocrine physiology occur during nonendocrine illnesses. For example, one commonly recognized manifestation is the euthyroid sick syndrome. Studies in adults show that the hypothalamic–pituitary–adrenal axis responds to stress with increased ACTH and increased cortisol secretion. Androstenedione levels may be increased compared to healthy individuals, but the ratio of cortisol to androstenedione is not significantly altered (66). This suggests that the increased androstenedione reflects increased adrenal steroidogenesis. In contrast, DHEAS and DHEA levels are generally lower (67). In situations of stress in which increased ACTH results in increased cortisol synthesis and secretion, adrenal androgen secretion does not increase (68). Testosterone levels are lower in men while estrogen levels may increase in women. The lower testosterone levels presumably represent decreased testicular testosterone secretion while the estrogen levels may reflect increased peripheral conversion of androstenedione.

Potential explanations for the pattern of adrenal steroidogenesis include increased rate of steroidogenesis, increased 3β-hydroxysteroid dehydrogenase activity, decreased 17β-hydrosteroid dehydrogenase activity, and increased aromatization (69). In an adult study, the magnitude of both central and peripheral suppression of the reproductive axis is correlated with acute disease severity (70).

The immune system, the hypothalamic–pituitary–adrenal axis, and the hypothalamic–pituitary–gonadal axis interact. With severe acute illness, the negative feedback of the hypothalamic–pituitary–adrenal axis is altered in that dexamethasone is less effective in suppressing cortisol than in healthy individuals. In addition, following a bolus infusion of human corticotropin-releasing hormone (hCRH), cortisol secretion was greater in sick individuals, despite greater basal ACTH and cortisol levels, than in healthy individuals (71). A study showing estrogenic regulation of the human CRH gene in a transient transfection system suggests one possible mode of communication between the hypothalamic–pituitary–gonadal axis and the hypothalamic–pituitary–adrenal axis. Further, this mechanism may form a basis for the gender differences observed in immune function such as with autoimmune disorders (72).

REFERENCES

1. Miller WL. Molecular biology of steroid hormone synthesis. *Endoc Rev* 1988;9:295–318.
2. Zuber MX, Simpson ER, Waterman MR. Expression of bovine 17α-hydroxylase cytochrome P450 cDNA in nonsteroidogenic (COS-1) cells. *Science* 1986;234:1258–1261.
3. Sizonenko PC, Paunier L. Failure of dehydroepiandrosterone enanthate to promote growth. *J Clin Endocrinol Metab* 1986;62:1322–1324.
4. Griffin JE. Androgen resistance: the clinical and molecular spectrum. *N Engl J Med* 1992;326:611–618.
5. French FS, Lubahn DB, Brown TR, Simental JA, Quigley CA, Yarbrough WG, Tan JA, Sar M, Joseph DR, Evans BA, et al. The molecular basis of androgen insensitivity. *Recent Prog Horm Res* 1990;46:1–38.

6. McPhaul MJ, Marcelli M, Tilley WD, Griffin JE, Wilson JD. Androgen resistance caused by mutations in the androgen receptor gene. *FASEB J* 1991;5:2910–2915.
7. Abraham GE. Ovarian and adrenal contribution to peripheral androgens during the menstrual cycle. *J Clin Endocrinol Metab* 1974;39:340–346.
8. Anderson DC. Sex hormone–binding globulin. *Clin Endocrinol* 1974;3:69–95.
9. Bolton NJ, Tapanainen J, Koivisto M, Vihko R. Circulating sex hormone–binding globulin and testosterone in newborns and infants. *Clin Endocrinol* 1989;31:201–207.
10. Belgorosky A, Rivarola MA. Progressive increase in nonsex hormone–binding globulin-bound testosterone from infancy to late prepuberty in boys. *J Clin Endocrinol Metab* 1987;64:482–485.
11. Belgorosky A, Rivarola MA. Progressive increase in nonsex hormone-binding globulin-bound testosterone and estradiol from infancy to late prepuberty in girls. *J Clin Endocrinol Metab* 1988;67:234–237.
12. Forest MG, Cathiard AM, Bertrand JA. Evidence of testicular activity in early infancy. *J Clin Endocrinol Metab* 1973;37:148–151.
13. DePeretti E, Forest MG. Unconjugated dehydroepiandrosterone plasma levels in normal subjects from birth to adolescence in human: the use of a sensitive radioimmunoassay. *J Clin Endocrinol Metab* 1976;43:982–986.
14. Forest MG, Cathiard AM. Pattern of plasma testosterone and Δ^4-androstenedione in normal newborns: evidence for testicular activity at birth. *J Clin Endocrinol Metab* 1975;41:977–980.
15. Winter JSD, Hughes IA, Reyes FI, Faiman C. Pituitary–gonadal relations in infancy: 2. Patterns of serum gonadal steroid concentrations in man from birth to two years of age. *J Clin Endocrinol Metab* 1976;42:679–686.
16. Parker CR Jr, Leuono KJ, Carr BR, Hauth J, MacDonald PC. Umbilical cord plasma levels of dehydroepiandrosterone sulfate during human gestation. *J Clin Endocrinol Metab* 1982;54:1216–1220.
17. Corbier P, Dehennin L, Castanier M, Edwards DA. Sex differences in serum luteinizing hormone and testosterone in the human neonate during the first few hours after birth. *J Clin Endocrinol Metab* 1990;71:1344–1348.
18. Donaldson A, Nicolini U, Symes EK, Rodeck CH, Tannirandorn Y. Changes in concentrations of cortisol, dehydroepiandrosterone sulphate and progesterone in fetal and maternal serum during pregnancy. *Clin Endocrinol* 1991;35:447–451.
19. Sakai LM, Baker LA, Jacklin CN, Shulman I. Sex steroids at birth: genetic and environmental variation and covariation. *Dev Psychobiol* 1992;24:559–570.
20. Carson DJ, Okuno A, Lee PA, Stetten G, Didolkar SM, Migeon CJ. Steroid concentrations in amniotic fluid: normal fetuses, fetuses with congenital adrenal hyperplasia due to deficiency, fetuses with Klinefelter's Syndrome. *Am J Dis Child* 1982;36:218–225.
21. Westney L, Bruney R, Ross B, Clark JFJ, Rajguru S, Ahluwalia B. Evidence that gonadal hormone levels in amniotic fluid are decreased in males born to alcohol users in humans. *Alcohol Alcohol* 1991;26:403–407.
22. Byrne GC, Perry YS, Winter JSD. Steroid inhibitory effects upon human adrenal 3 beta hydroxysteroid dehydrogenase activity. *J Clin Endocrinol Metab* 1986;62:413–418.
23. Reyes FI, Boroditsky RS, Winter JSD, Faiman C. Studies on human sexual development II. Fetal and maternal serum gonadotropin and sex steroid concentrations. *J Clin Endocrinol Metab* 1974;38:612–617.
24. Molsberry RL, Carr BR, Mendelson CR. Simpson ER. Human chorionic gonadotropin binding to human fetal testes as a function of gestational age. *J Clin Endocrinol Metab* 1982;55:791–794.
25. Harada N, Ogawa H, Shozu M, Yamada K, Suhara K, Nishida E, Takagi Y. Biochemical and molecular genetic analyses on placental aromatase (P-450$_{AROM}$) deficiency. *J Biol Chem* 1992;267:4781–4785.
26. Berkovitz GD, Lee PA, Brown TR, Migeon CJ. Etiologic evaluation of male pseudo-hermaphroditism in infancy and childhood. *Am J Dis Child* 1984;138:755–759.
27. Lee PA, Mazur T, Danish R, Amrhein J, Blizzard RM, Money J, Migeon CJ. Micropenis: I. Criteria, etiologies, and classification. *Johns Hopkins Med J* 1980;146:156–163.
28. Lee PA, Hoffman WH, White JJ, Engel RME, Blizzard RM. Serum gonadotropins in cryptorchidism: an indicator of functional testes. *Am J Dis Child* 1974;127:530–533.
29. Lee PA, Brown TR, Latorre HA. Diagnosis of the partial androgen insensitivity syndrome during infancy. *JAMA* 1986;255:2207–2209.

30. August GP, Grumbach MN, Kaplan SL. Hormonal changes in puberty: III. Correlation of plasma testosterone, LH, FSH, testicular size, and bone age with male pubertal development. *J Clin Endocrinol Metab* 1972;34:319–326.
31. Lee PA, Jaffe RB, Midgley Jr AR. Serum gonadotropin, testosterone and prolactin concentrations throughout puberty in boys: A longitudinal study. *J Clin Endocrinol Metab* 1974;39:664–673.
32. Hopper BR, Yen SSC. Circulating concentrations of dehydroepiandrosterone and dehydroepiandrosterone sulfate during puberty. *J Clin Endocrinol Metab* 1975;40:458–461.
33. Lee PA, Migeon CJ. Puberty in boys: correlation of plasma levels of gonadotropins (LH, FSH), androgens (testosterone, androstenedione, dehydroepiandrosterone and its sulfate), estrogens (estrone and estradiol) and progestins (progesterone and 17-hydroxyprogesterone). *J Clin Endocrinol Metab* 1975;41:556–562.
34. Sizonenko PE, Paunier L. Hormonal changes in puberty III: Correlation of plasma dehydroepiandrosterone, testosterone, FSH, and LH with stages of puberty and bone age in normal boys and girls and in patients with Addison's disease or hypogonadism or with premature or late adrenarche. *J Clin Endocrinol Metab* 1975;41:894–904.
35. Lee PA, Xenakis T, Winer J, Matsenbaugh S. Puberty in girls: correlation of serum levels of gonadotropins, prolactin, androgens, estrogens, and progestins with physical changes. *J Clin Endocrinol Metab* 1976;43:775–784.
36. Ghizzoni L, Virdis R, Ziveri M, et al. Adrenal steroid, cortisol, adrenocorticotropin, and β-endorphin responses to human corticotropin-releasing hormone stimulation test in normal children and children with premature pubarche. *J Clin Endocrinol Metab* 1989;69:875–880.
37. Kreitzer PM, Blethen SL, Festa RS, Chasalow FI. Dehydroepiandrosterone sulfate levels are not suppressible by glucocorticoids before adrenarche. *J Clin Endocrinol Metab* 1989;69:1309–1311.
38. Pang S, MacGillivray M, Wang M, et al. 3α-androstanediol glucuronide in virilizing congenital adrenal hyperplasia: a useful serum metabolic marker of integrated adrenal androgen secretion. *J Clin Endocrinol Metab* 1991;73:166–174.
39. Richards RJ, Svec F, Bao W, Srinivasan SR, Berenson GS. Steroid hormones during puberty: racial (black–white) differences in androstenedione and estradiol. The Bogalusa Heart Study. *J Clin Endocrinol Metab* 1992;75:624–631.
40. Ibanez L, Potau N, Virdis R, Zampolli M, Terzi C, Gussinye M, Carrascosa A, Vicens-Calvet E. Postpubertal outcome in girls diagnosed of premature pubarche during childhood: increased frequency of functional ovarian hyperandrogenism. *J Clin Endocrinol Metab* 1993;76:1599–1603.
41. Temeck JW, Pang S, Nelson C, New MI. Genetic defects of steroidogenesis in premature pubarche. *J Clin Endocrinol Metab* 1987;64:609–617.
42. Siegel SF, Finegold DN, Urban MD, McVie R, Lee PA. Premature pubarche: etiological heterogeneity. *J Clin Endocrinol Metab* 1992;74:239–247.
43. Siegel SF, Lee PA, Rudert WA, Swinyard M, Trucco M. Phenotype/genotype correlations in 21-hydroxylase deficiency. *Adolesc Pediatr Gynecol* (in press).
44. Urban MD, Lee PA, Plotnick LP, Migeon CJ. The diagnosis of Leydig Cell tumors in childhood. *Am J Dis Child* 1978;132:494–497.
45. Lee PA, Kowarski A, Migeon CJ, Blizzard RM. Lack of correlation between gonadotropin and adrenal androgen levels in agonadal children. *J Clin Endocrinol Metab* 1975;40:664–669.
46. Sklar CA, Kaplan SL, Grumbach MM. Evidence for dissociation between adrenarche and gonadarche: studies in patients with idiopathic precocious puberty, gonadal dysgenesis, isolated gonadotropin deficiency, and constitutionally delayed growth and adolescence. *J Clin Endocrinol Metab* 1980;51:548–556.
47. Cutler GB, Loriaux DL. Adrenarche and its relationship to the onset of puberty. *Fed Proc* 1980;39:2384–2390.
48. Counts DR, Pescovitz OH, Barnes KM, et al. Dissociation of adrenarche and gonadarche in precocious puberty and in isolated hypogonadotropic hypogonadism. *J Clin Endocrinol Metab* 1987;64:1174–1178.
49. Lee PA, Gareis FJ. Gonadotropin and sex steroid response to luteinizing hormone-releasing hormone in patients with premature adrenarche. *J Clin Endocrinol Metab* 1976;43:195–197.
50. Lee PA, Xenakis T, Winer J, Matsenbaugh S. Independence of gonadotropin and adrenal androgen secretion. *Andrologia* 1978;10:369–372.
51. Urban MD, Lee PA, Gutai JP, Migeon CJ. Androgens in pubertal males with Addison's Disease. *J Clin Endocrinol Metab* 1980;51:925–929.

52. Wu FCW, Brown DC, Butler GE, et al. Early morning plasma testosterone is an accurate predictor of imminent pubertal development in prepubertal boys. *J Clin Endocrinol Metab* 1993;76:26–31.
53. Ohzeki T, Manella B, Gübelin-DeCampo C, Zachmann M. Salivary testosterone concentrations in prepubertal and pubertal males: comparison with total and free plasma testosterone. *Horm Res* 1991; 36:235–237.
54. Lee PA, Gisriel DL. Correlation of gonadotropins with unbound testosterone during puberty in males. *Horm Res* 1980;12:130–136.
55. Lee PA. Acne and serum androgen during puberty. *Arch Dermatol* 1976;112:482–484.
56. Forbes GB, Porta CR, Herr BE, Griggs RC. Sequence of changes in body composition induced by testosterone and reversal of changes after drug is stopped. JAMA 1992;267:397–399.
57. Apter D, Vihko R. Endocrine determinants of fertility: serum androgen concentrations during follow-up of adolescents into the third decade of life. *J Clin Endocrinol Metab* 1990;71:970–974.
58. Urban MD, Lee PA, Migeon CJ. Adult height and fertility in men with congenital virilizing adrenal hyperplasia (CVAH). *N Engl J Med* 1978;299:1392–1396.
59. Siegel SF, Finegold DN, Murray PJ, Lee PA. Assessment of clinical hyperandrogenism in adolescent girls. *Adolesc Pediatr Gynecol* 1992;5:13–20.
60. Siegel SF, Lee PA. Polycystic ovary syndrome. *Curr Opin Pediatr* 1993;5:400–406.
61. Rosenwaks Z, Lee PA, Jones GS, Migeon CJ, Wentz AC. An attenuated form of congenital virilizing adrenal hyperplasia. *J Clin Endocrinol Metab* 1979;49:335–339.
62. Migeon CJ, Rosenwaks Z, Lee PA, Urban MD, Bias WB. The attenuated form of congenital adrenal hyperplasia as an allelic form of 21-hydroxylase deficiency. *J Clin Endocrinol Metab* 1980;51:647–649.
63. Lee PA, Rosenwaks Z, Urban MD, Migeon CJ, Bias WB. Attenuated forms of congenital adrenal hyperplasia due to 21-hydroxylase deficiency. *J Clin Endocrinol Metab* 1982;55:866–871.
64. Siegel SF, Finegold DN, Lanes R, Lee PA. ACTH stimulation tests and plasma dehydroepiandrosterone sulfate levels in women with hirsutism. *N Engl J Med* 1990;323:849–854.
65. Lee PA, Migeon CJ, Bias WD, Jones GS. Familial hypersecretion of adrenal androgens transmitted as a dominant, non-HLA linked trait. *Obstet Gynecol* 1987;69:259–264.
66. Wade CE, Lindberg JS, Cockrell JL, Lamiell JM, Hunt MM, Ducey J, Jurney TH. Upon-admission adrenal steroidogenesis is adapted to the degree of illness in intensive care unit patients. *J Clin Endocrinol Metab* 1988;67:223–227.
67. Luppa P, Munker R, Nagel D, Weber M, Engelhardt D. Serum androgens in intensive-care patients: correlations with clinical findings. *Clin Endocrinol* 1991;34:305–310.
68. Hauffa BP, Kaplan SL, Grumbach MM. Dissociation between plasma adrenal androgens and cortisol in Cushing's disease and ectopic ACTH producing tumor: relation to adrenarche. *Lancet* i: 1984;1373.
69. Spratt DI, Longcope C, Cox PM, Bigos ST, Wilbur-Welling C. Differential changes in serum concentrations of androgens and estrogens (in relation with cortisol) in postmenopausal women with acute illness. *J Clin Endocrinol Metab* 1993;76:1542–1547.
70. Spratt DI, Cox P, Orav J, Moloney J, Bigos T. Reproductive axis suppression in acute illness is related to disease severity. *J Clin Endocrinol Metab* 1993;76:1548–1554.
71. Reincke M, Allolio B, Würth G, Winkelmann W. The hypothalamic–pituitary–adrenal axis in critical illness: response to dexamethasone and corticotropin-releasing hormone. *J Clin Endocrinol Metab* 1993;77:151–156.
72. Vamvakopoulos NC, Chrousos GP. Evidence of direct estrogenic regulation of human corticotropin-releasing hormone gene expression: potential implications for the sexual dimorphism of the stress response and immune/inflammatory reaction. *J Clin Invest* 1993;92:1896–1902.

Androgenic Disorders,
edited by G. P. Redmond.
Raven Press, Ltd., New York © 1995.

6

Pathophysiology of Polycystic Ovarian Syndrome

Walter Futterweit

Department of Medicine, Division of Endocrinology and Metabolism, The Mount Sinai School of Medicine, New York, New York 10029.

The pathogenesis of polycystic ovarian syndrome (PCOS) is a matter of great controversy and debate. The heterogeneity and the confounding multifactorial causes in patient presentation makes it difficult to assign a single unifying hypothesis. It is clear, however, that there is no controversy regarding the histopathology of the polycystic ovary which has been well described (1,2). There are a number of clinical entities which can induce polycystic ovaries. Thus the anatomical changes seen in polycystic or multicystic ovaries are not unique, and the morphology of the ovaries as well as the diagnostic utilization of pelvic ultrasonography indicate a sign and not a specific diagnosis (3). During the last 10 years there have been outstanding contributions to the understanding of neuroendocrine, steroidogenic, as well as systemic and local factors in folliculogenesis including the role of insulin and related proteins. Controversies as to the exact role of the various pathophysiological events in the genesis of the PCOS are not likely to be resolved in the very near future. All of the proponents of major hypotheses have reported data that claim to substantiate their views. It is apparent that there are distinct subsets of patients with PCOS where a basic pathophysiological dysfunction is primary and a cascade of events then lead to a syndrome termed PCOS. The unifying thread is an abnormal ovary that is hyperandrogenic. To further confound the problem of identifying a specific and all-inclusive trigger event of PCOS, there has not as yet been a unified definition of PCOS (4). The importance of defining specific diagnostic criteria for PCOS is essential in understanding its clinical perspective and pathogenesis including possible polygenic states of what is certainly a complex group of diverse disorders. The purpose of this review is to examine the various possible mechanisms involved in the pathogenesis of this frequent and heterogeneous syndrome.

TABLE 1. *Various phenotypes of PCOS*

Sensitivity to androgens
Body weight (BMI), body composition, and fat distribution
Pattern and intensity of biochemical abnormalities
   gonadotropins
   steroids
     ovarian
     adrenal
     combined ovarian and adrenal disorders
   insulin concentration and insulin-resistance
   prolactin
Genetic factors
   intraovarian
   intra-adrenal
   intraovarian and intra-adrenal steroidogenic disorders
   obesity, body fat distribution, insulin resistance
Environmental factors
   nutrition
   psychosocial and stress (psychoneuroendocrine)

Modified from ref. 5.

OVERVIEW OF POLYCYSTIC OVARIAN SYNDROME

Defining PCOS

Phenotypes

It is well acknowledged that one of the major difficulties in the understanding of the pathogenesis of PCOS is the great variability of clinical and biological manifestations.

Various phenotypes may occur as a result of significant differences between patients with PCOS (5), including those in Table 1.

Modified Definition and Criteria for PCOS

In attempting to define the syndrome, one may utilize the approach based on a modified consensus of the NIH–NICHD Conference on PCOS in April 1990 (5) (Table 2). Furthermore, by defining diagnostic criteria of PCOS, one may then

TABLE 2. *Modified definition of PCOS: major and minor criteria*

Major criteria
   chronic anovulation
   hyperandrogenemia
   clinical signs of hyperandrogenism
   exclusion of other etiologies
Minor criteria
   Insulin resistance
   Perimenarchal onset of hirsutism and obesity
   Elevated LH/FSH ratio
   Ultrasonographic evidence of PCOS
   Intermittent anovulation associated with hyperandrogenemia (free testosterone, DHEAS)

classify the different subgroups with a view to better evaluate the pathogenesis of each of these subgroups, assess the accuracy of published research, and provide data necessary for formulating specific therapy.

The Scope and Frequency of PCOS

Clearly, the definitions include one or more of the major criteria, all of which are clinical. Despite abnormalities in ovarian morphology, gonadotropin secretion, and insulin action, these abnormalities, although frequently present, are not necessary for a definition of the syndrome. There is often a familial incidence of PCOS (6–10), but the genetics is not well understood (11).

The scope and frequency of the some of the major as well as minor criteria, as well as innovative observations and reviews, may be seen in the context of a number of important publications published in the last 10 years (7,12–40). PCOS accounts for 75% of patients with anovulatory infertility (41,42), 30% to 40% of secondary amenorrhea, and 85% to 90% of women with oligomenorrhea (43). Between 60% and 70% of patients with PCOS are hirsute (44,45), and both hirsute and nonhirsute women have hyperandrogenism (41). Parenthetically, the clinical and biochemically heterogeneous nature of PCOS is underscored by the fact that some women with all the typical clinical symptoms including morphologic evidence of polycystic ovaries may have normal serum luteinizing hormone (LH) or testosterone (T) levels. In 610 patients with PCOS studied with pelvic ultrasonography, 19 were noted to have similar findings (W. Futterweit, H.C. Yeh: *unpublished data*), which also underscores the variability of clinical course and findings at the time of initial study.

Heterogeneity in Presentation

Usual Types of Presentation

The woman with anovulation, onset of menstrual dysfunction since time of puberty, who presents with hirsutism or cystic acne with laboratory evidence of hyperandrogenism and an elevated serum LH/FSH (follicle-stimulating hormone) ratio is quite certain to have PCOS, once the usual exclusion criteria are met (46). This type of patient is often obese and may be concerned about her fertility potential. There is often a genetic history of similar complaints in a first degree family member. It is the author's experience that a genetic role is present in 25% to 30% of "classic" patients with PCOS as defined by major criteria (*unpublished data*). Laboratory studies often indicate a high normal serum T and more often an elevated level of free T, with or without other androgen abnormalities (29,47–49). On the other hand, the presence of hirsutism in an Oriental woman would be unusual and the major criteria would consist of chronic anovulation with hyperandrogenemia. Indeed, the absence of hirsutism in PCOS has been well described (22,50). This may occur with intermittent anovulation and/or parity (44,51) in the presence of documented hyperandrogenemia and possible inappropriate gonadotropin secretion (IGS).

Subtle Manifestations

Clinical signs of hyperandrogenism leading the patient to seek medical advice may be quite subtle. For example, the occurrence of overt changes such as cystic acne and oily skin in a woman in her late twenties or early thirties, androgenetic alopecia with diffuse thinning of hair in the crown area of the scalp (46,50,52,53), or intermittent anovulation and dysfunctional bleeding (44,46,53,54) actually meet some of the major criteria, and there also may be minor criteria that are helpful in establishing the presence of the syndrome. The purpose in stressing this is clear: There should be no all-inclusive list of criteria for PCOS, since there are obvious difficulties in applying any of the above criteria to a particular patient. The criteria that are stressed are guides in defining the likelihood that certain signs and symptoms as well as laboratory studies will be properly applied to each subject under study. This may lead one to avoid the all-inclusive generic term PCOS, and allow a more appropriate subgrouping of the subjects studied. These would include those with hyperprolactinemia (55,56), "lean" patients with or without insulin resistance, patients with regular ovulatory cycles, women with unusual stress and psychoneuroendocrine disturbances (37,57), and those identified as having a major adrenal component in the pathogenesis of PCOS (30).

Exclusion of Nonclassical Congenital Adrenocortical Hyperplasia

It is of major importance to exclude nonclassical forms of congenital adrenocortical hyperplasia (CAH), because the manifestations may be entirely similar to those of PCOS patients without an adrenal enzymatic defect (40,58). An adrenocorticotropin (ACTH)-stimulation test is used to exclude nonclassical forms of CAH while imaging studies, [e.g., ultrasonography and computed tomography (CT) scan (59,60)] may also be used, particularly when the clinical history indicates rapid progression of virilization, so as to exclude an androgen-secreting tumor of the adrenal or ovary (61–64).

The necessity of excluding nonclassical congenital adrenal hyperplasia (NCCAH) is underscored by important clinical observations (65). The clinical presentation as well as ultrasonographic findings of PCOS and CAH are frequently indistinguishable. The patient may have ovarian abnormalities as well as IGS, and subtle insulin resistance (IR), all secondary to an adrenal defect. There is an overlap in the clinical presentation of nonclassical 21-hydroxylase or late-onset 3β-hydroxysteroid dehydrogenase (3β-HSD) deficiency and that of PCOS (47,65,66). Hirsutism, acne, menstrual dysfunction, infertility (22,47,58,65) and androgenetic alopecia (52) are manifestations of both. Ultrasonographic features of polycystic ovaries are found frequently in nonclassical 21-hydroxylase CAH and 3β-HSD deficiency as well as in some patients with 11β-hydroxylase deficiency (40,67). Abnormal response to gonadotropin-releasing hormone (GnRH) similar to PCOS occurs frequently in nonclassical CAH (68). It is of interest that while adrenal androgens alter hypothalamic–ovarian dynamics, high dosage androgen therapy does not alter the adrenal steroidogenesis of ovulatory women as measured by the adrenal androgen response to ACTH (69).

Ultrasonography in PCOS

Criteria

The ancillary application of ultrasonography may be helpful in identifying suspected or subtle cases of the syndrome. Furthermore, the study may be useful in identifying neoplasms of the ovaries (70) or adrenals which may lead to morphologic changes of PCOS. The basic sonographic features are those of multiple (five to ten) developing follicles measuring 5 to 8 mm in diameter mostly distributed around the periphery of the ovary (41,71) and an increased amount of stroma (31). There is no basis for an arbitrary separation of polycystic ovaries into normal and enlarged ovaries (22), and studies indicate that the clinical and biochemical picture does not vary as a function of the ovarian size (72).

Correlation with Clinical Features of PCOS

There is a significant correlation between menstrual dysfunction and the presence of PCOS as judged by ultrasound and that determined by clinical and hormonal criteria (41,73). Ultrasonographic evidence of polycystic ovaries has been reported in 87% of anovulatory women, 26% of women with amenorrhea, and 87% of hirsute women with regular cycles (41). The diagnosis of PCOS in the latter study was supported by the finding of at least one of several endocrine markers of PCOS, that is, an increased LH/FSH ratio and/or evidence of hyperandrogenism. A study by Polson et al. (23) of 257 unselected healthy patients aged 18 to 36 years demonstrated that 23% had evidence of polycystic ovaries. This high incidence in a normal population is a striking finding. Of those with ultrasonographic evidence of polycystic ovaries, most had some irregularity of menses and/or increased body hair. Thus patients who had not sought medical advice for mildly irregular menses and/or hirsutism had ultrasonographic findings of polycystic ovaries, and some had an elevated serum LH level. Those with regular menses had a 7% incidence of polycystic ovaries on ultrasound, and of these only two were nonhirsute. Thus there appears to be a distinct subgroup of the heterogeneous PCOS spectrum. Hereditary, psychoendocrine, as well as nutritional components may also play important roles in the pathogenesis of the syndrome in the group of women studied.

The morphologic findings of ultrasonography of the ovaries may be nonspecific in that they indicate changes often seen in any anovulatory state, and which indeed are the rule in prepubertal girls. Despite the nonspecificity of the ultrasonographic study, it yields much information regarding size, the nature of the follicles and stroma, the state of the endometrium, the response to therapy, and possible associated ovarian neoplasms that may be present in up to 15% of patients with PCOS

(44,70). The correlation of the morphologic findings of polycystic ovaries with clinical criteria for PCOS generally has been convincing (23,72,74). A diagnosis based on ultrasonographic criteria, however, should not be made in the absence of defined criteria.

MAJOR HYPOTHESES OF PATHOGENESIS OF PCOS

In the heterogeneous syndrome PCOS, the common clinical features of oligomenorrhea, with or without hirsutism, may represent a final common pathway for a number of pathological entities. The most commonly held hypotheses (perspectives, or "schools") are categorized in Table 3. These include a primary central defect of abnormal gonadotropin secretion resulting in increased ovarian androgen production, the influence of an androgenic ovarian or adrenal environment on the ovary resulting in ovarian hyperandrogenism that may result in GnRH–LH dysfunction, inherent ovarian abnormalities in folliculogenesis, and/or enzymatic defects, genetic factors, and the effects of hyperinsulinism and their modulation by insulin-like growth factors (IGFs) on the ovary.

All of the above hypotheses have had some experimental support. In an excellent summation, Crowley stressed the well-known inherent bias of most investigators in defining their hypotheses regarding the location of the primary event for this syndrome (75). To date there has not been a report relating the natural history of PCOS in a large number of women. It is therefore apparent that even a simple question as to whether it may be transitional or fixed has not yet been forthcoming. Clinical and experimental data often do not state specific criteria for the diagnosis of PCOS, or the genetic or ethnic background of the patients studied, leaving the potential of a possible bias in the study and any genetic factor in the reported study unanswered. Furthermore, the time when studies were done (e.g., following progestin withdrawal or following spontaneous menses) have not always been carefully documented (75). Undoubtedly there has been a recent trend to strictly define more frequently the subsets of PCOS, and this will be a great help in understanding the complex entity of PCOS as well as in reducing the frequent number of published discordant results.

TABLE 3. *Hypotheses of primary defect in patients with PCOS*

Neuroendocrine
    abnormalities of gonadotropin secretion
    miscellaneous neuroendocrine dysfunction affecting GnRH
Ovarian
Ovarian–adrenal
Genetic factors associated with the above
Insulin and mediation of insulin action

PATHOPHYSIOLOGY OF NEUROENDOCRINE AND GONADOTROPIN ABNORMALITIES

In the neuroendocrine model of PCOS, the various factors that influence GnRH as well as the pulse abnormalities of LH are believed to be primary in the pathogenesis of this syndrome.

What neuroendocrine abnormalities may be demonstrated in patients with PCOS? What evidence supports or negates the hypothesis that these changes are primary, rather than secondary to an abnormal steroidal milieu and lack of normal ovarian cyclicity? This has been the subject of much study, controversy, and speculation. One may attempt to group these hypotheses into two major categories: (a) gonadotropin abnormalities, and (b) neuroendocrine changes resulting in an altered pattern of GnRH release. The hypotheses proposed by a number of investigators may be further subdivided into specific putative neuroendocrine defects that attempt to define the site of the dysfunctional neuroendocrine system (Table 4).

The neuroendocrine mechanisms that govern basal and cyclic gonadotropin secretion are present within the median basal hypothalamus (MBH), the conductor of normal menstrual cyclicity. The primary structure in the MBH is the arcuate nucleus, which mediates control of gonadotropin secretion. Normal gonadotropin release is dependent on the release of GnRH from the arcuate nucleus area. It is the ability to modulate the basal discharge rate of the arcuate GnRH neuronal system that may explain the occurrence of a number of physiologic as well as pathophysiologic processes in PCOS (26).

Inappropriate Gonadotropin Secretion (IGS)

A frequent biochemical feature of women with PCOS is the inappropriately elevated secretion of LH and a low or low-normal FSH release resulting in an elevated serum LH/FSH ratio (22,73,76–87). The abnormal serum LH/FSH ratio (>3.0) (26) is present in 60% to 75% of patients with PCOS (18,47,77,79,80,84,85,88), and variability in sampling frequency or techniques of sampling may alter the ratio (89). The mean mid-follicular LH/FSH ratio of normal ovulatory women is 1.3 (1.0–1.6) (77,90,91). There are times when the clinical course of PCOS is such that a return to even intermittent ovulatory cycles may alter the ratio so that no apparent increase in serum LH is noted. Variability in the circulating levels of gonadotropins

TABLE 4. *Neuroendocrine abnormalities*

Inappropriate gonadotropin secretion (IGS)
Variability of elevated LH levels in PCOS
   pulsatility and amplitude data
Role of hypothalamus in PCOS
Role of inhibin
Hyperprolactinemia
Role of neurotransmitters (opioids, catecholamines, etc.)

over periods of time in PCOS have been well documented (30,86,92–94). The high circulating serum LH level is maintained by exaggerated pulsatile LH release either in amplitude or increased oscillations (frequency) (15,77,86,95–99). There is great variability in amplitude and pulsatility in PCOS, and daily excursions are so great that they often resemble those of normal cycling women or those seen in a spontaneous mid-cycle LH surge (81). The latter frequently occur following a rapid increase of endogenous circulating estradiol (E_2) (81).

Lobo et al. (100) demonstrated that LH bioactivity is elevated in almost all patients (95%) with PCOS, whereas serum immunoreactive LH may be increased in up to 70% of PCOS patients. The increase in the bioactive/immunoreactive LH ratio (mean, 4.5) as compared to normal cycling women (mean, 3.5) has led to the suggestion that a more biologically active form of LH is secreted by women with PCOS (100–104). This finding is of importance in the understanding of the pathogenesis of PCOS since even those women with PCOS who have normal circulating levels of LH usually demonstrate increased bioactive LH concentrations.

Fauser and associates (104) demonstrated that the immunoradiometric (IRMA) LH assays (using monoclonal antibodies) in PCOS women tend to be lower then those using classical radioimmune assays RIA. LH levels as measured by RIA may be overestimated in view of cross-reactivity with circulating alpha-subunits as well as LH isohormones of varying biological activity. These investigators found a fourfold increase in serum bioactive LH levels over control women in the early follicular phase of the menstrual cycle (104). The median ratio of bioavailable LH/IRMA-LH ratio of PCOS patients was almost five times that of normal controls. In contrast, the mean IRMA-FSH, RIA-FSH and bioavailable FSH levels, as well as the bioavailable FSH/IRMA-FSH ratio, in PCOS patients were similar to those in normal women. This underscores two major statements regarding PCOS: (a) A normal serum LH level, particularly if done randomly and using an IRMA technique, may be misleading and does not exclude the presence of PCOS; and (b) Serum FSH levels appear to be normal in PCOS regardless of their estimation, including bioassay as measured by induction of aromatase activity in cultured rat granulosa cells (104). This may lead some to believe that perhaps aberrant folliculogenesis resulting from defective FSH action may be a factor in PCOS.

Pathogenesis of Elevated LH Levels in PCOS

The pituitary gland is primarily involved in the negative feedback effect of estrogens (105), although hypothalamic participation may also occur. It has been clearly demonstrated that the characteristic biochemical abnormality of an IGS usually seen in women with PCOS has not been considered secondary to a defect in the negative-feedback effect of estrogen on gonadotropin release (86). It has been suggested that the positive feedback effect of E_2 is of greater importance and that its effect is exerted both at the pituitary gland and at a hypothalamic level. Results of estrogen infusion for 4 hours results in a rapid decrease of serum LH with an attenuation of LH pulses (86) and a reduction of frequency of LH release similar to that found in normal and hypogonadal women (81,106,107). The resumption of increased pulse amplitude of LH has been found to occur 3 to 4 hours after cessation of E_2 infusion (86). Administration of 100 mg clomiphene citrate daily for 5 days elicits increased LH and FSH levels qualitatively and quantitatively similar to those seen in normal cycling women receiving the drug. This indicates the presence of an intact positive-feedback mechanism of estrogen on LH release in PCOS (86). Pituitary sensitization to chronic estrogen exposure in PCOS is suggested by the clinical observation that a 24-hour-more-rapid positive feedback to oral estrogen frequently occurs in anovulatory patients with PCOS as compared to control subjects (77,108). Parenthetically, elevations in estrone (E_1) production via extraglandular aromatization of androstenedione (A) has been hypothesized to have a role in the disparity between the LH and FSH levels in PCOS, primarily by selective suppression of FSH (82). The fundamental question remains, however, as to whether the IGS seen in PCOS arises as a primary hypothalamic–pituitary defect or is secondary to dysfunctional ovarian and/or adrenal disorders whose altered milieu impacts on the GnRH generator. The use of GnRH analogs and the exogenous administration of GnRH provide insight into a possible primary role of the hypothalamic–pituitary axis in the pathogenesis of PCOS.

LH Pulse Frequency and Amplitude

The inappropriate pulsatile LH secretion resulting in elevated mean LH levels may be due to increased pulse frequency, increased pulse amplitude, or both. There is general agreement that there is an increased pulse amplitude in patients with PCOS (15,67,96,98,99,109,110). Determination of LH pulse frequency is crucial in that this reflects the activity of the hypothalamic GnRH pulse generator (111). An abnormally high LH pulse frequency in PCOS patients would strongly suggest the presence of a central component in the pathogenesis of this syndrome. The issue of pulse frequency is a key one because it has been demonstrated that an exact GnRH pulse frequency is essential for appropriate synthesis of the mRNA for LH (112). A lower than normal GnRH frequency results in an attenuated mid-cycle surge and anovulation (113). A number of studies have demonstrated an increased pulse frequency in PCOS (15,16,96,98,99). Rapid pulsatile GnRH administration every 30 minutes in the normal menstrual cycle results in a mean increase of LH and an increase of LH/FSH ratio resulting in a luteal phase defect (114) common in women with PCOS. Waldstreicher et al. (15) found consistent increased LH amplitudes and pulse frequency in patients with PCOS in comparison to those found in normal women in the early follicular phase (EFP), mid-follicular and late follicular phases of the menstrual cycle. This suggested an increase in the frequency of pulsatile secretion of GnRH. The studies were performed over 12 to 24 hours. This was in agreement with some investigators (86,98,115), while others have been unable to confirm these findings (109). The exact frequency of LH peaks is still controversial. Increased pulse frequency is present in perhaps 50% of patients with PCOS (97), while LH amplitude is characteristically elevated (77,97,99,109). In one study of hyperandrogenic anovulatory women, LH pulsatility correlated primarily with elevated E_1 levels (87). Clearly the establishment of subgroups by clinical and bio-chemical criteria is essential, and frequent serum LH sampling (every 10 minutes) is mandatory in order to assess the role of the hypothalamus, that is, the presence of increased LH pulsatility, in the pathogenesis of PCOS.

Not all investigators are convinced that an increased LH pulse frequency does exist in PCOS (109). Some data indicating increased pulse frequency in PCOS (98) may not have taken into account the time of the cycle in normal controls, fairly brief sampling of 4 to 6 hours, lack of controls, and the potentially confounding effect of a sleep-related nocturnal decline in LH pulse frequency in the early follicular phase of normal women (114,116). The nocturnal slowing of LH pulse amplitude, typical of the early follicular phase of normal cycling women, does not occur in PCOS (109). Kazer and associates (109) studied women with PCOS and normal women in the early follicular phase during waking hours, for 12 hours. These investigators found that elevations in LH that occur in PCOS are due primarily to increased LH pulse amplitude. The pulse frequency, however, was similar to that found in normal women in the early follicular phase of the menstrual cycle. They noted an incidence of one pulse of LH per hour in groups of women with PCOS, as well as in normal women in the early follicular and mid-follicular phases of the cycle. They speculate that increased LH pulse amplitude found in women with PCOS may perhaps reflect an increased GnRH pulse amplitude or enhanced pituitary sensitivity to GnRH which is present in PCOS (86). Pathophysiological alterations in GnRH pulse am-plitude have also been described to result in profound alterations in gonadotropins similar to those observed in PCOS (117). Thus the interpretation of data relating to the central role of pulse frequency in PCOS has not entirely been settled, although recent data by Hall et al. (16) indicate that in a select group of patients with PCOS, increased pulsatility of LH and free alpha-subunit (FAS) suggests strongly the pres-ence of enhanced response to GnRH as a pathogenetic factor in PCOS.

"Frequency" Hypothesis of PCOS

Experimental control of GnRH dosage and frequency in men with GnRH defi-ciency has led Hall and co-workers (16) to propose an alternative hypothesis for the abnormal gonadotropin dynamics in PCOS. In studies of five men with GnRH deficiency, increasing the pulse frequency of GnRH within a selected time frame resulted in a relative loss of gonadotrope responsiveness (desensitization), which was considerably more marked for FSH than LH. The mean LH levels rose pro-gressively during that time, resulting in a high LH/FSH ratio. With maintenance of increased frequency of GnRH administration over a 7-day time interval, LH respon-siveness did not continue to decrease but remained constant (118).

The "frequency" hypothesis as proposed by Hall and co-workers (16) states that the increased frequency of GnRH secretion in PCOS leads to increased levels of LH with normal levels of FSH. This follows a period of increased GnRH frequency. A modest increase in GnRH pulse frequency sustained for a period of time has been proposed to lead to partial pituitary desensitization and differential effects on LH and FSH. This negates any potential effect of inhibin in PCOS to account for low levels of FSH.

Another approach in confirming these findings of an increase in the frequency of pulsatile release of LH in patients with PCOS, was the utilization of FAS as an additional marker of GnRH secretion (16). The gonadotrope and thyrotrope have a common alpha-subunit, which is also secreted in an uncombined or free form, and its secretion is controlled by both thyrotropin-releasing hormone (TRH) and GnRH (118). Euthyroid women in the early follicular phase demonstrate that the endogenous pulses of FAS are more than 90% concordant with pulses of LH, and that pulsatile FAS secretion is abolished by administration of a potent GnRH antagonist (119). These data suggest that there is no total increase in the amount of GnRH secreted despite the increased frequency of pulsatility and amplitude of pulses in PCOS. Although tonic secretion of FAS may be controlled by TRH, the pulsatile component of FAS appears to be primarily regulated by GnRH (16). Since FAS has a shorter half-life than LH (120), the study of FAS is advantageous in women with PCOS where the pulses are frequent. A concordance of pulses of FAS and LH was noted in women with PCOS, suggesting the high-frequency secretion of GnRH in PCOS (16). Thus an increased frequency of GnRH secretion in women with PCOS was demonstrated by Hall and co-investigators using two different neuroendocrine markers (16,121).

In a recent study by Berga and co-workers (122), increased pulse frequency in nine hyperandrogenic anovulatory women was described by comparing the 24-hour secretory pattern of LH and alpha-subunit. Mean pulse frequency of both LH and alpha-subunit was increased in these nine women compared to similar-aged and body-weight–matched control eumenorrheic women in the mid-follicular phase. Basal increased levels of LH and alpha-subunit were noted in the hyperandrogenic anovulatory women, in whom responses of both markers were exaggerated to administration of exogenous GnRH. The response of FSH in the hyperandrogenic women was similar to that in normal control subjects. Finally, there are data indicating that decreasing the frequency of LH pulses in anovulatory women with PCOS by administration of exogenous estrogen and progesterone for 3 weeks results in a normalization of the LH/FSH ratio (99). This is important evidence for the role of the increased GnRH pulse generator activity in PCOS. Although there appears to be a critical role for the increased GnRH pulse frequency in the pathogenesis of PCOS, the question still remains as to whether the increase is primary or secondary to abnormal steroidogenesis of ovarian or adrenal origin. The latter may not only enhance the GnRH pulse generator leading to increased LH secretion but may alter FSH secretion leading to IGS.

Experimental Model of "Unabated Gonadotropin Secretion"

An interesting experimental model in the rat which closely mimics that of polycystic ovaries is described by Bogovich (123). Her gonadotropin-induced model of PCOS demonstrates the following: (a) the primary role of an unabated gonadotropin stimulation in the development of the follicular cysts appears to be of greater importance than the relative serum concentrations of gonadotropins in determining the development of follicular cysts; (b) the stage of differentiation of the ovary does not appear to have a major role in the etiology of polycystic ovaries; (c) unabated stimulation by FSH and LH-like activity are sufficient to induce ovarian follicular cysts in the rat; and (d) the induction and stimulation of follicular aromatase activity need not be suppressed during initial induction of ovarian cysts. Thus the concept of unabated gonadotropin stimulation has been considered by some groups to be a possible primary pathogenetic mechanism rather than the relative serum concentration of LH. This experimental concept and the finding of elevated levels of bioactive LH in PCOS further support a central pathogenetic mechanism in PCOS in instances where circulating LH levels may not be increased. A somewhat modified model has been utilized to assess the role of hyperinsulinism in the development of follicular cysts (124).

The Hypothalamus and Its Role in the Pathogenesis of PCOS

There are a number of studies which suggest a central hypothalamic role in the genesis of PCOS. It has been suggested that circadian rhythmicity of LH may be defective in PCOS. In a study of pubertal patients with presumed PCOS, a desynchronization was found of the nocturnal LH secretory pattern compared to that of normal girls (125). This suggested that a developmental abnormality of hypothalamic GnRH secretion may be a major feature of this disorder. These teenage patients had an LH surge once a day that was of normal duration but desynchronized from the normal sleep period, occurring 7 to 8 hours later during the day than it should. This only involved LH, while the cortisol and prolactin profiles were normal. It was suggested that desynchronization of the LH clock from the sleep period may result in failure of an LH surge to occur, resulting in anovulation. Similar results were found by Porcu (126) who studied 12 adolescent women with high or normal levels of LH. A deranged circadian rhythmicity of LH, however, was found in only the high-LH group of five women. These studies suggest that an abnormal chronobiological LH secretion does occur in some adolescent women and that this derangement may be related to the development of PCOS. However, in several of these subjects there was spontaneous normalization of LH within 1 to 2 years. Thus the exact role of this abnormality is still uncertain.

In one report, the initiating event appeared to have been a luteinizing hormone–secreting pituitary microadenoma, since surgical removal of the pituitary adenoma resulted in a "cure" of the polycystic ovary syndrome (127).

Another reported abnormality in PCOS women is a frequent alteration in the circadian rhythm of gonadotropin secretion. Normal women have a reduced pulsatile LH secretion at night during the early follicular phase of the menstrual cycle (128), while this is absent in women with PCOS (109). An abnormal diurnal rhythm in LH secretion has also been reported in adults with PCOS (18). The exact role of chronobiological derangements in the pathogenesis of PCOS is as yet uncertain.

Although ultrasonographic features of PCOS may be present in women with weight loss–related amenorrhea (129–131), the hypothalamic disturbance is not associated with an increased ovarian stroma or biochemical features of PCOS. Occasionally, bilaterally enlarged ovaries may be noted in these women (129). Some patients with weight loss–related amenorrhea may have a history of erratic menses long before the onset of their eating disorder (131). An interesting report has demonstrated a surprising incidence of eating disorders in ultrasonographic-proven PCOS patients, with one-third having eating disorders, including a 6% incidence of bulimia nervosa compared to 1% of women attending an endocrine clinic with a variety of organic endocrinopathies (57). While this may implicate a hypothalamic etiology in the pathogenesis of the disorder in a distinct subset of patients with PCOS, further confirmatory data are necessary to assess the implications of these findings.

Ultrasonographic findings of PCOS may be been seen in patients with low serum LH levels (111,129). The persistence of morphologic abnormalities in the ovaries in the setting of low gonadotropins does not support the idea of a primary central defect in some subsets of patients with PCOS.

GnRH Responsiveness in PCOS

LH Hyperresponsiveness to GnRH

A more consistent finding than the often variable level of serum LH in women with PCOS is the frequently demonstrated enhanced pituitary sensitivity to administration of GnRH. There are clear data indicating that the positive feedback effect of estrogen on LH is operative to cause the exaggerated LH release in PCOS (83,86). The duration of estrogen exposure may be of more importance than the dose in determining pituitary gonadotropic activity (132). Even a small bolus of 10 μg GnRH in PCOS subjects causes a four-fold release of LH compared to that observed in normal cycling women in the early follicular phase of the menstrual cycle (133). Normal ovulatory women require a full 150 μg GnRH to achieve a maximum response of LH. The heightened pituitary sensitivity to GnRH appears to depend on the basal LH level and is most pronounced in those women with high serum LH levels (78,86). In several studies of women with PCOS having normal serum LH levels at the time of GnRH testing, the LH response was relatively normal or less hyperresponsive than those with elevated LH levels (92,134–136).

An important consideration is that the pituitary response of LH to GnRH in women with PCOS may mirror peripheral levels of E_1 and E_2 (83,86). A correlation between elevation of serum LH and that of free non–sex hormone–binding globulin (SHBG)–bound E_2 has been reported (137).

One of the widely held hypotheses is that the augmented response of LH is secondary to abnormal pituitary feedback by circulating estrogens and androgens. Despite this attractive hypothesis, some investigators have been unable to reproduce this abnormality by infusion of either class of steroids (82,138).

FSH Levels and Response to GnRH

The response of serum FSH to 150 μg GnRH is similar to that seen in normal ovulatory women, but the FSH response is diminished when low dosage GnRH is injected (86,132,135). This may be explained by greater sensitivity of FSH than of LH to the inhibitory (negative-feedback) effects of estrogen (82,137,139). Defective FSH secretion appears to be part of the pathogenesis of PCOS, since clomiphene citrate or low-dose FSH administration frequently results in ovulatory cycles (86,140–142).

Normal serum levels of FSH in PCOS compared to controls have been noted (104,143). This is in keeping with normal immunoreactive inhibin levels in the peripheral blood (115) and follicular fluid (143) of patients with PCOS. Normal systemic bioactivity of FSH suggests the concept of intraovarian dysregulation in PCOS (143).

To summarize: The most frequently found gonadotropin abnormalities in PCOS are:

1. an elevated LH/FSH ratio (IGS)
2. increased LH pulse amplitude and possibly frequency
3. exaggerated response of LH to GnRH
4. altered diurnal rhythm of LH secretion.

These may vary among different studies, indicating different selection criteria for patients chosen from a heterogeneous population for study. This is quite evident in the literature; some groups select only patients with elevated LH values (15,16) others do not (100). It is clear that pooled data from different centers is difficult to interpret in view of different patient selection criteria, including PCOS phenotypes. It would be of interest to determine whether the data of Hall and associates (16) also apply to those women with PCOS who have a normal LH/FSH ratio at time of testing, or whether, if a change in ratio does occur in an individual, the results of the pulsatility studies also vary.

Hyperprolactinemia in PCOS

Frequency of Hyperprolactinemia in PCOS

There is a subset of women with PCOS with hyperprolactinemia, some of whom have associated galactorrhea (55). Some reports have described the presence of hyperprolactinemia in up to one-third of PCOS patients (55,56,144–147). In a review of the literature of 394 patients with PCOS, 27% were found to be hyperprolactinemic (55). It is difficult to discern whether the hyperprolactinemia in PCOS women is a cause or an effect and whether it may reflect a central pathogenetic factor in this group of patients with PCOS. There are ample data supporting the hypothesis that the estrogenic feedback to the pituitary may sensitize lactotrope cells (145,148). Most reported studies are confined to establishing the diagnosis of PCOS and then finding prolactin (PRL) elevations in a number of these patients. A large series of hyperprolactinemic patients should be evaluated clinically and statistically so as to allow an analysis of the frequency of PCOS in women with elevated serum PRL concentrations. Intermittent elevations of serum PRL are not uncommon and this adds to the confounding variability of classifying PCOS women as being hyper-prolactinemic or not.

Dopamine Deficiency Hypothesis

Clinically, it is apparent that most studies of hyperprolactinemic patients with PCOS indicate a normal or reduced basal level of serum LH (55). The frequently noted elevation of serum LH seen in the majority of patients with PCOS often does not apply to the hyperprolactinemic subgroup. In a study of 556 patients with PCOS, the 11% of patients who were hyperprolactinemic usually did not demon-strate elevated gonadotropin levels (13). This suggests that the same hypothalamic dysfunction causing an increased LH/FSH ratio and elevation of serum PRL does not appear to be operative in this subset of patients with PCOS. Conflicting data from earlier studies by Luciano and associates (56) revealed that PCOS patients with elevated serum PRL levels (mean 43 ± 8 ng/mL) had baseline serum LH levels similar to those in nonhyperprolactinemic subjects. Basal levels of FSH were reported as being lower in the hyperprolactinemic patients than nonhyperprolac-tinemic women with PCOS. Similarly, the enhanced pituitary sensitivity to GnRH characteristic of women with PCOS was preserved (55,56) and was similar to that of nonhyperprolactinemic patients with PCOS (56). These findings could not be attributed to differences in circulating estrogen levels since the serum levels of E_1 and E_2 were similar in both groups (56).

The clinical study reported by Luciano and associates (56) is consistent with the hypothesis that the pathogenesis of PCOS may be related to a central deficiency of dopaminergic activity at the basal hypothalamus. It is also hypothesized that en-hancement of adrenal androgen production by hyperprolactinemia may increase ex-traglandular estrogen production, leading to a reduction of hypothalamic dopamine, (DA) resulting in enhancement of pituitary lactotropes but in some instances also an increased LH production (149).

Initial studies by several investigators suggested a central abnormality of DA regulation in PCOS patients. Exaggerated suppression of LH in PCOS women with elevated LH levels by high-dose DA infusion (5 µg/kg·min) (150,151) was consis-tent with this hypothesis. The hypothesis of a dopamine deficiency had also been suggested to explain decreased levels of the urinary metabolite homovanillic acid in the urine (152).

A logical method of testing this hypothesis was the possibility of modulating GnRH–LH dynamics by dopamine agonist therapy such as bromocriptine. This has produced conflicting results. A reduction of serum LH by dopamine agonists was documented by some investigators (153–157) and refuted by others (158,159).

Significant reductions of LH and T were found in PCOS women treated with bromocriptine by Falaschi and associates (156). Only 20% or so of patients demonstrated reduction of hirsutism and menstrual dysfunction in these studies.

Evidence Against the Dopamine Hypothesis

The hypothesis that inadequate hypothalamic secretion of DA is an important pathogenetic factor in causing elevated LH levels in most patients with PCOS has been questioned by subsequent studies. Rosen and Lobo (158) studied the effects of disulfiram, a compound that increases hypothalamic levels of DA via inhibition of conversion of DA to norepinephrine (NE), and found that it did not affect mean LH levels or pulsatile LH secretion in normal women and in three out of five women with PCOS. These data suggest that inadequate hypothalamic secretion of DA is not a significant pathogenetic component in most instances of PCOS. Barnes and co-workers (159) demonstrated that when PCOS subjects were matched for weight and serum estradiol levels, the degree of LH suppression achieved via infusion of DA was similar in both PCOS and normal controls studied in the mid-follicular phase of the menstrual cycle. The normoprolactinemic subjects with PCOS and the normal cycling women received intravenous DA in 2 doses (0.5 and 4 μg/kg·min) followed by 10 mg intravenous metoclopramide (MCP) (a DA receptor antagonist). In patients with PCOS, the decrease in LH was similar with both low and high DA doses (Fig. 1) (159), suggesting that the sensitivity to DA in women with PCOS is not increased. Serum PRL and TSH responses to DA were also similar in PCOS and normal women, with both groups showing a significant decrease. After MCP treatmeht, serum LH did not change in the PCOS or normal women, but the serum PRL level increased two-fold more in PCOS patients than in normal controls (149). The significantly increased PRL response to MCP in PCOS women suggests that brain DA may be increased in a number of PCOS patients compared to normal women. Alternatively, one must also consider that the exaggerated PRL response to MCP in PCOS patients may be the result of chronic hyperestrogenism.

The data of Barnes and associates (159) make it difficult to accept the hypothesis that central DA deficiency causes the inappropriately elevated LH secretion in most PCOS patients when MCP blockade of endogenous DA does not increase either the bioactive or immunoreactive LH in PCOS and normal women (159,160). As for the role of unbound serum estradiol as a possible factor in the development of hyperprolactinemia in this subset of PCOS women, it is of interest that almost 50% of PCOS patients with normal basal levels of PRL hyperrespond with increased PRL levels after GnRH stimulation (148).

Convincing evidence against a major disturbance related to DA in PCOS comes from studies of treatment of women with PCOS with bromocriptine. No changes in LH secretion were noted after 1, 2 and 12 months of treatment with bromocriptine (161,162). Furthermore, Buvat et al. (163) did not see any hormonal or clinical improvement in 55 women with PCOS treated in a double-blind study for 6 months.

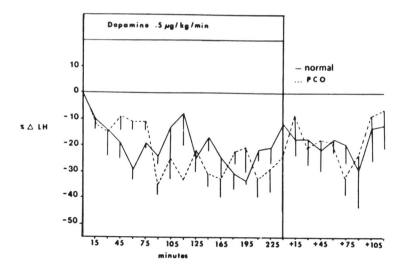

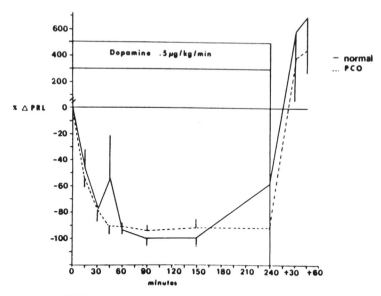

FIG. 1. Mean (± SEM) percent change in serum LH during low dose dopamine (DA) infusion (0.5 μg/kg·min) in normal and PCOS women (*top panel*). Mean percent change in serum prolactin (PRL) during low dose DA infusion in normal women and PCOS patients (*bottom panel*). (From ref. 159, with permission.)

Approximately one-half of the women with PCOS did show some reduction in LH which was not accompanied by a significant reduction of T. Most investigators concur that the use of DA agonist therapy should be reserved for the hyperprolactinemic subset of PCOS women. The generally negative results with such therapy in normoprolactinemic patients with PCOS raises doubts about the validity of the DA hypothesis as an important pathophysiological abnormality in PCOS (22). It appears that if any DA-related dysfunction of LH secretion exists in PCOS, it is limited to a relatively small subgroup of patients with PCOS. There may be a minor influence of DA deficiency on LH, probably occurring in those women with PCOS exhibiting the highest LH levels (37).

Thyrotropin–Releasing Hormone (TRH) Test in PCOS

Conflicting data have appeared in the literature regarding the response of PCOS patients to TRH, with some series demonstrating an exaggerated PRL response (56,145,149,155), while other studies have noted a normal PRL response to TRH (164).

Possible Association with Development of Pituitary Prolactinomas

The association of pituitary prolactin-secreting adenomas with PCOS has been described by several groups (56,165–170) and this may result from an inherent hypothalamic–pituitary abnormality or secondary to chronic hyperestrogenism. The cases that have been described usually follow number of years of documented PCOS and have included pituitary macroadenomas as well as microadenomas (165,166).

Inhibin and PCOS

Recent studies indicate that serum immunoreactive inhibin levels in anovulatory women with PCOS are similar to those of normal women (115,171) in the early or mid-follicular phase of the menstrual cycle (115). No primary defects in ovarian inhibin secretion in women with PCOS have been demonstrated in either the basal or the gonadotropin-stimulated (exogenous or endogenous) state (115). Furthermore, serum estradiol and inhibin rise in parallel in response to exogenous gonadotropins. The data of Buckler and associates (115) support the hypothesis that inhibin is FSH driven. Inhibin secretion may thus be considered a circulating marker of FSH action on the ovary and an important indicator of follicular viability. This is in agreement with earlier studies suggesting that ovarian inhibin activity depends on follicular viability rather than on follicle size (76,172).

Clearly, there is strong evidence showing that inhibin is produced by the granulosa cell of the ovarian follicle (173). Further, immunohistochemical studies indicate follicular granulosa cells are the source of inhibin (174). In a recent study (175) the immunohistochemical localization of inhibin α-, βA-, and βB-subunits were described in PCOS. Yamoto and co-workers (175) demonstrated that unlike normal ovaries, the granulosa cells in multicystic follicles of PCOS exhibited negative immunostaining for α-subunit and positive staining for βA- and βB-subunits. In contrast, the hyperplastic thecal and stromal cells exhibited positive staining for all three subunits. The findings suggest (175) that thecal and stromal cells in PCOS may produce both androgens as well as inhibin under chronic LH stimulation. The sustained hypersecretion of androgens by the thecal compartment may be augmented by the presence of hyperinsulinemia and possibly by an increased action of insulin-like growth factors (12). The novel theory of an enhanced effect of LH on the thecal–stromal cell production of inhibin warrants further study. The reader is referred to additional in vitro studies (173,174,176) of the possible role of inhibin in PCOS.

Endogenous Neurotransmitters and GnRH Modulation in PCOS

The role of opioids and other neurotransmitters and their effect on GnRH modulation have yet to be defined in PCOS. A number of references address their possible pathogenetic role in PCOS (152,160,177–187). Whether opioids are at least partially responsible for the hyperinsulinemia and insulin resistance in PCOS remains to be clarified. Similarly, the role of NE and serotonin on the GnRH–LH system in normal and PCOS women has not as yet been defined.

Summation of Neuroendocrine and Gonadotropin Hypotheses in the Pathogenesis of PCOS

There is clear evidence that a disordered gonadotropin secretion plays a critical role, perhaps a primary role, in the pathogenesis of PCOS. The weight of evidence indicates aberrant GnRH activity in this syndrome. Clearly, desensitization of LH secretion with GnRH agonists leads to a cessation of ovarian steroidal production with no change in adrenal secretion. The exact nature of the alteration leading to an inappropriate gonadotropin secretion in this heterogeneous disorder is still conjectural. Despite many data relating primary hypothalamic defects in the pathogenesis of PCOS, the possibility that these may result as a secondary phenomenon to an abnormal steroidal milieu can not be excluded. Estrogens (probably the unbound fraction) play a major role in the modulation of GnRH secretion and probably in the genesis of the almost uniformly elevated levels of bioactive LH present in women with PCOS. Regardless of the primary or secondary nature of the GnRH abnormality, the consensus of evidence favors an association with abnormalities of LH pulse amplitude and most likely pulse frequency. Modulation of the GnRH pulse generator may be reflected by varying subsets of PCOS, including those reflecting central effects of hyperprolactinemia, opioids, and catecholamines as well as those reflecting weight-related hypothalamic dysfunction. The consequences of increased LH as well as the elevated bioavailable LH may be amplified at the ovarian level, which further augments ovarian hyperandrogenism leading to a cascade of events perpetuating the gonadotropin abnormality. The heterogeneity of PCOS subsets makes it likely that several of these mechanisms apply.

PATHOPHYSIOLOGY OF OVARAN DYSFUNCTION IN PCOS

Overview

The role of ovarian or adrenal steroidogenesis in contributing to the increased androgen pool and the resulting extraglandular conversion of androgens to estrogens in the pathogenesis of PCOS appear to be important aspects in the perpetuation of the entity. The enhanced LH secretion undoubtedly is a factor leading to ovarian hyperandrogenism, but is the IGS primary or secondary to the steroidogenic milieu? One should consider, for example, that the pathogenesis of a patient with idiopathic hirsutism (hyperandrogenemia with normal menstrual cyclicity) is different from that of a patient with hyperthecosis. The consensus is that these are two extremes of PCOS, which is undoubtedly made up of a number of different subsets and phenotypes with different pathogenetic mechanisms. The common expression of all these subsets is ovarian hyperandrogenism. This section will review the various models, hypotheses, and studies which attempt to explain its pathogenesis. Inherent in any review is the well-known fact that in vitro and in vivo animal experimental models do not always apply to the human model. It is the purpose of this section to review studies relating to the genesis of ovarian hyperandrogenism, the role of the adrenal cortex, aberrant folliculogenesis, and the modulating effects of the insulin/IGF/IGFBP (IGF–binding protein) system in the pathogenesis of PCOS. Some of the experimental in vitro studies will be summarized briefly and cited so as to make the concepts more compact. Detailed descriptions of hyperinsulinemia, insulin resistance, and ovarian hyperandrogenism, and the confounding additive factor of obesity in PCOS, will be discussed in a later section.

Role of Estrogens and Androgens on the Hypothalamus in PCOS

In what way are the estrogen levels that are produced in PCOS different from the levels found in normal ovulatory women? Measurement of estradiol (E_2) concentrations in PCOS are generally similar to those of women in the mid-follicular phase of the menstrual cycle. Estrone (E_1) production rates, however, are increased 3 to 4 times above normal levels in PCOS, mostly via increased peripheral (extraglandular) aromatization of A (188), particularly in women with increased body weight (83). The reversal of the circulating E_2/E_1 ratio is characteristic of PCOS women.

The mechanism of an altered hypothalamic–pituitary response to estrogens in PCOS has been considered to some extent previously. Estrogens clearly exert a positive and negative feedback on LH release. A positive feedback enhances the frequency and/or amplitude of GnRH secretion, while the estrogen-associated negative feedback results in a greater sensitivity of pituitary FSH than LH to circulating estrogens. Augmented pituitary sensitivity to GnRH resulting in enhanced LH release correlates with basal levels of E_1 and E_2 (86). Thus the clinical observation that there is increased pituitary sensitivity to GnRH during the late follicular phase of the menstrual cycle, as well as enhanced pituitary response to GnRH following estrogen administration, offers evidence of an altered peripheral feedback set-point. In studies of women with PCOS, a direct correlation between serum LH/FSH levels and mean serum E_2 levels (15) as well as free nonSHBG–bound E_2 has been reported (137). The increased free nonSHBG–bound E_2 in PCOS (137) appears to be a factor in altering the pituitary sensitivity to GnRH. Thus smaller subthreshold pulses which may not normally be followed by LH secretion can result in detectable LH pulses (189). It is clear that peripheral estrogens, resulting from extraglandular conversion of the major ovarian androgen A, may be a contributory, albeit not the major, factor in the pathophysiology of the characteristic IGS of PCOS. This probably results in the preferential inhibitory feedback of chronic acyclic estrogen production on FSH as compared to LH release.

Acute administration of T and dihydrotestosterone (DHT) does not appear to result in the IGS in PCOS (138) or in normal women (190). Clinical and experimental studies indicate that hyperandrogenemia may not cause inappropriate LH release (191). The role of chronic androgen exposure as a causative mechanism in the IGS of PCOS, however, is controversial. Studies suggesting that enhanced LH release occurs secondary to androgens have been reported in virilizing adrenal and ovarian tumors (192,193). Ovulatory women receiving chronic exogenous T therapy in preparation for sex reversal surgery demonstrate a heterogeneous response, including some with an increase in the LH/FSH ratio (194). Reversal of the IGS by surgical removal of an ovarian tumor has been described (192). An elevated LH/FSH ratio may be also frequently found in a significant number of patients with late onset (nonclassical) 21-hydroxylase deficiency (58,67,195,196). There are no hard data proving that IGS may be induced by a primary steroidal abnormality or chronic androgen excess. A number of investigators, however, have data which they believe suggest that primary dysfunction of the ovaries and/or adrenals are the primary events leading to secondary changes in the activity of the GnRH pulse generator.

Ovarian Hyperandrogenism—The Common Thread

Consideration of the complex nature of ovarian folliculogenesis and steroidogenesis is essential for an understanding of the pathogenesis of PCOS. Despite the heterogeneity of PCOS, the various models proposed for the development of the syndrome must include ovarian hyperandrogenism as the common thread. Whether certain investigators champion a primary central hypothalamic–pituitary defect (15, 16,125,183), a primary ovarian (14,197,198) and/or adrenal steroidogenic defect (30,199), or a defect relating to insulin resistance (12,35,200), the basic constant is still an abnormal ovary that is secreting excessive androgens. Thus, for example, patients who have an adrenal enzymatic defect and/or a significant adrenocortical contributory factor usually develop the morphological and biochemical changes of polycystic ovaries. An adrenal contribution is characterized by elevated serum levels of dehydroepiandrosterone sulfate (DHEAS), which may also be present in association with elevated serum levels of T and free T (201,202). It appears that most PCOS patients will, after a varying time interval, have a gonadotropin-dependent form of ovarian hyperandrogenism which episodically or cyclically perpetuates the IGF. Proposed mechanisms include disordered folliculogenesis with a paucity of granulosa cells, dysregulation of steroidogenesis, hyperinsulinism, insulin resistance, obesity, IGFs and their binding proteins, and others.

There are ample data which confirm the hypothesis that PCOS is gonadotropin-dependent because inhibition of gonadotropin secretion with a GnRH-agonist markedly reduces ovarian androgen secretion (203–205). Biochemically the hyperandrogenism of PCOS is usually characterized by an increase in serum free T (29,47,48,206,207) frequently associated with IGS. Hyperandrogenemia is also often manifested by an increase in total T, which frequently indicates that the hyperandrogenemia is of ovarian origin. The increase in T and free T may be episodic, however, and an abnormal level may be missed on isolated sampling (208). The sampling technique may be improved by drawing three specimens at 6 to 18 minute intervals and pooling them. This may avoid the pulsatile episodic fluctuations such as are seen in serum T as well as LH (89).

The initiation of ovarian hyperandrogenism in PCOS arises from heterogeneous disorders that directly increase one of three variables: (a) the LH/FSH ratio, (b) the intraovarian concentrations and ratio of androgens to estrogens, or (c) the process of follicular atresia. An increase in any of these three variables can then induce changes in the others. For example, in instances where the LH/FSH abnormality may not be obvious, the initiating factor may be abnormalities of androgen production, particularly in the ovary, or by disorders which arrest follicular maturation causing follicular atresia. Disorders characterized by hyperinsulinism or insulin resistance probably initiate PCOS through the latter mechanisms (18), and recent studies indicate amplification of LH action via the insulin/IGF system (209–211).

Estrone Hypothesis

Much controversy surrounds the role of the adrenal cortex in the pathogenesis of the hyperandrogenism in PCOS. This follows the observation that frequently, adrenal 17-ketosteroid hyperresponsiveness occurs on ACTH testing. This is similar to the adrenal response to ACTH at the time of puberty (81,199). The term exaggerated adrenarche has been applied to a possible initiating role of the adrenals leading to the development of PCOS (81,199,212,213). Virilizing tumors may also lead to changes of polycystic ovaries (214), as well as the initiating events seen in patients with CAH, who frequently may present with PCOS (40,58,66,67,144,215,216). Eighty percent of women with CAH have co-existent morphologic PCOS (217). The proponents of an adrenal basis for the majority of patients with PCOS have proposed an estrone hypothesis (30). This model proposes that increased secretion of substrate A by the adrenals leads to increased estrogen concentrations, mainly E_1, through its peripheral aromatization mostly in adipose tissue. A schematic outline of steroidogenesis is depicted (Fig. 2) (76). Furthermore, elevated androgens and/or obesity decrease the SHBG concentration resulting in increased free estrone which may sensitize the pituitary to alter the LH/FSH ratio resulting in increased LH stimulation of ovarian androgens (30). The increased LH stimulates thecal cell A production and results in an associated deficient granulosa cell activity, thereby perpetuating the vicious cycle of PCOS. Therapeutic intervention with dexamethasone reduces A, which is followed by a reduction of the hyperestronemia and its attendant effect on pituitary gonadotropins (30).

The inherent weaknesses of the estrone hypothesis follow as a result of several observations (21,99):

1. Exogenous E_1 administration fails to increase circulating LH in PCOS and normal women (82).
2. There are distinct subsets of patients with PCOS who do not demonstrate elevated LH levels or IGS (79).
3. GnRH agonist treatment clearly defines the role of the ovary as a source of androgens in most patients with PCOS while no effect of treatment is noted on the adrenal androgens DHEA or DHEAS. Thus increased ovarian androgen levels are produced in a significant number of patients with PCOS independent of adrenal androgen production (203).
4. Utilization of a test dose of nafarelin in PCOS women demonstrates enhanced ovarian androgen steroidogenesis of the delta-4 pathway leading to increased circulating levels of E_1. This negates some of the impact of peripheral aromatization of the adrenal source of A leading to hyperestronemia (218).
5. Selective ovarian and adrenal catheterization data define the ovaries as the major site of androgens in higher androgenic women (219,220).
6. Estrogens may increase adrenal androgen production in vivo and in vitro (220).

The evidence indicates that if E_1 is a factor in perpetuating the IGS of PCOS, it is not the primary pathogenetic mechanism.

The Adrenal Factor in the Pathogenesis of PCOS

The fact that adrenal androgen concentrations are increased in a significant number of women with PCOS continues to raise the question as to whether the adrenal gland contributes to the pathogenesis. DHEAS, a 17-ketosteroid with a total pro-

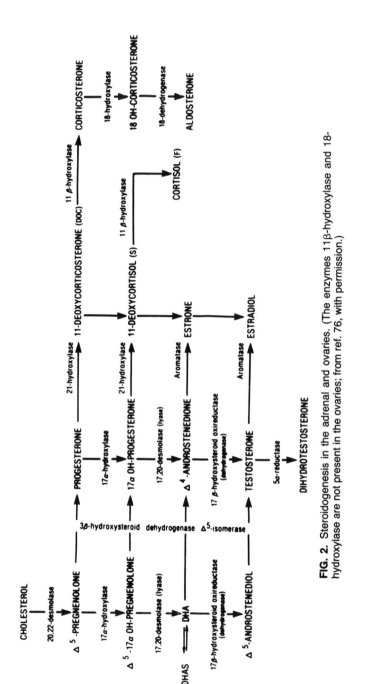

FIG. 2. Steroidogenesis in the adrenal and ovaries. (The enzymes 11β-hydroxylase and 18-hydroxylase are not present in the ovaries; from ref. 76, with permission.)

duction rate of greater than 10–15 mg/day, and almost exclusively of adrenal origin, is elevated in 50% or more of cases of PCOS (221,222). Its low metabolic clearance and long half-life makes it a valuable marker of adrenal androgen activity. DHEAS may also be increased in some patients with CAH, Cushing's syndrome, and hyperprolactinemia. A serum level greater than 700 µg/dL is suggestive of an adrenal tumor (64), and a CT scan of the adrenal may diagnose adrenal adenomas as small as 1 cm in diameter (59,60,64).

It is of interest to note the higher two-fold mean uptake of iodocholesterol by the adrenal glands of patients with PCOS than those of normal women (223). Ovarian visualization does not occur in these patients. This confirms that increased adrenal androgen production occurs in PCOS in addition to the ovarian T and A production. Most dexamethasone (DXM)-suppression studies have suggested excessive adrenal androgen production in many hirsute women (207,224,225), although not all agree (206). Interpretation of the suppression data is open to dispute because of evidence demonstrating that high or prolonged doses of glucocorticoids may have an inhibitory effect on gonadotropin secretion, thereby also suppressing ovarian androgen secretion (222,226,227).

GnRH agonist administration does not suppress the DHEAS level (203), suggesting adrenal androgen secretion is independent of pituitary–ovarian function in PCOS. Hyperresponsiveness of the 17-ketosteroid A to low dose ACTH stimulation was shown in 50% of women with PCOS (228). Prolonged ACTH stimulation (229) in PCOS causes increased levels of DHEA and other adrenal steroids. DXM-suppressed hyperandrogenism in PCOS has been considered to be related to partial 3β-hydroxysteroid dehydrogenase (3β-HSD) deficiency (198,230). Pang and co-workers (230), defining strict criteria for its diagnosis by ACTH stimulation, noted a 12.5% incidence of 3β-HSD deficiency in hirsute women, while the author's experience with ACTH testing of over 350 patients with PCOS has yielded a 4% frequency suggestive of a partial defect. (W. Futterweit; *unpublished data*). Lucky and co-investigators (231) found that hyperresponsiveness of plasma 17-ketosteroids to ACTH testing in hyperandrogenic women occurs in a pattern suggesting a relatively inefficient 3β-HSD activity in association with an increased C-17,20-lyase (desmolase) activity. This pattern closely resembles that seen in normal pubertal adrenal maturation (adrenarche) (232). The pattern of DHEA response to ACTH may explain the exaggerated adrenal response, rather than a putative adrenal androgen–stimulating hormone (AASH) (233,234). The increase in DHEA accounts for the increase in DHEAS via the sulfokinase activity of the zona reticularis, which continues to be developed at that time. Exaggerated adrenarche (18) may be caused by hyperplasia of the zona reticularis or possibly dysregulation of cytochrome P-450c17α that forms adrenal as well as ovarian androgens. Increased adrenal androgen production in many PCOS women occurs in the absence of overt dysfunction of the ACTH–cortisol axis and measurements of plasma ACTH have been in the normal range (235).

Site of Hyperandrogenism in PCOS: Ovarian vs. Adrenal

Adrenal Suppression Studies

Correlation between the results of selective ovarian and adrenal venous catheterization and the glucocorticoid suppression test has been notoriously poor (207,236). Short-term glucocorticoid suppression does not allow for suppression of androgens in hyperandrogenemic women (206,237,238), suggesting that the ovary is the predominant source of androgens in these women. In contrast to studies using short-term glucocorticoid administration, the use of glucocorticoids for longer periods of time demonstrates that a majority of women with androgen excess have some degree of suppressible adrenal androgen hypersecretion (239,240). It remains to be determined whether there is a distinct change in the IGS with glucocorticoid therapy in hyperandrogenic women. A possible effect of glucocorticoids on LH release in hyperandrogenic women has been described (241). This was noted in hirsute women with elevated serum T levels after chronic administration of 7.5 mg prednisone for 3 months. No effects were seen in either acute suppression studies with 2.0 mg DXM for 2 days, or in women with normal T levels (241). The mechanism of the suppressed LH levels in the hyperandrogenic women receiving chronic glucocorticoid treatment is not clear. It is theoretically possible that one of the effects of DXM may be suppression of the production of a pro-opromelanocortin (POMC) fragment other than ACTH that is responsible for androgen secretion. Thus it may reverse the cycle initiated by adrenal androgen excess, including its conversion to E_1 (242).

Selective Venous Catheterization Studies

A number of techniques, studies, and reports have focused on the role of the adrenal cortex in hyperandrogenism and PCOS in particular. Definition of the biochemical localization of the hyperandrogenism in PCOS, and the frequency of involvement of the ovaries, adrenals, or combined roles of both organs, have been studied in detail with the use of a variety of studies manipulating hormonal secretion from both sites, as well as by direct selective venous catheterization data from the ovaries and adrenal glands. Kirschner and Jacobs (207) utilized combined ovarian and adrenal venous catheterization to determine the site of the hyperandrogenemia in 13 hirsute women. They noted that all had elevated T production rates. Nine of the 13 patients had an ovarian source of the hyperandrogenism, while a combined adrenal and ovarian source was noted in the other four patients. They concluded that the major source of androgens was the ovaries. In a subsequent study, Kirschner and co-workers (220) studied 44 hirsute females with elevated T production rates and demonstrated that the major source of T was ovarian, either a direct ovarian secretion of T or a result of peripheral aromatization from ovarian secretion of A. Nearly half of the hirsute women who demonstrated DXM suppression of plasma T and A of at least 50% after 4 to 5 days of 2 to 4 mg DXM daily had an ovarian venous effluent of T and A higher than that found in their adrenal veins. The ovarian effluent of androgens was similar to the group of women who failed to suppress plasma androgens after DXM. The women who did not suppress following DXM characteristically had higher plasma levels of T as well as a higher T production rate than those women who suppressed their androgens at least 50% following DXM administration. These studies underscored previous difficulties in dynamic biochemical testing where an adrenal etiology was assigned as the site of excessive androgen production. The data of Kirschner and co-workers (200) suggested a direct effect of glucocorticoids on ovarian androgen production in hyperandrogenic women confirming earlier data of in vitro studies (243). Although the data of Kirschner and co-workers are impressive, there has been some concern regarding the lack of normal controls (207), calculation of the androgen secretion rates (244), and lack of combined ovarian and adrenal hyperandrogenism in the subjects studied.

Additional selective venous catheterization studies in hyperandrogenic women confirming the observations by Kirschner and coworkers have been reported (236, 245,246). The adrenals were identified, however, as a site of hyperandrogenemia in 20 hirsute women with PCOS in another catheterization study (247). Most of the women in the latter study demonstrated a combined ovarian and adrenal hypersecretion of testosterone.

In a large series of bilateral ovarian and adrenal catheterization studies performed in 60 androgenized women with no evidence of any functioning neoplasm, Moltz and associates (244) found a combined ovarian and adrenal excess in 41%, pure ovarian excess in 27%, and pure adrenal excess in 12%. Twenty percent of these women had normal ovarian and adrenal venous androgen concentrations. These investigators suggested that catheterization be reserved for (a) instances when there is a suspicion of neoplastic hyperandrogenism when noninvasive methods are incapable of identifying a lesion, or (b) when serum T levels exceed 150 ng/dL or serum DHEAS is greater than 670 ng/dL.

The inherent difficulties in selective venous catheterization sampling was stressed by Wentz and associates (248):

1. Frequently difficult cannulation of right adrenal vein and left ovarian vein.
2. Episodic nature of adrenal androgen secretion.
3. Iatrogenic increase in adrenal androgen secretion by stress.
4. Increased ovarian secretion in ovary containing a dominant follicle or a corpus luteum.
5. A 5% complication rate including venous thrombosis, extravasation of contrast medium, and hematoma formation around the adrenal gland (249), including adrenal hemorrhage.
6. Possible effects of radiation exposure in young patients.

It appears that the use of selective venous catheterization sampling in PCOS or virilizing disorders is generally unnecessary. Successful sampling of all four glands occurs in only about 45% of patients subjected to this technically difficult procedure (61). It should primarily be employed in instances when modern imaging techniques are inconclusive in detecting small virilizing adrenal or ovarian neoplasms, or in other hyperfunctional adrenal or ovarian states when clinically warranted.

Evidence for Intraovarian Site of Androgen Production

Further evidence that there is an inherent intraovarian mechanism associated with PCOS follows from clinical observations of patients subjected to bilateral wedge resection (250,251). The menses frequently become regular and pregnancy may follow after the transient reduction of hyperandrogenism. The intraovarian factors which may be responsible for some of the favorable results achieved with this now virtually discarded therapeutic modality are (a) increased local intraovarian blood flow allowing increased gonadotropin delivery to the follicles, and/or (b) an acute localized reduction of androgenic tissue which decreases local inhibitory effects of androgens on folliculogenesis (250). The favorable results obtained with bilateral ovarian wedge resection occur more often when the wedge resection is made deep into the medullary–hilar region of the ovaries (44,197). Laparoscopic punch biopsies or point cauterization of the ovaries has replaced ovarian wedge resection as a surgical option for unresponsive PCOS patients. Greenblatt and Casper (252) noted a drop in circulating T and A with a nadir at 3 to 4 days postoperatively. Ovarian surgery resulting in a reduction of T and A in patients with androgen excess strongly suggests that the ovaries are the main source of androgens in PCOS (237).

More confirmatory data suggesting a frequent ovarian source of hyperandrogenism is that administration of DXM does not suppress circulating free T to normal levels in PCOS (253). The coincidence of plasma T and LH pulsations (254) as well as the decline of ovarian androgen production (T and A) with combination estrogen –progestin therapy (91,253) is further evidence that the ovaries produce excess androgens in PCOS (222). There are data suggesting that oral contraceptive steroid therapy may also exert an influence on adrenal androgen production in normal as well as hyperandrogenic women (255–257). Suppression of plasma ACTH by oral contraceptive therapy has also been described by Carr and co-workers (255).

Compelling arguments for the presence of ovarian hyperandrogenism in PCOS are in selective suppression studies of pituitary–ovarian function by GnRH agonists. Treatment with a GnRH agonist for 1 month resulted in a mean plasma T level falling to the castrate range (203). The mechanism is one of pituitary desensitization of gonadotropes to further GnRH stimulation. Following GnRH administration to women with PCOS, the ovarian hormone levels of T, A, E_1, and E_2 were similar to those observed in oophorectomized women (203). In contrast, DHEA, DHEAS, and cortisol secretion levels were unaffected. This gave direct proof that in most instances of PCOS, the ovary is the primary source of excessive A and T production. Injection of a test dose of 100 μg of nafarelin, a GnRH agonist, yielded results that strongly suggest a significant ovarian source of the hyperandrogenism (218).

Because T and A are increased in PCOS while E_2 is not (48,206,207,258), the possibility that ovarian androgens are inefficiently converted to estrogens has been studied extensively. Primary ovarian enzymatic defect as a cause of PCOS is uncommon (18,19). There are rare cases of congenital 3β-hydroxysteroid dehydrogenase deficiency (3β-HSD) presenting as PCOS (259,260). There also have been reports of ovarian 17-ketosteroid reductase deficiency (261,262). This enzyme converts A to T and E_1 to E_2 in the ovary and adrenal cortex. Women with primary amenorrhea, virilization, and bilaterally enlarged ovaries have been described and it appears that the defect is probably transmitted as an autosomal recessive trait. The features of this defect, namely, an elevated serum level of A and E_1 with a normal or elevated T concentration (via extraglandular conversion of A to T), are further enhanced by human chorionic gonadotropin (hCG) stimulation testing. The ratio of serum A/T is exaggerated by hCG testing. There is no suppression of A, T, or their production rates with DXM testing. In the report by Toscano et al. (262), the 17-ketosteroid reductase deficiency was found in two of 43 women with PCOS. They also described oligospermia and gynecomastia in siblings of two affected patients who presented with PCOS. The inherited nature of this disorder is apparent from the clinical and biochemical findings which may include altered A/T ratios in affected male siblings.

Dysregulation of Cytochrome P-450c17α Hypothesis

Introduction

It may be hypothesized that the androgenic intraovarian environment associated with follicular atresia found in PCOS may result as a primary event or a secondary phenomenon, or that follicular maturational arrest results in follicular atresia. Most in vitro studies of PCOS ovarian follicular fluid and isolated thecal and stromal cells demonstrate increased amounts of T, A, and DHEA (260,263). Initial considerations of the in vitro studies appear to be compatible with steroidogenic defects, particularly 3β-HSD or aromatase deficiency. It is clear, however, that the functional aromatase deficiency (secondary to the gonadotropin secretory abnormalities) present in cultured granulosa cells of patients with PCOS, are typically reversed by administration of FSH in vitro (176). The latter finding suggests that the aromatase deficiency found in PCOS is usually secondary to the gonadotropin abnormalities and not intrinsic in the ovary. Aromatase deficiency may also be secondary to follicular atresia from a variety of causes (18,19). In view of the reduced capacity of atretic follicles to convert A and T to estrogen, the development of an androgenic follicular microenvironment (172,264) leads to polycystic ovaries.

A novel hypothesis was introduced five years ago which deserves detailed attention. The frequent finding of an inefficient 3β-HSD defect combined with an enhanced 17α-hydroxylase and 17, 20-lyase activity on ACTH testing of women with PCOS prompted Rosenfield and co-investigators (14,265) to propose dysregulation of cytochrome P-450c17α of the ovaries and adrenals as a pathogenetic model for gonadotropin-dependent ovarian hyperandrogenism in PCOS. The dual action of the single enzyme, cytochrome P-450c17α, converts both progesterone and pregnenolone to 17-hydroxyprogesterone (17-OHP) and 17-hydroxypregnenolone (17-Preg), respectively, by 17α-hydroxylation. Furthermore, the C-17, 20-lyase (17, 20-desmolase) activity of this enzyme is expressed by the cleavage of the 21-C androgens to the C-l9 androgens A and DHEA (Fig. 3, Fig. 4) (14,19). The model of Rosenfield and associates (14) proposes that functional ovarian hyperandrogenism is the common denominator of PCOS via abnormal regulation (dysregulation) of P-450c17α which is present in the ovarian thecal-interstitial-stromal cells. Any factor that increases intraovarian androgens or causes premature follicular atresia can result in ovarian hyperandrogenism (Fig. 5) (21).

The model also attempts to account for instances of extraovarian hyperandrogenemia (e.g., congenital adrenal hyperplasia, virilizing tumors), which are associated with morphologic and biochemical changes of polycystic ovaries (3,21,58,66, 67,192,215,266) (Fig. 5). Identical histopathological findings to those of women with PCOS have also been demonstrated following chronic exogenous administra-

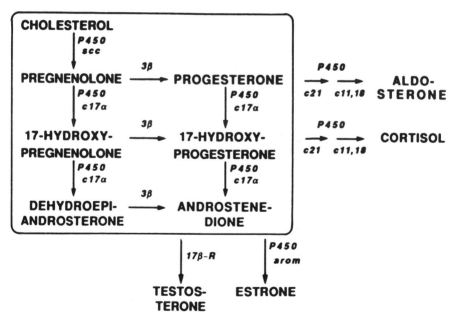

FIG. 3. Schematic outline of major steroidogenic pathways including the enclosed area which contains the core steroidogenic pathway utilized by the gonads and the adrenal gland. P450 , cytochrome P450; scc , side chain cleavage; c17α, c21, c11, c18, arom (aromatase) designate the sites of action of specific P450 enzymes. The non-P450 enzymes are 3β-hydroxysteroid dehydrogenase/delta5-isomerase (3β) and 17β-reductase (17β-R). (From ref. 14, with permission.)

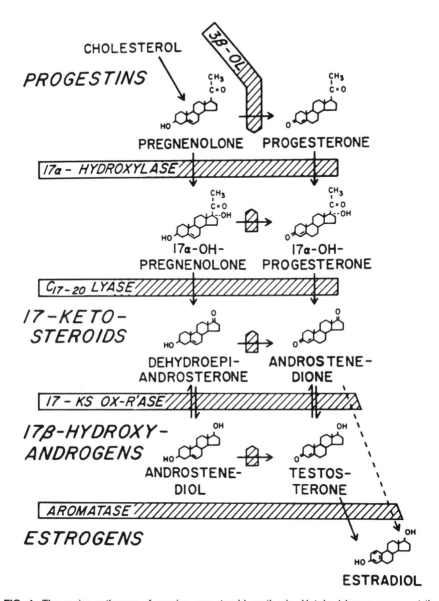

FIG. 4. The major pathways of ovarian sex steroid synthesis. *Hatched boxes* represent the enzyme steps. Estrone, the intermediate from androstenedione by an alternate pathway (*dotted line*) by which aromatase precedes 17-ketosteroid oxireductase activity, is not shown. 3β-ol, 3β-hydroxysteroid dehydrogenase; 17-KS ox-r'ase , 17-ketosteroid oxireductase. (From ref. 19, with permission.)

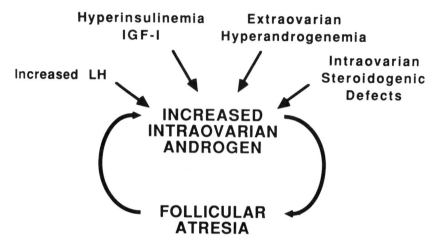

FIG. 5. Pathophysiology of PCOS as functional ovarian hyperandrogenism. PCOS arises from a number of heterogeneous entities which either increase intraovarian androgen concentrations or cause premature follicular atresia. An increase in either can cause abnormalities in the other in a to-and-fro manner. (From ref. 21, with permission.)

tion of testosterone to female-to-male transsexuals prior to sex-reversal surgery (267,268). This indicates that chronically elevated levels of testosterone lead to the characteristic morphologic features of polycystic ovaries (269), as well as to the potential for complications such as uterine endometrial hyperplasia (267). On the other hand, exogenous administration of testosterone for 6 months to ovulatory women prior to sex reversal surgery does not alter adrenal steroidogenesis (69).

Nafarelin (GnRH Agonist) Testing—The Biochemical Model

In order to test the proposed model of dysregulation of steroidogenesis (14,218, 265,270), PCOS patients with ovarian hyperandrogenism were tested with the GnRH agonist nafarelin (218). Nafarelin was administered to eight oligomenorrheic women with PCOS whose plasma free T did not suppress following DXM (48). Following administration of DXM 0.5 mg q.i.d. for 4 days to five PCOS and nine control women studied in the early follicular phase of the menstrual cycle, 100 μg nafarelin was given subcutaneously and blood samples were drawn every 4 hours for 24 hours (218). Patients with PCOS had a masculinized pituitary–gonadal response to nafarelin (218). The response of the PCOS women resembled that of men with both groups having an exaggerated early response of serum LH and lesser response of FSH. The steroidogenic response was also similar to that seen following hCG injection to men (271). These responses of LH and FSH were followed by significantly greater responses of PCOS women in plasma 17-OHP (>220 ng/dL; >6.4 nmol/L) and A levels 16 to 24 hours after the administration of nafarelin than those found in normal women (Fig. 6) (218). These findings occurred in the PCOS

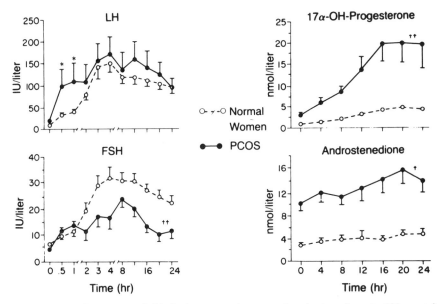

Fig. 6. Hormonal response of 17α-hydroxyprogesterone and androstenedione to 100 μg sub-cutaneous nafarelin in nine normal women and five women with PCOS after dexamethasone treatment. *, $p < 0.05$ for the comparison with normal women of the response at different times. † indicates a $p < 0.01$ and †† indicates $p < 0.02$ for the comparison with normal women of the areas under the response curve. The values are mean ± SEM. (From ref. 218, with permission.)

subjects whether they were pretreated with DXM or not. The significantly enhanced 17-OHP secretion as well as that of A and E_1 suggests increased activity of both 17α-hydroxylase and 17,20-lyase (i.e., cytochrome P-450c17α) in the delta-4 pathway of women with PCOS compared to control subjects (Fig. 7) (265). The enhanced ovarian androgen and E_1 secretion following nafarelin argues against the estrone hypothesis proposed by others (30). Likewise, no pattern suggestive of an ovarian partial 3β-HSD or 17-ketosteroid reductase deficiency was demonstrated (14,218,270,272).

Model as Applied to Adrenal Androgenic Hyperfunction in PCOS

Alterations of enzymes that have been proposed by other investigators as pathogenetic mechanisms in PCOS may now be examined in a new perspective (19):

a. 3β-hydroxy-delta-5-steroid dehydrogenase (3β-HSD): It has been estimated that 10 to 40% of hirsute women have a hyperresponse of various delta-5-steroids to ACTH (198,201,202,231). In the study of PCOS women by Barnes and associates (218) it was concluded that instances of true 3β-HSD deficiency were rare. Dysregulation of the androgen-forming enzyme 17-hydroxylase/17, 20-lyase was postulated to be the enzymatic defect in most women with PCOS accounting for the

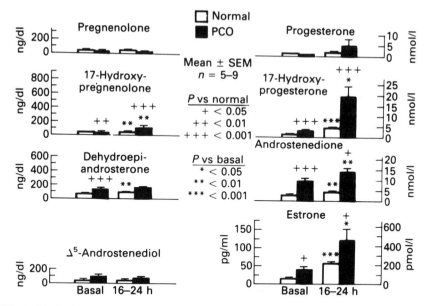

FIG. 7. Maximal steroid level responses before and at 16–24 hours after administration of 100 µg nafarelin. There were nine normal women studied in the follicular phase and five women with PCOS. Treatment with dexamethasone 2.0 mg daily was begun 4 days prior to testing and continued for 24 h following injection of nafarelin. The schematic representation is in accordance with the steroidogenic pathway, and the delta5-path on the left and the delta4-pathway on the right. Statistical data are present in the figure. (From ref. 265, with permission.)

ACTH hyperresponsiveness of the delta-5 pathways (14,218) rather than an inherent 3β-HSD defect.

b. 17-hydroxylase/17,20-lyase: A single P-450 enzyme, P-450c17α, has both 17-hydroxylase and 17,20-lyase activity. As stated previously, it is the initial step converting progesterone (P) first to 17-OHP and then to A. In the delta-5 pathway, it converts pregnenolone to 17-Preg, and then to DHEA (Fig. 4). Increased activity of this enzyme in PCOS has been attributed to dysregulation of P-450c17α, and it is the common endpoint in the pathogenesis of the great majority of patients with PCOS (14,19,265,270). This results in a greater 17-OHP/A ratio in women with PCOS after nafarelin compared to normal women. This hypothesis combines the adrenal and ovarian abnormalities seen in PCOS into a common mechanism.

Intrinsic abnormalities in the regulation of P-450c17α in the adrenal cortex may also explain the adrenal 17-ketosteroid hyperresponsiveness to ACTH (14,229) suggestive of a partial 3β-HSD deficiency in about 10% to 40% of hirsute patients with PCOS (14,19,198,228,231,272,273). Some have speculated that this may be an exaggerated adrenarche associated with the peripubertal onset of symptoms (14,81, 199,212,231,274) or it may be an adrenal form or factor in PCOS (19,30).

Another possibility for adrenal androgenic hyperfunction in many hirsute women including those with PCOS may be one wherein adrenal P-450cl7α and/or 17-lyase activity may be abnormally up-regulated, similar to a dysregulation of ovarian P-450c17α (14). An increase in adrenal 17-lyase activity occurs during adrenarche with both in vivo and in vitro studies characterized mainly by a rise in adrenal DHEA (232,275). Adrenarche requires a selective activation in the expression of both the 17-lyase and 17α-hydroxylase activity of the cytochrome P-450c17α enzyme. Furthermore, the efficiency of 17α-hydroxylase and 11β-hydroxylase rises while that of 3β-HSD falls during adrenarche (232,275,276) with an associated rise in sulfokinase activity (277). The coexistent ovarian and adrenal hyperresponsiveness to their respective tropic hormones (e.g., nafarelin or ACTH) may be due to a similar type of hyperactive dysregulation of P-450c17α in both glands leading to increased secretion of 17-ketosteroids (14,232,265,270). There may be a regulatory defect resulting in overactivity of 17-lyase in both the delta-5 and delta-4 pathways and 17α-hydroxylase in the delta-5 pathway, without having to invoke an enzymatic defect in steroidogenesis (265).

Model as Applied to LH Activity

Although the P-450c17α activity is increased in PCOS, it is somewhat inefficient compared to that of normal women. Although both 17-OHP and A are increased after nafarelin, the 17-OHP response in PCOS is greater resulting in an elevated 17-OHP/A ratio compared to normal ovulatory women (265). This is secondary to increased efficiency of the 17α-hydroxylase enzyme. Where the levels of LH are elevated, there is inhibition of P-450cl7α starting with a relative decrease (down-regulation) of 17, 20-lyase compared to 17α-hydroxylase activity (14).

Abnormal regulation of intraovarian androgen can be a manifestation of increased LH secretion. If the primary defect in a major group of women with PCOS is a hypothalamic–pituitary disorder resulting in LH hypersecretion, one may expect evidence of P-450c17α dysregulation. In vitro experiments indicate that small doses of LH increase the activity of P-450c17α in thecal cells while higher levels of LH inhibit P-450c17α. Inhibition begins with a relative decrease in 17,20-lyase activity compared to 17-hydroxylase activity (14). The investigators postulate that in the subset of PCOS patients where LH abnormalities are not overtly present, there is dysregulation of androgen secretion with increased activity of ovarian P-450c17α (14,265,270). This can occur secondary to intrinsic enzymatic defects or as a result of endocrine, paracrine, or autocrine factors which modulate the ovarian androgen response to LH.

The results of the nafarelin and DXM suppression tests correlate strongly. The data of Rosenfield and co-workers (265) suggest an ovarian cause of hyperandrogenism in two-thirds of cases of PCOS, an adrenal cause in two-thirds, with a mixed ovarian–adrenal origin in one-third.

Associated Factors in the Proposed Model Requiring Further Corroboration

The above model by Rosenfield and co-workers is appealing, but as the authors state, there are variables which as yet have to be defined more fully and which probably have to be incorporated into their model:

1. The role of FSH in stimulating steroidogenesis in granulosa cells.
2. The role of long-loop negative feedback of estradiol on release of FSH.
3. A putative short-loop (paracrine) negative-feedback effect of estrogen on the 17, 20-lyase activity of theca-interstitial cells (TIC) (278). Is there a role for T in the regulation of P-450c17α?
4. The synergism of hyperinsulinemia and LH in stimulating androgen secretion by theca cells. Does insulin prevent down-regulation of LH receptors by LH (14)?
5. The specific roles of the paracrine regulatory effects of insulin, IGF-I, and testosterone.
6. The role of the intraovarian androgenic environment on enzymatic activities and formation of estrogens.
7. The roles of inhibin and activin in affecting LH-stimulated or IGF-I–stimulated androgen production (279).

The hypothesis of dysregulation of P-450c17α not only provides the link between ovarian and adrenal hyperandrogenism in PCOS, but possibly also between hyperinsulinemia and ovarian hyperandrogenism. It is evident that insulin is involved in regulation of steroidogenesis. The effect of growth factors as well as insulin may be involved in the dysregulation of P-450c17α in PCOS. Insulin receptors are present in human granulosa as well as thecal cells (280). The insulin concentrations found in hyperandrogenic women are synergistic with LH in stimulation of androgen secretion by theca from both hyperandrogenic and normal women (12,278,281). The mechanism of this synergism may perhaps be secondary to a possible effect of insulin preventing down-regulation of LH receptors by LH (14). Thus in hyperinsulinemic women, insulin may potentiate the effect of LH on P-450cl7α and cause ovarian hyperandrogenism even in PCOS subsets where LH levels are not elevated.

The role of IGF-I appears important in that in vitro studies have demonstrated that it stimulates androgen secretion by human and rat thecal cell cultures by acting synergistically with LH (281). This augmentation is associated with induction of receptors for LH and prevention of the reduction in the number of LH receptors by LH (282). IGF-I levels are elevated in the follicular fluid of PCOS ovaries compared to levels in similar-sized follicles in normal women (283). Thus one can hypothesize that abnormal production of IGF-I by granulosa cells may result in increased sensitivity of P-450c17α to LH and be a major pathogenetic factor leading to ovarian hyperandrogenism (14,19). New data relating that the prevalence and gene expression of IGF-II in human ovaries is greater than that of IGF-I (33) have to be taken into account, and reassessment of the role of autocrine/paracrine factors in the ovaries remains to be delineated.

There are data demonstrating that IGF-I (and probably IGF-II) serves as a potent up-regulator of P-450 aromatase gene expression and synthesis in human granulosa cells and luteinized granulosa cells, and that this is enhanced in the presence of FSH and hCG (284,285). A paracrine role for IGF-I in the small antral follicle is suggested by the finding of IGF-I receptors in human granulosa cells as well as in thecal cells (33).

The dysregulation of P-4S0c17α in PCOS may also be secondary to other factors in the regulation of ovarian steroidogenesis such as the inhibin–activin family of proteins. In human thecal cells, inhibin further stimulates LH-induced and IGF-I–induced thecal androgen production (286). Activin, on the other hand, inhibits LH-stimulated or IGF-I–stimulated androgen production (279). According to the proposed model, the dysregulation of P-450cl7α in PCOS may occur due to an overproduction of inhibin relative to activin by the granulosa cells.

In summary, this model proposes that PCOS is a functional state of ovarian hyperandrogenism characterized by thecal cell hyperresponsiveness of 17-OHP and A. This does not result from an inherent enzymatic deficiency but from enhanced 17α-hydroxylase activity, with a stimulated but relatively inefficient 17-lyase activity resulting from dysregulation of the androgen-forming enzyme cytochrome P-450c17α. The abnormal regulation (dysregulation) of P-450c17α activities is probably the pathogenetic factor in most PCOS patients and may arise from either excessive LH stimulation or increased bioactive LH, or via escape from desensitization to LH. The latter may result from an inherent ovarian defect in the paracrine feedback mechanisms by which ovarian androgen and estrogen synthesis are regulated. Modulation of intraovarian androgen formation is accomplished by intrinsic intraovarian feedback at the levels of 17α-hydroxylase and 17,20-lyase activity, both of which are activities of cytochrome P-450c17α (272). Testosterone and estradiol appear to inhibit the activities of cytochrome P-450c17α, while IGF-I, inhibin, and insulin stimulate its activity (Fig. 8) (272).

Aberrant Folliculogenesis in PCOS

Overview

Folliculogenesis is clearly dependent on a number of interdependent processes including gonadotropins, adequacy of steroidogenesis, the factors regulating cytochrome P-450 aromatase, and the role of the intraovarian microenvironment (34). In this section, a review of the present state of knowledge of folliculogenesis and the complex interplay of gonadotropins, steroids, and IGFs and their binding proteins will be presented. (The role of insulin will be detailed in a later section). Central again is the question of whether the proposed intraovarian pathogenetic mechanisms in PCOS suggest inherent defects or whether they are secondary to perturbations of the hypothalamic–pituitary unit.

Under normal circumstances, one cohort follicle in the ovary acquires the unique capacity to synthesize large quantities of E_2. This process occurs according to the

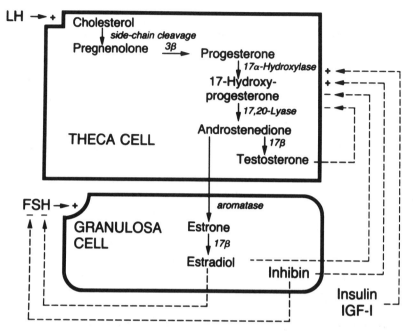

FIG. 8. Schematic representation of major factors regulating ovarian and estrogen biosynthesis. LH-induced androgen biosynthesis by theca–interstitial cells is normally coordinated with FSH-stimulated estrogen synthesis by granulosa cells to modify any hypersecretion of either, according to the two-gonadotropin, two-cell model of ovarian steroidogenesis. There is intraovarian feedback modulation at the levels of 17α-hydroxylase and 17,20-lyase, both of which are activities of cytochrome P-450c17α. Estradiol and inhibin are examples of FSH-stimulated hormones that may exert counterregulatory paracrine effects on the cytochrome P-450c17α enzymes, while also exerting long-loop negative feedback inhibition of FSH secretion. Inhibitory factors (*minus signs*) as well as stimulatory effects (*plus signs*) are noted. Inhibin, insulin, and IGF-I stimulate cytochrome P-450c17α activities. 3β-3β-hydroxy-delta5-steroid dehydrogenase; 17β, 17β reductase. (From ref. 272, with permission.)

"Two-cell Two-Gonadotropin Principle" (34) (Fig. 8). In response to LH, the TIC synthesize and secrete A which diffuses across the basal lamina into the granulosa cells where it is aromatized to E_2 in response to FSH stimulation. The newly synthesized E_2 is released both into the follicular fluid and into the circulation where it creates a permissive estrogenic microenvironment. As E_2 levels rise in the blood circulation, the predictable activities of FSH and LH follow, which ultimately results in ovulation (34).

In PCOS, the recruitment and growth to the small antral stages proceed normally with a normal number of primary follicles present (44,76,287), but the selection of dominant preovulatory follicles is lacking (288). Hughesdon (1) found that although the number of primordial follicles in polycystic ovaries was within normal range, the number of growing follicles at each stage of development (primary, secondary, tertiary, and early Graafian) was double that of normal ovaries. This suggests that the process of folliculogenesis is aberrant in PCOS, leading to the existence of large numbers of small, developing 4 to 7 mm Graafian follicles (cysts) (34). Some of the proposed mechanisms for the arrested follicular development are discussed below.

There are three major theories, among many, that attempt to explain the pathogenesis of PCOS (34): (a) the pathophysiologic mechanisms leading to inappropriately high LH levels result in aberrant folliculogenesis, whereby TIC become hyperactive and all cohort follicles die by atresia; (b) inappropriately reduced FSH activity in the follicular microenvironment leading to lack of expression of P-450 aromatase activity on the granulosa cells and aberrant folliculogenesis; and (c) IGF/insulin alterations in the follicular autocrine/paracrine system as well as the endocrine local effects of insulin and IGFs (34,289).

Gonadotropins and Steroidogenic Dysfunction

Unlike the normal ovary, there is a reduced capacity of the granulosa cells to proliferate in PCOS, resulting in impaired induction of P-450 aromatase. The decreased number of granulosa cells suggests that they lack adequate FSH stimulation to support their proliferation (34). The administration of FSH, however, to women with PCOS corrects the abnormality by stimulating mitosis in granulosa cells. Thus one can conclude that there is no difference in aromatase activity of granulosa cells from similar-size follicles of PCOS and normal ovaries. In addition to gonadotropins, growth factors modulate aromatase activity. Both insulin and IGF-I are mitogenic for granulosa cells and synergize with FSH to stimulate E_2 production (18).

Alterations in FSH receptor desensitization/down-regulation mechanisms may, however, be operable. These conclusions follow from in vitro data (290) which suggest that PCOS granulosa cells demonstrate (a) supersensitivity to FSH, (b) an inability to maintain a high rate of E_2 production when stimulated continuously with FSH, and (c) inability to produce large quantities of P-450 aromatase. Whether this is a direct effect of FSH or one controlled indirectly by production of regulatory molecules, such as growth factors, is unknown. For example, two mitogens, fibroblast growth factor (FGF) and epidermal growth factor (EGF), can stimulate mitosis in human granulosa cells in vitro (291). Also, premature entry of LH into the follicular fluid perturbs the selection process. Normally, when a dominant follicle is growing, LH is excluded from entry into the antral fluid until late in the follicular phase. Premature elevation of circulating LH/hCG in the the mid-follicular phase arrests the development of the dominant follicle by suppressing mitosis of granulosa cells (292,293).

Data relating to the levels of gonadotropins, E_2, A, IGF-I, and DHT in the small human Graafian follicles (34) are presented in Table 5.

To what extent are the TIC responsible for the absence of E_2 production by the PCOS follicle? Studies of the microenvironment of PCOS follicles reveal that the levels of A are in the normal range (Table 5) (34,294–296). There is no defect in the ability of LH to stimulate the synthesis of A by PCOS thecal cells. One is therefore

TABLE 5. *Endocrine microenvironment of small human graafian follicles*

4–7 mm Follicle	Hormone concentration					
	FSH (mIU/mL)	LH (mIU/mL)	IGF-I (ng/mL)	A (ng/mL)	E_2 (ng/mL)	DHT (ng/mL)
Normal dominant	2.5	ND	100	800	100–500	2
Normal atretic	ND	ND	100	800	10–50	2
PCOS	3.5	?	100	800	10–50	ND

Modified from ref. 34.
ND, not determined.

led to conclude that the P-450 aromatase is dysfunctional in the PCOS follicle. There are several theories which may account for the limited ability of the PCOS granulosa cells to aromatize A from the TIC to E_2 (17,34): (a) a reduced level of bioactive FSH in the microenvironment to induce P-450 aromatase gene expression, (b) absence of an active signal transduction system for FSH receptors in the granulosa cells, (c) the presence of an FSH inhibitor, and (d) the presence of P-450 aromatase inhibitor(s) that prevents the normal expression of P-450 aromatase activity.

Theory a. A reduction of FSH in the follicular fluid of PCOS ovaries is unlikely in view of bioassay measurements of FSH that indicate that they contain as much FSH as that found in the normal dominant follicle (Table 5) (290,294–296). In contrast to the finding that immunoreactive FSH rises within the microenvironment of the dominant follicle (297), the level of immunoreactive FSH was undetectable in atretic follicles.

Theory b. An absence of an active signaling system for FSH receptors in PCOS follicles is also unlikely (17). In vitro experiments have demonstrated that FSH produces marked increases in P-450 aromatase activity in PCOS granulosa cells, similar to or greater than size-matched dominant follicles of normal women (294). Furthermore, there is marked five-fold sensitivity of the PCOS granulosa cells to FSH compared to that of normal cells (284,294).

Theories c and d. There is a possible inhibitor of FSH in follicular fluid produced by granulosa cells which may block FSH signal transmission or block the activity of the P-450 aromatase enzyme itself. This could explain how the differentiation of granulosa cells in PCOS is blocked in the presence of normal levels of FSH activity in the follicular fluid and in the presence of a highly active FSH receptor and signal transmission system. The concept of FSH inhibitors in follicular fluid (298) has received new support from in vitro studies of rat granulosa cells indicating that FSH induction of P-450 aromatase in rat granulosa cells can be blocked by a polypeptide present in porcine follicular fluid (299). The FSH inhibitor appears to be a locally produced human growth hormone–dependent IGF binding protein (IGFBP), IGFBP-3 (300).

The granulosa cells of the ovarian follicle secrete several proteins into the follicular fluid which modify FSH secretion. Although related in structure, the activins and inhibins have opposite effects on pituitary FSH secretion (301,302), as well as on gonadal steroid synthesis (303). These are but several of many putative mechanisms regulating ovarian tissue by autocrine/paracrine mechanisms.

Thickening or fibrosis of the tunica albuginea is unlikely to be a factor in the pathogenesis of PCOS since follicle selection and ovulation can occur despite its presence (34). A possible factor may be hyperactivity of the fibroblasts in the theca interna (288) in that an increased thickness of the basal lamina may be present in PCOS. This can occur secondary to chronic hyperandrogenemia. This has been reported to occur in clinical studies of long-term treatment with testosterone, which also thickens the tunica albuginea (267,268).

In summary, an inhibitor, possibly an aberrant growth factor response in the PCOS microenvironment, may prevent the selection and development of a dominant follicle by blocking the physiologic responses of expressing P-450 aromatase enzyme activity of PCOS granulosa cells to FSH. This inhibitor may be an IGFBP, FSH agonist, FSH antagonist, growth factor, EGF (286), or other molecules. Although there is no evidence for a lack of FSH bioactivity in the PCOS antral follicle, there appears to be an alteration of the biologic action of FSH on granulosa cell differentiation (i.e., a disorder in folliculogenesis).

Growth Factors and Ovarian Steroidogenesis

Physiology and Effects of IGFs and IGFBPs

IGFs are pleotropic polypeptide modulators of many effects of cell physiology including proliferation, anabolic actions, and also the induction and maintenance of differentiation. The term insulin-like growth factors applies because they are characterized by a striking structural homology with proinsulin. The IGFs appear to be growth factors that have endocrine as well as autocrine/paracrine modes of action, and they are produced primarily by the liver. Locally produced IGFs, however, are considered to be important in the regulation of growth and differentiation of ovarian follicles (304).

Experimental studies of the rat follicle demonstrate that all five families of growth factors are expressed in the ovary: (a)IGF-insulin (305), (b) transforming growth factor-b (TGF-b) (306), (c) TGF-a EGF (307), (d) FGF (308), and (e) the cytokine systems (286).

The IGFs are circulating proteins bound to their receptors on the cell membrane and are almost entirely bound to high-affinity, soluble, IGFBPs in the circulation (309). The latter serve as a storage and delivery system to specific target sites for these peptides and preclude their interaction with their receptors, thereby modulating the IGF bioactivity. IGFBP-1 and IGFBP-3 have been isolated and characterized from humans. The liver is probably the main site for the production of IGFBPs, which are produced also by decidualized endometrium and granulosa cells (310). IGFBP-1 is the major binding protein in human amniotic fluid; IGFBP-2 is the major fetal/neonatal IGFBP and is found in the CNS; and IGFBP-3 is the major binding protein of adult serum (311). Both IGF-I and IGF-II have growth-promoting and insulin-like effects. The total level of IGF-I and IGF-II in human plasma is about 800 ng/mL, about 1,000 times that of insulin. Since recombinant human IGF-I is 6% as potent as insulin in producing hypoglycemia in healthy adults, circulating IGFs have the potential to contribute more than 50 times the activity of insulin. An important role of the IGF-IGFBP system in the counter-regulatory mechanisms of glucose appears appealing.

A major review of the IGFs has been published by Clemmons et al. (312). The following paragraphs summarize the major characteristics of IGF-I, IGF-II, IGFBP-1, and IGFBP-3.

IGF-I

Levels are growth hormone–dependent
Liver is the principal producer and is growth hormone–mediated, while in other tissues it is not entirely growth hormone–mediated
Pubertal rise noted, with a gradual decrease with aging
Increases in acromegaly
Decreased levels in fasting (via decreased binding of growth hormone to its hepatic receptor)
In vitro growth promotes insulin-like effects
Insulin enhances the growth hormone release of IGF-I
Influences proliferation and differentiation of granulosa cells in vitro (305) and in vivo (313)
Enhanced biologic activity in suppressed IGFBP-1 production state (e.g., insulin)
Follicular fluid concentrations similar to those in peripheral venous blood (33,314)
Suppressed with combination estrogen–progestin therapy in PCOS, unlike in normal women (49)

IGF-II

Levels are not growth hormone–dependent
Serum concentration is much greater than that of IGF-I
No pubertal rise demonstrated
No rise in acromegaly
Important in fetal growth and development
Greater intraovarian gene expression and concentration than IGF-I (33)
Higher follicular fluid concentrations than in peripheral venous blood (33,314)

IGFBP-1

Levels are independent of growth hormone secretion
Secretion is suppressed by insulin and probably glucose (in vitro)
Produced mainly by liver, and also in human granulosa cells

Insulin is a major regulator of its hepatic production

Increased by fasting, or low insulin production

Inversely related to insulin levels (315,316); insulinoma patients have very low levels that return to normal after removal of the tumor (311)

Secretion may be suppressed by IGF-I

Inhibits IGF-I in vitro

Acute modulator of IGF level (39)

Diurnal variation (increased at night, decreased during day) (317)

Increased levels with age, as IGF-I levels decrease with age

May sequester most of free IGF in the circulation, inhibiting its action

Increased with combination estrogen–progestin therapy in PCOS, unlike in normal women (49)

IGFBP-3

Growth hormone–dependent, and increased in acromegaly

Regulated by IGF-I

Likely to exert growth hormone–mediating effects via IGF-I

In normal adults has a $40 \times$ increased level over that of IGFBP-1

Has the highest affinity for IGF-I and IGF-II (not insulin)

Binds more than 95% of circulating IGF-I and IGF-II

Functions as a reservoir for long-term effects of IGF (39)

No relation to insulin or glucose effects

Liver and many other tissues produce it

Peak levels at puberty, then levels decrease with age

No diurnal variation

IGF-I and IGF-II have their own high-affinity receptors and bind very weakly to insulin receptors. There are two types of receptors for IGFs. Type I receptors are structurally similar to insulin receptors and mediate most of the known effects of IGF-I and IGF-II. Type II receptors are unrelated to the insulin receptor and have the highest affinity for IGF-I and IGF-II. Most of the effects of IGF-II including granulosa cell growth and differentiation are mediated by binding to the IGF-I receptor or insulin receptor, not the type II receptor (33,318).

Growth Factors (GFs) in Normal and PCOS Ovaries

Recent in vitro evidence supports the concept that growth factors IGF-I and IGF-II modulate to amplify or attenuate the biologic responses of the endocrine system, and is likely of importance in determining folliculogenesis including the P-450 aromatase activity of human granulosa cells (34,284). The extent of P-450 aromatase stimulation by IGFs appears equal to or greater than that of FSH, and both act synergistically to control the level of P-450 aromatase in granulosa cells (284). In normal follicles, IGFs play a role in the selection of the dominant follicle by enhancing the ability of FSH to induce granulosa cell differentiation (24,284,305).

Effects on Granulosa Cells

There is evidence indicating that gonadotropins may stimulate IGF-I production by granulosa cells (24,319). The latter, particularly those in small antral follicles (33), are also capable of producing IGF-I and contain receptors for IGF-I, suggesting that IGF-I may act on granulosa cells in an autocrine fashion. IGF-I has also been noted to enhance the induction of LH receptors by FSH in granulosa cells (320–322). An IGF-I effect in augmenting FSH-promoted biosynthesis of estrogen (322) and progesterone (323) has also been reported. The concentration of IGFBP in media is reduced after administration of FSH, suggesting an interplay of IGF and FSH at the local level (324). Reduction of the local levels of IGFBPs may increase the availability to free IGF to cell surface receptors. It is apparent from experimental studies that FSH hormonal action may be dependent in part on the bioavailability of granulosa cell–derived IGFs and their receptors with amplification of the gonadotropic signal (24).

Experimentally, the ovary displays the third highest level of IGF-I expression, with the liver and uterus being the most active (39). IGF-I is found in normal quantities in PCOS follicles, and at a concentration similar to that found in serum (283). PCOS follicles demonstrate a normal granulosa cell response of P-450 aromatase activity to IGF-I (284,294), indicating a fully functional IGF-I signal-transduction system associated with the IGF-I receptor. In normal human follicles, virtually all the IGF-I in the microenvironment is bound to the IGFBPs, most notably the small 34-kDa (34K) IGFBP (IGFBP-l) (325). IGF-I activity is modulated by low molecular weight binding proteins, that prevent IGF-I from binding to its receptor (326), thereby increasing the local concentration of free IGF-I. The production of this small IGFBP by human granulosa cells suggests a role of the granulosa cells in determining the amount of biologically active free IGF in the microenvironment (310,316,327). PCOS patients have been found to have an 80% decrease in the circulating level of this protein (328,329), as well as a reduced level of this IGFBP in their follicular fluid (FF) (330). Insulin is also able to stimulate target cells by binding to both insulin and IGF-I receptors (331). The data of Rutanen and associates (326) suggest that hyperinsulinemia in PCOS patients may be associated with decreased levels of the 34K IGFBP resulting in increased IGF-I receptor binding in the ovary, which may play an important pathogenetic role in the granulosa cell as well as enhancing androgen production by the thecal-interstitial and stromal cells in PCOS (12,281). The role of insulin in decreasing hepatic IGFBP-1 production may be of relevance in the pathogenesis of PCOS. The increased insulin/IGFBP-1 ratio is unassociated with changes in growth hormone (GH), IGF-I, IGF-II, or IGFBP-3 (17).

In vitro studies by Erickson and investigators (284) indicate that PCOS granulosa cells have enhanced sensitivity to FSH, a response that is dependent on the possible high level of IGF-I stimulation in the PCOS microenvironment. The finding of increased free IGF-I in PCOS follicles strengthens the view that this may be an important contributory factor in the development of hyperandrogenism in PCOS.

In a study comparing IGFBP profiles of the FF of atretic follicles in patients with PCOS to those of normal cycling women, there was no significant difference (332). Although IGFBP-1 was not detected in PCOS follicles, the amounts of IGFBP-2 and -4 in FF were greater in PCOS women (333), and this may act to sequester IGFs and block the IGF action on the granulosa cell folliculogenesis. In support of this hypothesis are in vitro studies indicating that IGFBPs may inhibit gonadotropin-stimulated rat granulosa cell steroidogenesis (299,334).

Effects on Theca–Interstitial Cells (TIC)

How can small Graafian follicles in PCOS produce such high levels of A? One possibility is that the 4 to 7-mm diameter PCOS follicles contain abnormally large numbers of TIC relative to normal follicles, and that this hyperplasia may be responsible for the hyperandrogenism (17). Morphometric studies of numbers of TIC or their mitotic rates in PCOS, however, are not abnormal. There is apparent hyperplasia of the TIC, and the thecal cells hyperrespond in PCOS as compared to normal (318). There may also be TIC resistance to LH-induced desensitization and down-regulation of receptors for LH. Both insulin and IGF-I may be important factors in the hyperactivity of TIC in PCOS. An important advance in this field occurred when it was discovered that the action of LH in humans can be amplified by insulin and IGF-I (12,32,235,311). Although excellent proof exists in animals there is no decisive proof that IGF-I promotes increased androgen production by human TIC. Clearly, the role of IGF-I and IGF-II and the binding proteins in normal and PCOS TIC must be further established by both in vitro and in vivo studies.

Selection process of the dominant follicle in the PCOS ovary may be inhibited by the hyperandrogenemia of the hyperactive TIC. Experimentally, T and DHT are atretagenic in rodents and their formation by high LH levels may form the basis for the persistent pattern of atresia in PCOS. There is no direct evidence, however, for this conclusion. A more likely hypothesis is that increased LH activity in PCOS may lead to the formation of other types of regulatory molecules, such as TIF growth factor, that disrupt selection (17).

Autocrine–Paracrine Role of GFs in Folliculogenesis of Normal and PCOS Ovaries

IGF-I and IGF-II are synthesized by the TIC and granulosa cells (335) with both present in FF of developing follicles (283). Recent data demonstrate that it is likely that intrafollicular IGF-I may be circulatory in origin (33). Receptors for IGF-I and IGF-II, as well as insulin, are expressed in human granulosa cells and TIC follicle cells (280,335–337). Receptors for IGF-I in human granulosa cells may serve an important function in the activity of both IGF-I and IGF-II (33). IGF-1 and insulin are capable of stimulating biologic responses in human TIC and granulosa cells (mitosis and E_2 production in granulosa cells) (284,294). Furthermore, FSH acts in synergy with IGF-I to control the level of biologic responses (284,294), and these mechanisms result in increased FSH sensitivity (284). IGF-I also acts in synergy with LH to further increase androgen production (27,211,281).

In humans, the IGF/insulin system is one of the best studied examples of a follicular growth factor system (27,32,39,210). In PCOS, emerging evidence supports the existence of an altered system that may impinge on ovarian function. What is known of the follicular IGF/insulin system in PCOS? (a) FF of PCOS follicles contains levels of IGF-I similar to those found in normal women (283), arguing against the cause of PCOS being a reduction of IGF-I in the microenvironment. There are no data regarding IGF-II and insulin in PCOS follicles. (b) IGF-I alone and in combination with normal bioactive concentrations of FSH is highly effective in stimulating E_2 synthesis in PCOS granulosa cells, and the responses are equivalent to those of normal women (289). The IGF-I receptor–signaling pathway in the granulosa cells therefore does not appear to be a pathogenetic cause of PCOS. (c) In vitro experiments suggest that the ability of the insulin receptor to function physiologically may be altered. Unlike in the normal human granulosa cells (338), insulin is incapable of stimulating E_2 synthesis in PCOS granulosa cells in vitro (294), possibly related to insulin resistance (IR). If one postulates a physiologic role of insulin in normal folliculogenesis, a defect in the insulin receptor–signaling pathway in the granulosa cell may be an important pathogenetic mechanism in PCOS (17).

One of the effects of high circulating insulin in women is a selective decrease in IGFBP-1 (339,340), and as mentioned previously in this section this binding protein is thought to be involved in determining the amount of free (biologically active) IGF-1 in body fluids. It follows that women with PCOS who are hyperinsulinemic have subnormal levels of IGFBP-1 in plasma (39,328,329,341) and in the FF (330, 333). The low FF concentration of IGFBP-1 may result in a higher concentration of free IGF-1, which may lead to abnormal granulosa cell differentiation in PCOS.

PCOS women demonstrate daytime (feeding) and night (fasting) hyperinsulinism in association with euglycemia, while an attenuation of IGFBP-1 and its circadian variation is present (39). The increased IGF-I/IGFBP-1 ratio in women with PCOS results in increased bioavailable IGFs which exert an endocrine mode of action on target cells (39). The latter include effects on ovarian theca-stromal granulosa cells as well as pituitary cells, augmenting GnRH-induced LH release in vitro (39,342).

One of the main lines of evidence that supports the role of growth factors in PCOS is the strong correlation between hyperinsulinemia and hyperandrogenism in women with this disease (17). According to the Barbieri et al. model (27), hyperandrogenism results from a direct hyperinsulinemic action on the ovarian interstitial tissue, TIC as well as hilar cells. In vitro experiments indicate that both insulin and IGF-I interact with receptors on these cell types to stimulate A and T production (27,32).

The peripubertal onset of PCOS is a well-known clinical finding in PCOS

(199,274). Transient IR develops during puberty in association with a rise in the secretion of insulin, IGF-I, and GH, and with reduced levels of SHBG and IGFBP (343). It has been speculated that increased pubertal adrenal androgen and extra-glandular conversion to estrogens leads to pituitary sensitivity to GnRH which may enhance gonadotropin action on ovary (exaggerated adrenarche hypothesis). Thus pubertal IR may serve as the link between the transition of hyperandrogenism from the adrenals to the ovaries (17). IR appears to extend beyond puberty in women susceptible to the development of PCOS. The ensuing compensatory hyperinsulin-ism inhibits IGFBP-1 and SHBG production by the liver (278), an effect which increases the bioavailability of IGF-I and sex steroids to target tissues (274). Ampli-fication of gonadotropin action in this model of pathogenesis of PCOS occurs be-cause circulating insulin and IGF-I can be delivered to the ovary, and IGF-I, and particularly IGF-II (33) and its IGFBP-1, are produced by the granulosa cells. The paracrine action of IGFs between granulosa cells and thecal cells prevails because IGFBPs may function as inhibitors of FSH action on the granulosa cells.

Summary of Role of GFs in Folliculogenesis

The interplay of insulin and IGFs also are appealing in perhaps clarifying some of the effects of hyperinsulinism in PCOS. Despite the ample data presented in this section, there are conflicting data which must be resolved (344). There is no con-crete evidence in human granulosa cells for major IGF-I gene expression. A recent study revealed a greater IGF-II gene expression than IGF-I in the human ovary (33). The source of IGF-I in human FF remains to be defined, but it may be derived from circulating IGF-I, although the ovarian interstitial cells may contribute to the intra-follicular pool (344). The presence of mRNA for IGF-II has been demonstrated in human granulosa cells that were obtained after superovulation therapy (33,345) as well as by other means (33). There are ample data indicating an endocrine as well as a paracrine/autocrine role of the GFs in folliculogenesis.

Growth Hormone

The clinical finding that GH facilitates ovulation induction in GH-deficient pa-tients as well as in patients receiving gonadotropins because of unresponsiveness to clomiphene citrate or gonadotropin therapy alone (321) has focused interest on pos-sible effects of GH on the ovarian IGF-IGFBP system. From the limited human experimental data available (346), there is no evidence of a change in the ovarian IGF-IGFBP system after the administration of GH (347). Serum IGF-I concentra-tions are often normal in women with PCOS while the serum GH level is usually reduced (39,348), although varying levels have been described (349,350). Low mean levels of GH have also been noted in lean women with PCOS (348). The mechanism of this is not clear. GH secretion may be reduced due to associated hyperinsulinism (351) or enhanced feedback at the pituitary level (341). The role of

GH in PCOS is not clear and further investigation of GH, IGFs, and somatostatin as pathogenetic factors in PCOS appear indicated.

PATHOPHYSIOLOGY OF OBESITY: A MAJOR PRIMARY OR SYNERGISTIC FACTOR IN PCOS?

Overview

Obesity is often associated with hyperandrogenism of various etiologies and is an aggravating factor in PCOS. Hyperinsulinemia and IR are frequently associated with hyperandrogenism in PCOS women, and insulin appears to be an important regulator of ovarian steroidogenesis both in vitro and in vivo. These findings have established the basis on which new hypotheses on the pathogenesis of PCOS have been developed (28). These mechanisms may explain (a) the frequent association between obesity and PCOS, and (b) the mechanisms by which obesity may cause or perpetuate the development of hyperandrogenism in PCOS. The hypothesis of a pathogenetic role of obesity in PCOS has been supported by clinical observations that weight loss can significantly improve both hyperandrogenism and hyperinsulinism and restore fertility in such women. It is difficult to refute the fact that initial treatment of the obese PCOS patient with stringent weight reduction effects improvement of many of the clinical and biochemical parameters of the disease. Caloric restriction in obese healthy women results in a fall in serum insulin concentration and possibly also a fall in IGF-I (352). Insulin receptors in obesity impact on the effectiveness of weight loss regimens (353). It has been demonstrated that a very low calorie diet (330 kcal/day) results in a highly significant increase in IGFBP-1 and SHBG concentrations in obese women with PCOS (354).

Physiological Role of Estrogens in Obesity

Obesity is often associated with increased estrogen production. The magnitude of A production and the extraglandular conversion of A to E_1 is related to excess body fat (188,355,356). Due to lowered SHBG levels, the concentration of free E_2 is increased at target tissues (357,358). In obese pre- and postmenopausal women, increased levels of estrone sulfate are found due to concurrent reduction of its metabolic clearance rate (MCR) and an increase in its production rate (PR) (359). This estrogen is an important reservoir of active hormones as it may be converted to $E_1 > E_2$ in several tissues, such as the hypothalamus, cerebral cortex, and endometrium (360,361). The influence of the circulating estrogens may be via peripheral and central mechanisms. E_2-mediated gonadotropin release is another mechanism (199) wherein high estrogen levels may generate inappropriate feedback signals at the hypothalamic–pituitary level modifying the dynamics of pulsatile LH release and circulating LH concentrations.

The albumin-bound fraction of E_2 is physiologically important in that it alters the MCR (137). Increased E_1 and other estrogens may be a factor in the inappropriate gonadotropin secretion seen in PCOS women by increasing GnRH sensitivity (133). In a study of 23 women with PCOS by Lobo and co-workers (137), the unbound physiologically active (nonSHBG-bound) E_2 levels were elevated, possibly due to the reduced SHBG secondary to obesity, hyperinsulinemia, or increased androgens. The increase in free E_2 (nonSHBG-bound) occurred in the presence of normal or low total serum E_2 levels and correlated with the high LH/FSH ratio of women with PCOS (137). Thus biologically active unbound free E_2 appears to have a positive feedback influence on LH.

Adipose Tissue as Source and Reservoir of Sex Steroids

Adipose tissue is an important site of active steroid production and metabolism. It possesses the aromatase enzyme system which allows circulating androgens to be converted to estrogens (362,363). The main androgen precursor of E_1 in adipose tissue is A (188). In vitro and in vivo studies have demonstrated a significant correlation between the rate of conversion of A to E_1 and the overall quantity of adipose tissue itself (364).

Adipose tissue also contains the enzyme 17β-hydroxysteroid dehydrogenase, which converts E_2 to E_1, A to T, and DHEA to A (356,364). There is ample proof that adipose tissue is an important tissue where androgens undergo active metabolic clearance and as a site of estrogen formation due to the presence of these enzymes. The androgens T and A show an active uptake by fat tissue, where concentrations are reached that are much higher than in any other tissues (363).

Endorphins and Obesity

Mechanisms for the increased opioid activity in obesity are still unknown. Unlike cortisol and β-lipotropin, elevated β-endorphin levels cannot be suppressed in obese subjects, unlike normal weight controls. The increased opioid activity appears to be neuroendocrine and partly independent of the hypothalamus (365).

Obesity, SHBG, Body Fat Distribution, and Androgen Metabolism

Simple obesity, not associated with obvious endocrine abnormalities, is associated with abnormalities in androgen metabolism. One of the major findings in obesity is that the concentrations of SHBG are usually lower than those found in normal weight women (366–368). SHBG levels are inversely correlated with body weight in both premenopausal and postmenopausal women (366,369). Since not all obese women have reduced levels of SHBG in spite of similar circulating androgen levels and similar degrees of excess body weight, it has been suggested that factors other than excess body weight may be involved in the regulation of SHBG synthesis and metabolism. There is firm evidence that in obesity, the decrease of SHBG may result as a direct effect of insulin on its hepatic production (370,371). The consequences of reduced SHBG are those of elevated levels of free estrogens (372) as well as nonSHBG-bound T (presumably free and biologically active). Decreased SHBG also results in increased MCRs of T and other androgens for which there is high binding affinity. Thus despite normal androgen plasma levels in some women with obesity, the enhanced turnover of androgens leads to increased tissue exposure (373).

Another factor in assessing the role of obesity and its metabolic consequences is the body fat distribution, which can be divided into the abdominal (android) and the peripheral (gynoid) types. The most widely used anthropometric method to define the two types of body fat distribution is the ratio between the waist (W) and hip (H) circumferences (WHR) (374). Women with PCOS frequently have an android distribution of fat (375). Several investigators have noted that that an increased WHR is associated with a progressive increase in glucose and insulin levels, and by higher insulin and glucose responses to an oral glucose challenge (376–379). Evans and coworkers (373) were the first to find an independent, inverse relationship between the WHR, SHBG values, and the percentage of free T levels in premenopausal women with wide ranges of body weight. This has subsequently been confirmed by other studies (369,378).

The maintenance of normal circulating levels of androgens in obesity suggests the presence of a regulatory feed-back mechanism which adjusts both the PR and MCR of these hormones to body size. Women with simple obesity have an increased androgen production but, because of the increased adipose tissue, androgens are not only cleared by the liver (380) but in adipose tissue as well, thereby reducing uptake by target androgen-sensitive tissues. This may offer an explanation as to why obese women may be protected to some extent against the biologic effects of hyperandrogenemia (28).

Obesity and PCOS

In Stein and Leventhal's original description, obesity, together with hirsutism and infertility, represented one of the characteristic signs of the eponymous syndrome (381). The correlation between obesity and infertility has been confirmed by well-documented studies (382,383). A significant correlation between the age of onset of obesity and the age of onset of oligomenorrhea or amenorrhea was found in obese women with PCOS (384). This confirmed the clinical impression of Yen (199) that one of the most characteristic features of women with PCOS was the premenarcheal onset of obesity.

Undoubtedly obesity is the most common cause of IR, independent of androgens. The incidence of obesity in PCOS is very common (2,13,51,199) and approximates 50% of PCOS women (44). Many women with PCOS are overweight before or during the time of menarche, leading to a reduction of SHBG (372). Since SHBG is the principal protein that binds DHT, T, and E_2, the resulting increased free T may lead to inhibition of follicular maturation which may induce anovulation and altered ovarian morphology (267–269). Obese adolescents with irregular cycles tend to demonstrate morphologic ovarian multifollicularity, anovulation, and high plasma LH and androgen levels (385,386). Compared to normal weight women with PCOS, obese women with PCOS demonstrate lower SHBG concentrations (13,20,367,387–389). Obesity has also been well characterized as a common feature in ovarian stromal hyperthecosis, which is a distinct and more severely virilized subset of PCOS (47).

The presence of obesity as one of several contributory factors in PCOS raises a number of interesting questions (28): (a) Do obese women with PCOS have different clinical and hormonal patterns compared to non-obese PCOS women, and do they represent a distinct subset with different pathophysiology? (b) Since LH hypersecretion represents one of the most important pathogenetic mechanisms of the syndrome (199,76), does obesity affect LH secretion or its peripheral effects, or is it associated with other factors capable of altering ovarian steroidogenesis by mechanisms which are independent of gonadotropin regulation? (c) Since obesity alters extraglandular androgen metabolism and may be regulated by many factors including hormones and nutrients, what are these factors and what is their role in determining obesity-related hyperandrogenism? (28)

It is now well documented that both obese and non-obese women with PCOS have contradictory data relating to hormonal differences (13,20,39,367,387,388, 390). No difference in the plasma LH and FSH levels, pulse amplitude and frequency, or response to GnRH was noted in the two groups (390). A more significant SHBG reduction, however, is present in obese PCOS women (20,367,387,388) as well as a lower A/E_1 ratio, than in the non-obese group (387). In an earlier study by Laatikainen and co-workers (391), obese women with PCOS were found to have decreased LH amplitude in comparison to lean women with PCOS. Additional data by Yen and associates (39) indicate that obesity may attenuate LH hypersecretion in PCOS and also augment a further reduction of IGFBP-1 in view of its hyperinsulinemic effect. There is a report indicating a slightly higher serum T concentration in obese women with PCOS (13), which may confirm the clinical observation that obese PCOS women are more likely to have menstrual dysfunction (392) and hirsutism than lean women with PCOS (31,389).

A significant reduction in serum GH in PCOS (39) in the presence of normal IGF-I levels suggests an alteration of the GH–IGF-I feedback axis in PCOS (39). In contrast, the reduction of LH hypersecretion in the presence of obesity, which was shown to be positively correlated to GH secretion, suggests neuroendocrine–metabolic aberrations distinct from as well as in common with lean PCOS subjects. It is the author's impression that obesity adds a significant synergistic factor in the genesis of PCOS, mostly via inherent abnormalities in obesity itself (Table 6).

TABLE 6. *Additive effects of obesity to the pathophysiology of PCOS*

Increased insulin resistance
Elevated basal levels of insulin
Reduction of hepatic synthesis of SHBG
Increased levels of free testosterone
Metabolic effects of the increased WHR
Reduction of IGFBP-1

HYPERINSULINEMIA, INSULIN RESISTANCE, AND HYPERANDROGENISM IN PCOS: EVIDENCE FOR A MAJOR ROLE IN PATHOGENESIS OF PCOS

Overview

The presence of hyperinsulinemia in PCOS not only provides insight into an important possible pathogenetic mechanism but has led to the observation that the metabolic long-term complications of PCOS may be substantial. Much of what has been written about this syndrome has stressed the reproductive dysfunction and complications, but realistically, the metabolic complications of hyperinsulinism are of greater magnitude (354,393,394). Data substantiate the hazard of obesity in PCOS in that 20% of obese PCOS women have impaired glucose tolerance or non–insulin-dependent diabetes mellitus (NIDDM) in their 20s and 30s (387). Basal increases in the hepatic glucose production and reduced suppression of hepatic glucose output by insulin appear to be seen only in obese PCOS women (20,387,395, 396). The negative impact of obesity on PCOS is of major epidemiologic importance, since impaired glucose tolerance is uncommon in non-obese women with PCOS (387,354).

Attempts to demonstrate the presence of defective degradation of insulin, insulin antibodies, or insulin receptor antibodies in PCOS have been unsuccessful (397). In the classic study by Burghen and co-workers (397) they first described the presence of hyperinsulinemia in PCOS, and they found that the degree of hyperandrogenism (serum T and A) and hyperinsulinemia were correlated.

Definition and Causes of Insulin Resistance

Hyperinsulinemia in PCOS appears to result from IR. The definition of IR is a state in which a normal insulin level results in a subnormal activity in glucose clearance. This results in hyperinsulinemia in patients with intact pancreatic function. Hyperinsulinemia itself down-regulates insulin receptors (353), resulting in postreceptor cellular desensitization (398). IR has a key role in the manifestation and pathogenesis of many disorders including hyperandrogenism, obesity, diabetes mellitus, and possible hypertension (399,400). There are a number of causes of IR and these have been summarized in a review article by Moller and Flier (399).

Effects and Mediation of Hyperinsulinism in PCOS

Intact insulin, rather than proinsulin or split proinsulin, is the dominant component of immunoreactive insulin in PCOS patients (401). Women with PCOS appear to have profound IR similar to or greater than that seen in patients with NIDDM

(20,402). It is speculated that the insulin levels in NIDDM are insufficiently elevated to produce ovarian hyperandrogenism (22).

Acanthosis nigricans (AN) in women with PCOS is an epiphenomenon that usually signifies the presence of associated hyperinsulinemia and IR (403,404). This may result from the action of insulin on IGF receptors in the skin. It is frequently seen with skin tags in the nape of the neck (*personal observation*). Some reports claim that the severity of AN and of hyperinsulinism appear to be correlated (405), but in view of the different clinical frequencies of AN in different ethnic groups, this is difficult to prove. Its incidence may vary considerably and most of the women are obese (387,403–408). The pathogenetic mechanism of hyperinsulinism in PCOS may involve both a decreased receptor number and postreceptor defects (405, 409,410). Controversy exists as to whether hyperinsulinemia and IR are in some way related to the presence of obesity or to other factors such as PCOS itself. Flier and co-investigators (407) found that obese PCOS women with AN had more hyperinsulinemia and IR than a weight-matched group of hyperandrogenized women without AN. These data were confirmed by Dunaif and co-workers (20, 387,390,408) who also observed that only obese women with PCOS were at risk for impaired glucose tolerance. However, Stuart et al. (406) observed that the degree of AN and hyperandrogenism were more closely correlated with insulin levels than with the degree of obesity, which suggests that IR in obese hyperandrogenized women with AN may not be due to the obesity alone. Thus, although women with PCOS and AN are usually obese, the precise nature of this association and the possible additive or causal role of obesity in hyperandrogenic states are still largely unknown (28). It is clear, however, that the association between IR and ovarian hyperandrogenism is not limited only to PCOS, but exists in other entities as well.

After the study of Burghen and co-workers (397), other investigators made similar findings documenting IR and hyperinsulinism in PCOS, (12,200,204,387,390, 403,411–417), in both obese and lean women with PCOS (20,367,411,418–420). The role of obesity in both hyperinsulinemia and hyperandrogenism in obese women with PCOS has been intensively investigated by comparing the fasting and glucose-stimulated insulin concentrations in obese and non-obese patients with PCOS. Most studies indicate that the fasting and postglucose insulin levels are significantly higher in the obese than in the non-obese group (20,387,388,390,413, 414,421). Refinements of studies of insulin sensitivity with the euglycemic hyperinsulinemic clamp technique (20) or the combined infusion of glucose, insulin, and somatostatin (414) demonstrate that obese women with PCOS have significantly higher insulin insensitivity (i.e., reduced insulin sensitivity) than their non-obese counterparts and thus a more severe insulin resistant state. Thus it is likely that the hyperinsulinemia and IR in PCOS are more common in the obese than in the non-obese group (422) and those with an increased WHR (390). Some of the above data confirm the aggravating synergistic effect of obesity in the expression of PCOS (423).

Serum insulin levels also have been reported to be normal in hyperandrogenic women with PCOS with normal menstrual cycles, suggesting that insulin insensitivity is a feature mainly of oligomenorrheic patients (422,424). Serum T and SHBG levels were similar in PCOS women with oligomenorrhea and in those with regular menses (424). Fasting and stimulated insulin levels as well as the WHR showed a negative correlation with insulin sensitivity. Testosterone did not correlate significantly with any variable, although a number of other groups of investigators have demonstrated a correlation between T and insulin levels (12,397,406,411–413) as well as free T (340,387,422). Is the observed hyperinsulinemia in most women with PCOS secondary to enhanced pancreatic insulin secretion, reduced catabolism, defective target-cell action, or a combination of these and other factors? It has been noted that IR in non-obese hyperandrogenic women is due to peripheral rather than hepatic resistance to insulin action (425). This was in accord with studies indicating a negative relationship between SHBG and serum insulin levels, but not insulin sensitivity (424), suggesting a direct inhibitory effect of insulin on SHBG production by the liver (370,371). Both insulin and IGF-I receptors have been identified in human ovarian stroma (280,426) and in animal granulosa cells (427). Insulin may stimulate ovarian androgen biosynthesis through binding to the IGF-I receptor (33,237,282).

IR in obese women usually is reversible and oligomenorrhea in PCOS often reverts to regular cycles with hypocaloric diets (367,406,411–413). Peripheral T, A, and DHEAS levels have been reported to be significantly decreased in obese PCOS women with caloric restriction (423,429–431). The reduction of androgens following weight loss in hyperandrogenic women is consistent, in part, with the hypothesis that weight loss causes a reduction of the hyperinsulinemia, which in turn reduces androgen concentrations (209). This is not the case in obese women with normal menses, where no changes in T or DHEAS were found (432). The reduction in SHBG may also be a factor in reducing hyperandrogenism in that it decreases the MCR of T and reduces free T (423). Clinically, some of the hirsutism may diminish and AN when present may gradually disappear (407,423, 430). It appears that the PCOS phenotype combined with insulin insensitivity predisposes a woman to oligomenorrhea and anovulation.

It has been stated previously that SHBG and IGFBP-1 are both synthesized by the liver. The insulin-dependent small molecular weight IGFBP-1 binds mainly to IGF-I, although its precise role in delivering IGF-I to peripheral tissues is poorly understood. Although sex steroids (T and E_2) modulate SHBG production, there is growing evidence that insulin plays a role in the regulation of SHBG and IGFBP-1 secretion (433). In vitro evidence for the regulation of SHBG and IGFBP-1 by insulin has been reported in human hepatocarcinoma G2 (Hep G2) cells (370,371). An oral glucose load induces a rapid increase in serum insulin levels resulting in a marked reduction in IGFBP-1 concentrations (329). There is a significant negative correlation of insulin with both binding proteins, SHBG and IGFBP-1 (311,434), that modulate the bioavailability of IGFs at their receptor sites (39). Increased SHBG and IGFBP-1 levels have been associated with decreased insulin concentrations (349). Further evidence supporting the role of insulin in the regulation of these two binding proteins comes from studies in pubertal children showing a decline in serum SHBG and IGFBP-1 associated with an increase in insulin concentrations (435). In boys the decline in SHBG may be explained by a rise in T, but in girls the decrease in SHBG, albeit smaller, suggests that insulin is responsible (343,372).

Most patients with PCOS do demonstrate inappropriate LH secretion (22,76, 199). Normal LH levels are found, however, in 20% to 40% of PCOS patients (31,76). Data of Grulet and associates (367) are similar to those of Dunaif and associates (20), demonstrating a decrease in insulin sensitivity of 25% to 37% in lean PCOS and 20% to 30% in obese PCOS when measured by the hyperinsulinemic euglycemic clamp technique. These have been confirmed by other groups (411,418). These results indicate that in PCOS, IR is frequently found independent of obesity (365). In evaluating the respective roles of LH and IR, Grulet and associates (367) noted an interesting correlation between insulin sensitivity and the LH level in both lean and obese women with PCOS. A clear reduction in insulin sensitivity occurred in the group of 23 women with PCOS who had low LH levels and demonstrated no differences in body mass index (BMI) and androgen or SHBG levels when compared to the 38 women in the high-LH group. It is possible that the IR of the low-LH group of PCOS women may have a different origin as reported by Peiris and associates (425). These results favor a complementary action of LH and insulin in the pathogenesis of PCOS.

Hyperinsulinemia before and after an oral glucose tolerance test (OGGT) may also occur in patients with PCOS in the absence of obesity, AN (204,411), and type of body fat distribution (436, 437). The use of the insulin-glucose clamp technique has demonstrated IR in PCOS to be independent of obesity or the fat-free mass (20). Hyperinsulinemia and IR persist despite long-term interruption of ovarian androgen secretion with a long-acting GnRH agonist (203). The persistence of hyperinsulinism and IR in patients whose ovaries were suppressed by GnRH-a treatment suggests that disordered insulin action is a possible intrinsic defect in PCOS which perhaps may be a factor leading to, rather than resulting from, ovarian hyperandrogenism.

Despite impairments in target tissue insulin sensitivity, most PCOS women present with a normal GTT (12,20,418,438). Ciaraldi et al. (439) demonstrated that the IR in PCOS may involve a novel mechanism of marked defects in glucose transport sensitivity without significant changes in receptor dynamics. Adipocytes obtained by biopsies of PCOS women demonstrated postbinding impairment of insulin receptor–mediated signal transduction, resulting in a marked decrease in insulin sensitivity, greater than that produced by obesity itself (395,439). This unique feature in PCOS is different from other IR states (399). The resulting hyperinsulinemia, probably arising at the time of puberty, may impinge on the ovarian IGF system (39). The pubertal hyperinsulinemia may also impact on hepatic IGFBP-1 production (339,340) and represent a pathogenetic factor in its genesis. The important question as to whether these mechanisms of IR also exists in ovarian cells of PCOS patients has not yet been resolved.

Hyperinsulinism and Hyperandrogenism: Which Causes Which?

Insulin resistance and hyperinsulinemia have been well documented in women with PCOS (204,397,411,413). Many investigators have demonstrated that insulin is an important factor in the regulation of ovarian steroidogenesis (338,440) and that hyperinsulinemia and hyperandrogenemia appear to be interrelated in women with PCOS (32,200,210,278,387). Two distinct points of view concerning the association between insulin resistance and hyperandrogenism have evolved: (a) Does hyperandrogenism have an impact on the hyperinsulinism of PCOS? and (b) Does the hyperinsulinemia cause or aggravate the hyperandrogenism in PCOS women?

Hyperandrogenism as a factor in the production of IR has been hypothesized since it was shown that administration of estrogens and progesterone caused remission of IR (441) and that IR was induced by administration of androgens (442,443). A number of other observations are of interest in that they support the hypothesis that hyperandrogenism perhaps is a factor in the pathogenesis of IR. A positive linear correlation between insulin and androgen levels has been demonstrated (373, 397,411,444). (This may also suggest that hyperinsulinemia is a causative factor in the production of ovarian hyperinsulinism.) Several investigators have demonstrated that women with central (android) obesity who have higher free androgen levels demonstrate a significantly higher degree of IR than weight-matched controls (373,377). Treatment with the antiandrogen spironolactone has been reported to reduce insulin and T concentrations in women with PCOS (444), suggesting that reduction of T improved insulin sensitivity. A recent study by Elkind-Hirsch and co-workers (445) noted that treatment of 12 hyperandrogenic patients with PCOS with a long-acting GnRH agonist for 6 weeks improved insulin sensitivity in mildly IR women while not having any effect on those with severe IR.

The observation that a transient IR is frequently noted at puberty also suggests a role of sex steroids in its genesis (446,447). Subtle IR may also be noted in some women with nonclassical 21-hydroxylase deficiency adrenocortical hyperandrogenism (446,447). The trigger mechanism of the hyperandrogenism and insulin insensitivity in these women is not clear.

A unique "experiment of nature" is the syndrome of hyperandrogenism, IR, and AN, which has been termed the HAIR-AN syndrome (209,403). Barbieri suggests that 5% of hyperandrogenic women have the HAIR-IN syndrome, particularly patients with hyperthecosis and those with serum total T levels greater than 100 ng/dL (209). The fact that two genetically different causes of IR (Kahn type A and type B IR) as well as other diverse sources of compensatory hyperinsulinemia secondary to IR result in hyperandrogenism is strong evidence that hyperinsulinemia causes hyperandrogenism (209,448,449). In most instances the source of the hyperandrogenism is ovarian in origin. Point mutations in the insulin receptor gene may result in the HAIR-AN syndrome and is the first example of a specific genetic analysis of ovarian hyperandrogenism (209,450). Studies have revealed DNA changes in the insulin receptor gene associated with the HAIR-AN phenotype (451,452). This leads one to suspect that it is possible for any acquired cause of insulin-receptor dysfunction to be associated with ovarian hyperandrogenism (209), often hyperthecosis (12,453,454). The presence of both insulin and IGF-I receptors in the human ovary allows IR to result in an increased interaction of insulin with IGF-I receptors leading to ovarian hyperandrogenism (209). This may allow the IR state to demonstrate its effect on carbohydrate metabolism while the ovaries may remain sensitive to the effects of insulin.

A number of additional studies have revealed contradictory results regarding the hypothesis that hyperandrogenemia may result in hyperinsulinemia (32). Chronic administration of androgens to female rhesus monkeys does not alter insulin sensitivity (455). The administration of synthetic androgens to men may not necessarily be extrapolated to results with endogenous androgens. It is currently believed that although some degree of IR may be secondary to androgens in some women, hyperinsulinemia and IR cannot be explained simply by elevated androgen levels. The genetic types of IR with insulin-receptor abnormalities, some of which include various mutations of the insulin receptor gene, are associated with marked hyperandrogenism (448,455). Suppression of hyperandrogenism via GnRH analogues (204,205,221,411) or antiandrogens such as cyproterone has failed to reduce the degree of hyperinsulinemia and IR in obese and non-obese women with PCOS (205,384,414,415). Reversal of hyperandrogenism in the HAIR-AN syndrome does not improve the IR (12). The normalization of hyperandrogenism due to congenital adrenocortical hyperplasia does not alter IR when present (456). Furthermore, the large concentration of T in men is not associated with significant or frequent hyperinsulinemia, and the incidence of IR in men and women appears to be the same. Administration of pharmacological doses of androgens to normal men has been shown not alter insulin sensitivity (457). In a study of women with ovarian hyperandrogenism, bilateral oophorectomy eliminated the hyperandrogenism but was not associated with a reduction of the hyperinsulinemia (454). This was also confirmed in reports by Annos and Taymor (453) and others (204,205).

Hyperandrogenism has been associated with numerous insulin resistant states (35). These include PCOS (397,411,413), Kahn type A and type B IR (extreme IR, AN and hyperandrogenism with the presence of an autoimmune disorders in Type B) (448,449), leprechaunism (458), lipoatrophic diabetes, and the HAIR-AN syndrome (403). It has been postulated that insulin may mediate the ovarian hyperandrogenism accompanying these IR states (27,32,403,459).

Although the existence of a relationship between IR and hyperandrogenism is well established (12,27,210,387,460), studies of the effect of experimentally induced increased circulating insulin levels on androgen concentrations in hyperandrogenic women have been conflicting. Using the euglycemic-hyperinsulinemic clamp technique (418,438,459,461–463), the OGTT (397,412,420,464), and the insulin tolerance test (465), conflicting data have been reported. A variable increase or unchanged A level (438,461,464), increased T (412,461,462), decreased androgen levels (459,466), and unchanged levels of androgens have been described (390,420,459,463,467).

A study of Nestler and co-workers (35) suggested a primary role for insulin in the causation of hyperandrogenism by administering diazoxide (inhibitor of insulin release in pancreatic β-cells) for 10 days to five obese IR PCOS women. A mean decrease of fasting serum insulin was noted after diazoxide administration with a marked reduction of serum insulin in response to an oral glucose load (Fig. 9) when

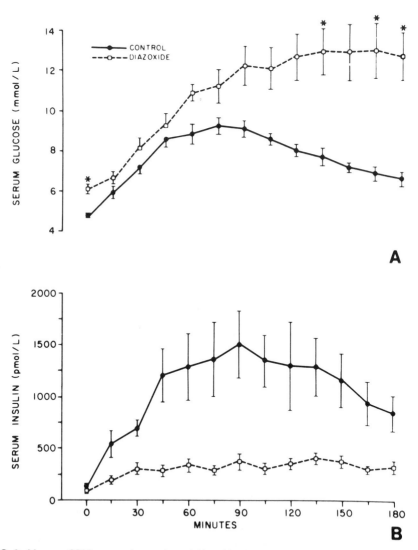

FIG. 9. Mean ± SEM serum glucose (panel A) and insulin (panel B) responses after 100 g oral glucose in five obese women with PCOS during the control study (*closed circles*) and after 10 days of oral diazoxide administration (300 mg/day) (*open circles*). * = $p < 0.003$ compared to control value at the same time point. (From ref. 35, with permission.)

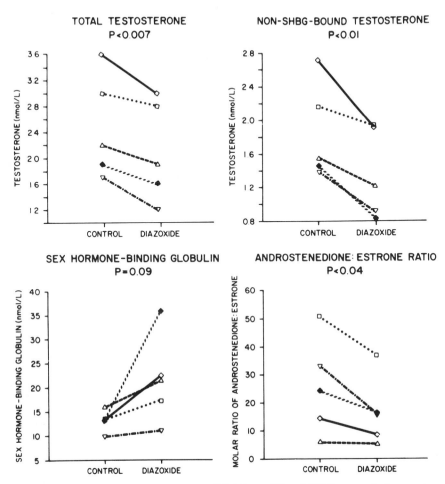

FIG. 10. The serum total testosterone, non-SHBG-bound T, and SHBG concentrations and molar ratio of serum androstenedione to estrone ratio in five obese women with PCOS during a control study and after 10 days of oral diazoxide administration. (From ref. 35, with permission.)

compared to the control study (35). It was also demonstrated that parallel to the reduction of insulin levels, there was a significant decrease in plasma T (total and nonSHBG-bound T) concentrations (Fig. 10), without any effect on the pulsatile secretion of LH and FSH or their response to GnRH injection (35). These effects were not noted in non-obese normal women, thus suggesting the importance of obesity as a predisposing factor. This also suggested that in normal women there may be a different sensitivity of steroidogenesis to the effects of insulin or that perhaps normal insulin concentrations do not play an important role in the regulation of androgen levels (468). The report of Nestler and co-workers (35) appears to be major evidence for a physiologic role for insulin in regulating steroidogenesis whereby a reduction of insulin levels in PCOS is associated with a reduction of androgen levels.

Clinical findings indicate that many obese normal women are hyperinsulinemic and yet not hyperandrogenic. This is an important observation that requires explanation and is not entirely resolved. One explanation may be that women with PCOS are genetically predisposed to the insulin stimulation effect of ovarian androgens; that is, a PCOS gene needs to be present if hyperinsulinemia is to exert an effect (the "iceberg" hypothesis) (468). The often familial nature of PCOS (7) suggests that this hypothesis may be valid.

Hyperinsulinemia, the Ovaries, and Adrenals: Possible Opposing Effects of DHEA/DHEAS and Testosterone?

There may be an alternative explanation as to why experimentally induced hyperinsulinemia may result in a rise of A levels in PCOS but not in normal women. One could speculate opposing effects of hyperinsulinemia on ovarian as opposed to adrenal A production. This theory is supported by several observations. Administration of insulin to normal men (most of the A is adrenal in origin) causes a reduction of serum A levels (35), while serum A is either unchanged or increased in normal women (406,438,461). In vitro studies suggest that insulin may affect different human steroidogenic tissues in different ways (468). In a study of a group of women with elevated levels of DHEA and DHEAS, who demonstrated an adrenal source of androgens, no IR was noted despite their obesity and the elevation of serum T (469). The insulin levels were inversely correlated with DHEAS (469).

In an in vivo study, Farah and co-workers (470) noted a positive correlation between the DHEA production rate and fasting insulin levels up to 40 μU/mL. When fasting insulin levels exceeded that level in women with PCOS and AN, the DHEA production rate decreased as the fasting insulin increased. A hyperinsulinemic euglycemic clamp study demonstrated a progressive decline of DHEA and DHEAS with increasing hyperinsulinemia (459,471). It is speculated that there is a decreased adrenal androgen production with increasing hyperinsulinemia via increased metabolic clearance of these androgens including A (35,459,464,469,470).

Similarly, other investigators have noted a negative correlation between fasting insulin and DHEA levels in PCOS (12,435), suggesting a functional role of insulin on circulating levels of DHEA. These groups hypothesize that the severity of the IR state that is associated with hyperandrogenemia is dependent on the origin of androgen excess. If this is true, then the ratio of DHEA and T (DHEA/T) may be an important indicator of insulin sensitivity of women in general, and of patients with hyperandrogenism in particular. There may be an opposing effect of DHEA/DHEAS and T on the regulation of insulin secretion and action. It is interesting to speculate that the combined insulin effects on inhibition of adrenal production of androgens is compensated for by enhanced ovarian androgen production in women.

There may possibly be an insulin-mediated depression of DHEA and DHEAS (471). It is possible that in instances of IR in PCOS the adrenal androgen suppressive effect is attenuated, which may contribute to the hyperandrogenism of women with PCOS. The impaired adrenal effect of insulin appears to represent another peripheral manifestation of reduction in insulin action in some women with PCOS (466).

In Vitro Effects of Insulin on the Ovary

The known in vitro stimulatory effects of insulin on the ovary are varied. Contradictory studies have emerged on the role of insulin on the aromatase activity of granulosa cells of normal women and those with PCOS (294,338). Stimulation of ovarian aromatase activity (211,338) and the augmentation of 5α-reductase activity (389) have been reported. These effects may reflect a synergistic effect mediated by IGF-I, IGF-II, and the IGF-I receptor, and to a lesser extent the insulin receptor itself. The known in vitro stimulatory effects of insulin on the ovaries have been reviewed by Schwartz and Diamond (440).

Insulin Resistance, Obesity, and Effect of Weight Reduction in PCOS

The probable synergistic effect of obesity in the pathogenesis of PCOS indicates the important role of weight reduction in the obese subject with PCOS in reducing the IR of PCOS and its potential health sequelae (429). Weight reduction in the obese PCOS woman potentially reverses a number of pathophysiological abnormalities including SHBG, free T, and others (409,423,429,430). Although obesity is a synergistic pathogenetic factor in the IR of PCOS, it is not the major one. As previously noted, this is underscored by the fact that non-obese women with PCOS often have IR (20,367,390,411,418).

Proposed Mechanism(s) of Ovarian-Induced Hyperandrogenism by Hyperinsulinemia

There are many data confirming a major role of hyperinsulinemia, a universal feature of IR states, via a direct stimulatory effect on ovarian steroidogenesis (12,27,32,403,449). These stimulatory effects of hyperinsulinemia on the ovaries may involve (a) enhanced steroidogenesis of androgens by TIC, (b) synergism with LH on ovarian steroidogenesis, (c) an effect on SHBG production by liver, and (d) the effects of IGF-I and IGF-II which may amplify the LH effect on the ovaries.

A large body of experimental evidence yields insight into the mechanisms involved in the production of hyperandrogenism by hyperinsulinemia. High-affinity insulin receptors have been demonstrated in ovarian granulosa cells, TIC, and stroma (27,32,33,210,472,473) where they stimulate androgen synthesis directly òr indirectly (210,474). The known in vitro stimulatory effects of insulin on the ovaries have been reported, with increased sensitivity to the effects of insulin in PCOS (27,278,440).

Insulin, SHBG, and IGF/IGFBP Modulation of Ovarian Androgen Production

The importance of insulin in the modulation of hepatic production of SHBG and thereby in the regulation of sex steroids has been noted previously. In vitro studies have demonstrated that insulin is capable of inhibiting the production of SHBG in human hepatoma (Hep G2) cell line culture (370). SHBG is reduced in hyperandrogenemia, in obesity (367,475), and in hyperprolactinemic states (476). The frequently reduced SHBG concentration in PCOS women results in an increased fraction of free T and E_2 (477). It appears, however, that the modest elevations of androgens in PCOS have relatively minor effects on the SHBG. Raising plasma T levels of hypogonadal women to levels of 126 mg/dL causes SHBG concentrations to fall by only 8.5% (478). In contrast, PCOS patients with similar T levels and much higher E_2 levels have SHBG levels that are 42% lower than those of normal women (477). These observations were confirmed by Nestler (468) who found that administration of a GnRH agonist did not significantly change SHBG concentrations in obese women with PCOS in spite of a marked reduction of T and free T. A significant rise in SHBG was observed, however, when diazoxide was administered for 10 days to six obese women with PCOS who were pretreated with a long-acting GnRH agonist for 2 months to suppress ovarian androgen steroid production (475). While the depot GnRH-a treatment did not alter SHBG levels, the mean SHBG levels rose 32% following diazoxide inhibition of insulin release. These data confirm the role of hyperinsulinemia in reducing serum SHBG concentrations in obese women with PCOS independently of any effect on serum sex steroids. The specific role of hyperinsulinemia in obese PCOS women is strengthened by the fact that serum SHBG levels are lower than those found in normal men, despite the lower androgens and higher estrogen levels in PCOS (370). It is clear that hyperinsulinemia exerts an effect on SHBG production independent of any possible sex steroid effect, and this is an important factor in the pathogenesis and perpetuation of the PCOS.

An additional effect by which insulin may influence androgens is by an effect on the low molecular weight IGFBP which may be synthesized in the ovarian cells (310) and is regulated by insulin itself. The IGFBP can be inhibited by insulin administration (479) and has been noted to be inversely correlated with insulin levels in women with PCOS (480). Since IGFBP acts as an inhibitor of IGF-1 production (481), its decrease in hyperinsulinemic states favors an increase in androgen production by increasing the intraovarian concentrations of IGF-1, which in turn, with its IGF-I receptor, represents a significant amplifier of LH-induced androgen synthesis (278).

Paradox of Insulin Action on Ovary in Insulin Resistance

The obvious question which is puzzling to investigators studying the effects of insulin on the PCOS ovary is the paradox of how can the ovary remain sensitive to insulin, when classical target organs for insulin such as liver, fat, or muscle are insulin resistant and do not respond in a normal fashion to insulin (210)?

The cellular mechanisms by which insulin might express its effect on androgen homeostasis in obese women with PCOS are not fully known (32). It is likely that different mechanisms exist wherein the classic insulin receptor could mediate its effects on hyperandrogenism other than those responsible for glucose transport (210). This may explain how an individual may have IR in terms of glucose transport and still be sensitive to the actions of insulin on sex steroids and SHBG (35).

One of the major reasons for the insulin-induced ovarian hyperandrogenism is the synergistic effect of insulin with LH (210), possibly via an up-regulation of LH receptors (27,338,367). Several important in vitro studies address the possible effects of insulin being mediated by IGF-I receptors (281,337).

Insulin-->Decreases synthesis of SHBG--->Increased Free T
LH and Insulin = = = = = = = = =>Hyperandrogenism
LH------------>(stromal and thecal luteinization)
= = = = = =>follicular atresia

The intrafollicular androgenic environment leading to follicular atresia (278) reduces granulosa cell estrogen production. A schematic outline of hypothetical mechanisms of hyperandrogenism in insulin resistant states is depicted (Fig. 11) (36,210). The role of insulin on the ovary is significant in that it affects a number of processes including stimulation of steroidogenesis in TIC and stroma, the up-regulation of gonadotropin receptors and possibly such key steroidogenic enzymes as aromatase (32,211,338).

What is the receptor mechanism responsible for the mediation of insulin effects in the ovaries of IR women? Characterization of insulin receptors in the human ovary has found them to exhibit most of the classical features of insulin receptors found in other tissues (280,426). One of the first groups of investigators to propose the hypothesis that insulin may not act through its own receptor but through that of others in its ovarian hyperstimulation effect in instances of extreme IR was that of Taylor and associates (449). Some of the proposed receptors mediating the effect of insulin in ovaries of IR women are IGF-I receptors (33,280,304,426). These receptors have been demonstrated in human granulosa and stromal cells (210,280). IGF-I is produced in the ovary and may serve as an important factor in granulosa cell differentiation and in follicular development (305,482). IGF-I is a potent stimulator of steroidogenesis, perhaps more so than insulin (305,318,483,484). IGF-I (as well as IGF-II) functions by binding to a specific receptor for IGF-I that is similar to the insulin receptor and also possesses tyrosine kinase activity.

The concept of the effects of insulin and binding to IGF-I receptors is summarized in several studies (32,211,305,485). The mediation of IGFs, as well as the

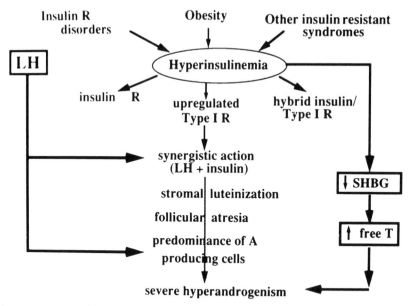

FIG. 11. Hypothetical mechanisms of hyperandrogenism in insulin-resistant states. (From refs. 36 and 210, with permission.)

presence of hybrid insulin/IGF-I receptors, in the production of ovarian hyperinsulinism may be an important pathogenetic factor in women with PCOS (486,487).

Thus it appears that insulin may act on the ovary to induce hyperandrogenism via a number of mechanisms including the insulin receptor, the type I IGF receptor, or a hybrid insulin type I receptor in ovarian stroma (Fig. 11) (36,210) which may be differentially up-regulated. Hyperinsulinemia synergizes with LH, promoting stromal luteinization and follicular atresia, resulting in ovarian hyperandrogenism (36).

It has been suggested that factors other than insulin, for example, gonadotropins or sex steroids, may protect ovarian insulin receptors from down-regulation by insulin in premenopausal women (488). If this mechanism does indeed exist, insulin receptors could be down-regulated by hyperinsulinemia in some tissues (e.g., liver, fat, muscle) rendering them IR, while at the same time insulin receptors could be preserved in other tissues such as the ovary, allowing these tissues to remain sensitive to insulin (210).

Summation

IR is often associated with hyperandrogenism and is frequently found in obese and non-obese women with PCOS. There are several mechanisms which may implicate the role of IR in the pathogenesis of PCOS:

1. The increased LH secretion and/or activity may possibly be related to some extent to the hyperinsulinemia in that in vitro data indicate that insulin, in vitro,

can enhance GnRH-induced LH secretion from cultured pituitary cells (39,342, 489). This has not been confirmed as yet in vivo.

2. LH and insulin can synergize resulting in ovarian hyperandrogenism in vitro (39,281), and there appears to be a greater synergism between LH and IGF-I than insulin (281,305,320,337).

3. There is in vivo evidence that hyperinsulinemia may up-regulate type I IGF receptor (211), further enhancing the effect of insulin and IGF-I on the ovary.

4. Hyperinsulinemia inhibits SHBG liver production in PCOS resulting in increased free T.

5. Hyperinsulinemia inhibits IGFBPs which allows for higher free levels of IGFs (36,39,311,328,329,427).

Interpretation of data relating the effects of reducing hyperandrogenemia and noting the presence or absence of correlation with insulin sensitivity is hampered by the heterogeneity of responses of the diverse patients with PCOS. It has been suggested by some investigators that hyperandrogenic women should be divided into subgroups (209,412,417,445). These may include (a) women with IR, very high levels of insulin, and minimally elevated LH and (b) those with no IR and normal insulin levels with elevated LH (417). Those hyperandrogenic women with IR may have minimal elevation of serum LH similar to the subgroup proposed by others relating to LH levels (79,85). Perhaps studies of the role of androgen suppression in hyperandrogenic women with PCOS (445) should be done after dividing patients into 3 subgroups: (a) those with significant IR, (b) those with established criteria defining mild IR, and (c) non-IR subjects. Basically, just as a baseline LH level may mirror the response to its tropic hormone GnRH, basal insulin level (and IR status) may be found to correlate with insulin sensitivity modulation studies in women with PCOS. Therefore, more exact definition of the type of hyperandrogenic patients studied would be invaluable in defining the interaction of insulin and androgens, as well as the roles of various modalities (caloric restriction, combination estrogen–progestin therapy, long-acting GnRH agonists, antiandrogens, and others) in possibly modifying the hyperinsulinism when present. This has, of course, important therapeutic and long-term health implications in the treatment of this disorder.

The fact that many studies in animal models have been performed and indicate an important role for IGF-I in the modulation of insulin action and in the pathogenesis of ovarian hyperandrogenism in IR states must be re-examined in the light of recent studies by El-Roeiy and associates (33). They clearly demonstrate that IGF-II is the major and most abundant growth factor with gene expression in the whole human ovary, with important function in the development of the dominant follicle. It appears to exert its effect via the IGF-I receptor, rather than its own receptor. There is now fairly strong evidence that there may well be an endocrine as well as an autocrine/paracrine role of the IGF system in follicular maturation (36,314,490). Since the control of biologic expression of IGFs is dependent on their regulatory effects by IGFBPs, further studies defining localization of the IGFBPs is necessary and should be forthcoming. Clearly, circulatory (extraovarian) IGF-I may impinge on the human follicular mechanism as well as local and extraovarian IGF-II, but much more data are needed to piece together the complex role of IGFs and their binding proteins in the pathogenesis of PCOS.

Genetics of PCOS

A genetic basis for PCOS may exist and its role in the pathogenesis of PCOS has to be fully defined. Clinical observations by a number of observers including Goldzieher (44) and Givens and associates (6) indicate that a family history is frequently present for hirsutism, menstrual dysfunction, or cystic ovaries. Since PCOS is heterogeneous, with many different diagnostic criteria, it is likely that there is genetic heterogeneity in some PCOS women as well (11), while others may have no genetic basis for their disease. Once appropriate diagnostic criteria are strictly applied, one may utilize classic segregation analysis and deduce the mode of inheritance, namely monogenic or polygenic (11). Clinical studies of PCOS have demonstrated that there is a varying incidence and phenotypic expression present in kindred of affected subjects with PCOS (6–10,491–498). Some studies strongly indicate familial aggregates of PCOS particularly in women with hyperthecosis (6,7,9,492,498). An autosomal dominant pattern has been suggested in some families (6,7,10,494, 498), by a specific morphologic definition of the disease (e.g., hyperthecosis) or what is considered a possible phenotype of male kindred obligate carriers of affected probands with PCOS (7,10,494,497).

Marked variability of phenotypic findings within and among families of women with PCOS was noted by Givens (7). He concluded that each family was unique but afforded a basis for forming the following conclusions:

1. There is dominant transmission in PCOS.
2. The type and degree of expression of the disorder are variable. Precocious adrenarche as well as a high incidence of spontaneous recurrent early miscarriages (499,500) have been reported.
3. There is abnormal gonadotropin secretion and testicular function in some male kin of women with PCOS.
4. Associated disorders, including diabetes mellitus, hyperinsulinemia, obesity, hypertension, and ischemic heart disease, are present with variable incidence.

Evaluation of pedigree data do not allow a clear genetic explanation for PCOS. Both autosomal and X-linked patterns have been invoked to explain the familial nature of this disorder. The available pedigree data do not distinguish between these modes of inheritance (8,491,492,494,496). In a literature review of chromosomal studies of 189 women with polycystic ovaries, 13 had a variety of sex chromosomal abnormalities, consisting of mosaics of the number of X chromosomes found (495).

The evaluation of genetic studies in PCOS is inherently difficult because few studies indicate ethnic background, attempts to exclude an adrenal etiology, or careful historical information on the male phenotype. There now have been three studies demonstrating an association between PCOS and premature male balding (10,494, 497). In the study by Carey and co-investigators of 10 families of women with PCOS (10), premature male pattern baldness (MPB) (age < 30 years) was assessed in male first-degree relatives. Eight of 18 males demonstrated this phenotypic sign, similar to the incidence found in previous studies describing this sign (494,497). The incidence of MPB in non–PCOS related families has been described as 7% (494,497). If MPB is taken as a male phenotype for obligate male carriers, then one may conclude that PCOS is consistent with autosomal dominant inheritance (10, 494), with almost full penetration (10).

There is disagreement as to what is considered the female and male phenotype in published genetic studies (11). Other genes may be involved, for example, those modifying the expression for obesity where a genetic tendency has been described (501). Many obese normal women are hyperinsulinemic and yet not hyperandrogenic. The reason for this has not as yet been explained. As previously mentioned, one explanation is that women with PCOS are genetically predisposed to insulin stimulation of ovarian androgens. This states that a PCOS gene needs to be present ("iceberg" hypothesis) if hyperinsulinemia is to exert an effect on ovarian hyperandrogenism (468).

It appears that new advances in the identification of the gene or genes responsible for some of the subsets of PCOS may yield much information about the genetics and pathophysiology of PCOS. It is likely that genetic heterogeneity exists in view of the existence of many entities which manifest the PCOS (11). The study of defined populations of PCOS, including ethnic background and the presence or absence of IR, may be informative as a basis for elucidating specific gene defects in this complex entity.

CONCLUSIONS

The pathogenesis of PCOS is inherently difficult to ascertain in view of the many subsets and different phenotypes that have been described. One may conclude, however, with a fair degree of certainty, that there are at least two major pathogenetic mechanisms involved. Each may be unique in establishing a cause of the syndrome or may be combined with the other. They are (a) an inherent defect in the regulation of gonadotropins with the formation of an altered LH/FSH ratio (IGS), and (b) an inherent defect in an altered regulation of folliculogenesis and/or ovarian steroidogenesis. The latter may be related to (a) hyperinsulinemia, or (b) autocrine/paracrine abnormalities of the ovaries which amplify the effect of LH in inducing ovarian hyperandrogenism.

The final common pathway unquestionably involves ovarian hyperandrogenism which in turn results in a cascade of events which further perpetuate the IGS, lead to formation of follicular atresia, amplify the effect of LH on ovarian hyperandrogenism via the insulin/IGF system, and promote a vicious cycle which reduces the effectiveness of FSH on granulosa cell function leading to an androgenic microenvironment.

The synergistic effect of obesity in further aggravating these mechanisms is important but not primary. Obesity does suppress SHBG and effectively reduces the peripheral aromatization of androgens to E_1, which perhaps may also have a role, albeit minor, in the pathogenesis of the IGS. There must be a major priority in the treatment of the obese woman with PCOS to encourage caloric restriction in that the hyperinsulinemia, SHBG, and some of the hyperandrogenemia is altered favorably.

The genetics of PCOS will be an important aspect of new advances in the pathogenesis of PCOS. Clinically there is a distinct familial incidence in many women with this syndrome. The question of a dominant mode of inheritance remains to be answered and further studies of specific female and male phenotypes are indicated. Studies under way may demonstrate a specific gene or several genes involved in the insulin resistance of PCOS and/or their susceptibility to hypothalamic or ovarian dysfunction.

In conclusion, the author views PCOS as one of two major subsets. The first involves a central nervous system–hypothalamic GnRH defect which may or may not be associated with a genetic factor. The second involves a host of ovarian and/or adrenal defects associated with hyperinsulinism and an altered autocrine/paracrine dysfunction which probably is associated with a higher incidence of obesity and genetic defects. Defects in the latter group are capable of amplifying the LH effects on the ovary even in the presence of normal LH levels, and are particularly important in their synergistic effect on the almost uniformly increased levels of bioavailable LH found in women with PCOS. Only by defining these heterogeneous patients with distinct criteria and phenotypes will important contributions in this area be forthcoming with a clearer explanation as to their pathophysiology.

ACKNOWLEDGMENT

I am grateful for the technical assistance rendered by Mr. Richard Weiss in the preparation of this manuscript.

REFERENCES

1. Hughesdon PE. Morphology and morphogenesis of the Stein-Leventhal ovary and of so-called "hyperthecosis." *Obstet Gynecol Surv* 1982;37:59–77.
2. Goldzieher JW, Green JA. The polycystic ovary. I. Clinical and histologic features. *J Clin Endocrinol Metab* 1962;22:325–338.
3. Givens JR. Polycystic ovaries—sign, not a diagnosis. *Semin Reprod Endocrinol* 1984;2:271–280.
4. Zawadski JK, Dunaif A. Diagnostic criteria for polycystic ovary syndrome: toward a rational approach. In: Dunaif A, Givens JR, Haseltine FP, Merriam GR, eds. *Polycystic ovary syndrome.* Cambridge, MA: Blackwell Scientific, 1992;377–384.

5. Bringer J, Lefebvre P, Boulet F, Grigorescu F, Renard E, Hedon B, Orsetti A, Jaffiol C. Body composition and regional fat distribution in polycystic ovarian syndrome. In: Tolis G, Bringer J, Chrousos GP, eds. *Intraovarian regulators and polycystic ovarian syndrome: recent progress on clinical and therapeutic aspects*. New York: Annals NY Academy of Sciences 1993;687:115–123.

6. Givens JR, Wiser WL, Coleman SA, Wilroy RS, Andersen RN, Fish SA. Familial ovarian hyperthecosis: a study of two families. *Am J Obstet Gynecol* 1971;110:959–972.

7. Givens JR. Familial polycystic ovarian disease. *Endocrinol Metab Clin North Am* 1988;17:771–783.

8. Cooper HE, Spellacy WN, Prem KA, Cohen WD. Hereditary factors in the Stein-Leventhal syndrome. *Am J Obstet Gynecol* 1968;100:371–387.

9. Judd HL, Scully RE, Herbst AL, Yen SSC, Ingersol FM , Kliman B. Familial hyperthecosis: comparison of endocrinologic and histologic findings with polycystic ovarian disease. *Am J Obstet Gynecol* 1973;117:976–982.

10. Carey AH, Chan KL, Short F, White D, Williamson R, Franks S. Evidence for a single gene effect causing polycystic ovaries and male pattern baldness. *Clin Endocrinol (Oxf)* 1993;38:653–658.

11. Simpson JL. Elucidating the genetics of polycystic ovary syndrome. In: Dunaif A, Givens JR, Haseltine FP, Merriam GR, eds. *Polycystic ovary syndrome*. Cambridge, MA: Blackwell Scientific; 1992;59–69.

12. Barbieri RL, Smith S, Ryan KJ. The role of hyperinsulinemia in the pathogenesis of ovarian hyperandrogenism. *Fertil Steril* 1988;50:197–212.

13. Conway GS, Honour JW, Jacobs HS. Heterogeneity of the polycystic ovary syndrome: clinical, endocrine, and ultrasound features in 556 patients. *Clin Endocrinol (Oxf)* 1989;30:459–470.

14. Rosenfield RL, Barnes RB, Cara JF, Lucky AW. Dysregulation of cytochrome P450c17α as the cause of polycystic ovary syndrome. *Fertil Steril* 1990;53:785–791.

15. Waldstreicher J, Santoro NF, Hall JE, Filicori M, Crowley WF Jr. Hyperfunction of the hypothalamic–pituitary axis in women with PCOD: indirect evidence for partial gonadotroph desensitization. *J Clin Endocrinol Metab* 1988;66:165–172.

16. Hall JE, Taylor AE, Martin KA, Crowley WF Jr. Neuroendocrine investigation of polycystic ovary syndrome: new approaches. In: Dunaif A, Givens JR, Haseltine FP, Merriam GR, eds. *Polycystic ovary syndrome*. Cambridge, MA: Blackwell Scientific; 1992;39–50.

17. Erickson GF, Yen SSC. The polycystic ovary syndrome. In: Adashi EY, Leung PCK, eds. *The ovary*. New York: Raven Press; 1993:561–579.

18. Barnes RB. Polycystic ovary syndrome and ovarian steroidogenesis. *Sem Reprod Endocrinol* 1991;9:360–366.

19. Barnes R, Rosenfield RL. The polycystic ovary syndrome: pathogenesis and treatment. *Ann Intern Med* 1989;110:386–399.

20. Dunaif A, Segal KR, Futterweit W, Dobrjansky A. Profound peripheral insulin resistance, independent of obesity, in polycystic ovary syndrome. *Diabetes* 1989;38:1165–1174.

21. Cara JF, Rosenfield RL. Androgens and the adolescent girl. In: Sanfilippo JS, ed. *Pediatric and Adolescent Gynecology*. Philadelphia: WB Saunders; 1994:250–277.

22. Goldzieher JW, Young RL. Selected aspects of polycystic ovarian disease. *Endocrinol Metab Clin North Am* 1992;21:141–171.

23. Polson DW, Adams J, Wadsworth J, Franks S. Polycystic ovaries: a common finding in normal women. *Lancet* 1988;1:870–872.

24. Adashi EY. The intraovarian insulin-like growth factor system. In: Adashi EY, Leung PCK, eds. *The ovary*. New York: Raven Press, 1993:319–335.

25. Adashi EY, Resnick CE, D'Ercole AJ, Svoboda ME, Van Wyk JJ. Insulin-like growth factors as intraovarian regulators of granulosa cell growth and function. *Endocr Rev* 1985;6:400–420.

26. Adashi EY. Hypothalamic–pituitary dysfunction in polycystic ovarian disease. *Endocrinol Metab Clinics North Am* 1988;17:649–666.

27. Barbieri RL, Makris A, Randall RW, Daniels G, Kistner RW, Ryan KJ. Insulin stimulates androgen accumulation in incubations of ovarian stroma obtained from women with hyperandrogenism. *J Clin Endocrinol Metab* 1986;62:904–910.

28. Pasquali R, Casimirri F. The impact of hyperandrogenism and polycystic ovary syndrome in premenopausal women. *Clin Endocrinol (Oxf)* 1993;39:1–16.

29. Mechanick JI, Dunaif A. Masculinization: a clinical approach to the diagnosis and treatment of hyperandrogenic women. In: Mazzaferri E, ed. *Advances in endocrinology and metabolism*. St. Louis: Mosby-Year Book, 1990;1:129–173.

30. McKenna TJ. Pathogenesis and treatment of polycystic ovary syndrome. *N Engl J Med* 1988;318: 558–562.
31. Franks S. Polycystic ovary syndrome: a changing perspective. *Clin Endocrinol (Oxf)* 1989;31:87–120.
32. Poretsky L, Kalin MF. The gonadotropic function of insulin. *Endocr Rev* 1987;8:132–141.
33. El-Roeiy A, Chen X, Roberts VJ, LeRoith D, Roberts CT Jr, Yen SSC. Expression of insulin-like growth factor-I (IGF-I) and IGF-II and the IGF-I, IGF-II, and insulin receptor genes and localization of the gene products in the human ovary. *J Clin Endocrinol Metab* 1993;77:1411–1418.
34. Erickson GF. Folliculogenesis in polycystic ovary syndrome. In: Dunaif A, Givens JR, Haseltine FP, Merriam GR, eds. *Polycystic ovary syndrome.* Cambridge, MA: Blackwell Scientific; 1992; 111–128.
35. Nestler JE, Barlascini CO, Matt DW, Steingold KA, Plymate SR, Clore JN, Blackard WG. Suppression of serum insulin by diazoxide reduces serum testosterone levels in obese women with polycystic ovary syndrome. *J Clin Endocrinol Metab* 1989;68:1027–1032.
36. Giudice LC. Insulin-like growth factors and ovarian follicular development. *Endocr Rev* 1992;13: 641–669.
37. Lobo RA. The role of neurotransmitters and opioids in polycystic ovarian syndrome. *Endocrinol Metab Clin North Am* 1988;17:667–683.
38. Suikkari AM, Jalkanen J, Koistinen R, Butzow R, Ritvos O, Ranta T, Seppala M. Human granulosa cells synthesize low molecular weight insulin-like growth factor-binding protein. *Endocrinology* 1989;124:1088–1090.
39. Yen SSC, Laughlin GA, Morales AJ. Interface between extra- and intraovarian factors in polycystic ovarian syndrome. In: Tolis G, Bringer J, Chrousos GP, eds. *Intraovarian regulators and polycystic ovarian syndrome: recent progress on clinical and therapeutic aspects.* New York: Annals NY Academy of Sciences (Vol 687); 1993:98–111.
40. New MI. Polycystic ovarian disease and congenital and late-onset adrenal hyperplasia. *Endocrinol Metab Clin North Am* 1988; 17:637–648.
41. Adams J, Polson DW, Franks S. Prevalence of polycystic ovaries in women with anovulation and idiopathic hirsutism. *Br Med J* 1986;293:355–359.
42. Hull MGR. Epidemiology of infertility and polycystic ovarian disease: endocrinological and demographic studies. *Gynecol Endocrinol* 1987;1:235–245.
43. Franks S, White DM. Prevalence of and etiological factors in polycystic ovarian syndrome. In: Tolis G, Bringer J, Chrousos GP, eds. *Intraovarian regulators and polycystic ovarian syndrome: recent progress on clinical and therapeutic aspects.* New York: Annals NY Academy of Sciences (Vol 687); 1993:112–114.
44. Goldzieher JW. Polycystic ovarian disease. *Fertil Steril* 1981;35:371–394.
45. Cheung AP, Chang RJ. Polycystic ovaries and other ovarian causes of hyperandrogenism. *Infertil Reprod Med Clin North Am* 1991;2:465–477.
46. Futterweit W, Mechanick JI. Polycystic ovarian disease: etiology, diagnosis, and treatment. *Compr Ther* 1988;14:12–20.
47. Futterweit W. Laboratory diagnosis and differential diagnosis of polycystic ovarian disease. In: *Polycystic ovarian disease.* New York: Springer-Verlag; 1984;113–135.
48. Hatch R, Rosenfield RL, Kim MH, Tredway D. Hirsutism: implications, etiology, and management. *Am J Obstet Gynecol* 1981;140:815–830.
49. Suikkari AM, Tiitinen A, Stenman UH, Seppala M, Laatikainen T. Oral contraceptives increase insulin-like growth-factor binding-protein-1 in women with polycystic ovarian disease. *Fertil Steril* 1991;55:895–899.
50. Rosenfield RL, Lucky AW. Acne, hirsutism, and alopecia in adolescent girls: clinical expressions of androgen excess. *Endocrinol Metab Clin North Am* 1993;22:507–532.
51. Futterweit W. Clinical features of polycystic ovarian disease. In: *Polycystic ovarian disease.* New York: Springer-Verlag; 1984:83–95.
52. Futterweit W, Dunaif A, Yeh HC, Kingsley P. The prevalence of hyperandrogenism in 109 consecutive female patients with diffuse alopecia. *J Am Acad Dermatol* 1988;19:831–836.
53. Young RL, Goldzieher JW. Clinical manifestations of polycystic ovarian disease. *Endocrinol Metab Clin North Am* 1988;17:621–635.
54. Deaton JL. Hyperandrogenism and uterine bleeding. *Infertil Reprod Med Clin North Am* 1991;2: 561–583.
55. Futterweit W. Hyperprolactinemia and polycystic ovarian disease. In: *Polycystic ovarian disease.* New York: Springer-Verlag; 1984:97–111.

56. Luciano AA, Chapler FK, Sherman BM. Hyperprolactinemia in polycystic ovary syndrome. *Fertil Steril* 1984;41:719–725.

57. McCluskey S, Evans C, Lacey JH, Pearce JM, Jacobs H. Polycystic ovary syndrome and bulimia. *Fertil Steril* 1991;55:287–291.

58. New MI. Nonclassical 21–hydroxylase deficiency. In: Dunaif A, Givens JR, Haseltine FP, Merriam GR, eds. *Polycystic ovary syndrome.* Cambridge, MA: Blackwell Scientific; 1992:145–161.

59. Karstaedt N, Sagel SS, Stanley RJ, Melson GL, Levitt RG. Computed tomography of the adrenal gland. *Radiology* 1978;129:723–730.

60. Korobkin M. Overview of adrenal imaging/adrenal CT. *Urol Radiol* 1989;11:221–226.

61. Faber K, Hughes CL Jr. Laboratory evaluation of hyperandrogenic conditions. *Infertil Reprod Med Clin North Am* 1991;2:495–509.

62. Pittaway DE. Neoplastic causes of hyperandrogenism. *Infertil Repr Med Clin North Am* 1991;2: 531–545.

63. Rittmaster RS. Evaluation and treatment of hirsutism. *Infertil Repr Med Clin North Am* 1991;2: 511–530.

64. Gabrilove JL, Seman AT, Sabet R, Mitty HA, Nicolis GL. Virilizing adrenal adenoma with studies on the steroid content of the adrenal venous effluent and a review of the literature. *Endocr Rev* 2: 462–470.

65. New MI. Nonclassical congenital adrenal hyperplasia and the polycystic ovarian syndrome. In: Tolis G, Bringer J, Chrousos GP, eds. *Intraovarian requlators and polycystic ovarian syndrome: recent progress on clinical and therapeutic aspects.* New York: Annals NY Academy of Sciences (Vol 687), 1993:193–205.

66. Lobo RA, Kletzky OA, Kaptein EM, Goebelsmann U. Prolactin modulation of dehydroepiandrosterone sulfate secretion. *Am J Obstet Gynecol* 1980;138:632–636.

67. Levin JH, Carmina E, Lobo RA. Is the inappropriate gonadotropin secretion of patients with polycystic ovary syndrome similar to that of patients with adult-onset congenital adrenal hyperplasia? *Fertil Steril* 1991;56:635–640.

68. Gangemi M, Benato M, Guacci AM, Menghetti G. Stimulation tests in adrenogenital syndrome induced by 21-hydroxylase deficit. *Clin Exp Obst Gynecol* 1983;10:127–130.

69. Futterweit W, Green G, Tarlin N, Dunaif A. Chronic high-dosage androgen administration to ovulatory women does not alter adrenocortical steroidogenesis. *Fertil Steril* 1992;58:124–128.

70. Futterweit W, Scher J, Nunez AE, Strauss L, Rayfield EJ. A case of bilateral dermoid cysts, insulin resistance, and polycystic ovarian disease: association of ovarian tumors with polycystic ovaries with review of the literature. *Mt Sinai J Med* 1983;50:251–255.

71. Yeh HC, Futterweit W, Thornton JC. Polycystic ovarian disease: ultrasonographic features in 104 patients. *Radiology* 1987;163:111–116.

72. Futterweit W, Yeh HC, Thornton JC. Lack of correlation of ultrasonographically determined ovarian size with age, ponderal index, and hormonal factors in 45 patients with polycystic ovarian disease. *Int J Fertil* 1987;32:456–459.

73. Fox R, Corrigan E, Thomas PA, Hull MGR. The diagnosis of polycystic ovaries in women with oligo-amenorrhea: predictive power of endocrine tests. *Clin Endocrinol (Oxf)* 1991;34:127–131.

74. Franks S. Morphology of the polycystic ovary. In: Dunaif A, Givens JR, Haseltine FP, Merriam GR, eds. *Polycystic ovary syndrome.* Cambridge, MA: Blackwell Scientific; 1992:19–28.

75. Crowley WF Jr, Hall JE, Martin KA, Adams J, Taylor AE. An overview of the diagnostic considerations in polycystic ovarian syndrome. In: Tolis G, Bringer J, Chrousos GP, eds. *Intraovarian regulators and polycystic ovarian syndrome: recent progress on clinical and therapeutic aspects.* New York: Annals NY Academy of Sciences (Vol 687), 1993:235–241.

76. Futterweit, W. Pathophysiology of polycystic ovarian disease. In: *Polycystic ovarian disease.* New York: Springer-Verlag; 1984:49–82.

77. Baird DT, Corker CS, Davidson DW, Hunter WM, Michie EA, Van Look PFA. Pituitary-ovarian relationships in polycystic ovary syndrome. *J Clin Endocrinol Metab* 1977;45:798–809.

78. Moltz L, Rommler A, Schwartz U. Peripheral steroid-gonadotropin interactions and diagnostic significance of double stimulation tests with luteinizing-hormone releasing hormone in polycystic ovarian disease. *Am J Obstet Gynecol* 1979;134:813–818.

79. Berger MJ, Taymor ML, Patton WC. Gonadotropin levels and secretory patterns in patients with typical and atypical polycystic ovarian disease. *Fertil Steril* 1975;26:619–626.

80. Moll GW Jr, Rosenfield RL. Plasma free testosterone in the diagnosis of adolescent polycystic ovary syndrome. *J Pediatr* 1983;102:461–464.

81. Yen SSC, Chaney C, Judd HL. Functional aberrations of the hypothalamic–pituitary system in polycystic ovary syndrome: a consideration of the pathogenesis. In: James VH, Serio M, Giusti G, eds. *The endocrine function of the human ovary*. New York: Academic Press; 1976:373–385.

82. Chang RJ, Mandel FP, Lu JKH, Judd HL. Enhanced disparity of gonadotropin secretion of estrone in women with polycystic ovarian disease. *J Clin Endocrinol Metab* 1982;54:490–494.

83. DeVane GW, Czekala NM, Judd HL, Yen SSC. Circulating gonadotropins, estrogens and androgens in polycystic ovarian disease. *Am J Obstet Gynecol* 1975;121:496–500.

84. Gambrell RD, Greenblatt RB, Mahesh VB. Inappropriate secretion of LH in the Stein-Leventhal syndrome. *Obstet Gynecol* 1973;42:429–440.

85. Givens JR, Andersen RN, Umstot ES, Wiser WL. Clinical findings and hormonal responses in patients with polycystic ovarian disease with normal versus elevated LH levels. *Obstet Gynecol* 1976;47:388–394.

86. Rebar R, Judd HL, Yen SSC, Rakoff J, Vandenberg G, Naftolin F. Characterization of the inappropriate gonadotropin secretion in polycystic ovary syndrome. *J Clin Invest* 1976;57:1320–1329.

87. Graf MA, Bielfeld P, Distler W, Weiers C, Kuhn-Velten WN. Pulsatile luteinizing hormone secretion pattern in hyperandrogenic women. *Fertil Steril* 1993;59:761–767.

88. Duignan NM, Shaw RW, Rudd BT, Holder G, Williams JW, Butt WR, Loga-Edwards R, London DR. Sex hormone levels and gonadotropin release in the polycystic ovary syndrome. *Clin Endocrinol (Oxf)* 1975;4:287–295.

89. Goldzieher JW, Dozier TS, Smith KD, Steinberger E. Improving the diagnostic reliability of rapidly fluctuating plasma hormone levels by optimized multiple-sampling techniques. *J Clin Endocrinol Metab* 1976;43:824–830.

90. Aono T, Miyazaki M, Miyake A, Kinugasa T, Kurachi K, Matsumoto K. Responses of serum gonadotrophins to LH-releasing hormone and oestrogens in Japanese women with polycystic ovaries. *Acta Endocrinol (Copenh)* 1977;85:840–849.

91. Givens JR, Andersen RN, Wiser WL, Fish SA. Dynamics of suppression and recovery of plasma FSH, LH, androstenedione and testosterone in polycystic ovarian disease using an oral contraceptive. *J Clin Endocrinol Metab* 1974;38:727–735.

92. Duignan NM. Polycystic ovarian disease. *Br J Obstet Gynaecol* 1976;83:593–602.

93. Coney PJ. Polycystic ovarian disease: current concepts of pathophysiology and therapy. *Fertil Steril* 1984;42:667–682.

94. Katz M. Polycystic ovaries. *Clin Obstet Gynecol* 1981;8:715–731.

95. Wentz AC, Jones GS, Sapp KC. Pulsatile gonadotropin output in menstrual dysfunction. *Obstet Gynecol* 1976;47:677–683.

96. Filicori M, Campaniello E, Michelacci L, Pareschi A, Ferrari P, Bolelli GF, Flamigni C. Gonadotropin-releasing hormone (GnRH) analog suppression renders polycystic ovarian disease patients more susceptible to ovulation induction with pulsatile GnRH. *J Clin Endocrinol Metab* 1988;66: 327–333.

97. Filicori M, Flamigni C. Hypothalamic–pituitary abnormalities in polycystic ovary syndrome. In: Dunaif A, Givens JR, Haseltine FP, Merriam GR, eds. *Polycystic ovary syndrome*. Cambridge, MA: Blackwell Scientific; 1992;31–50.

98. Burger CW, Korsen T, Van Kessel H, Van Dop PA, Caron FJM, Schoemaker J. Pulsatile luteinizing hormone patterns in the follicular phase of the menstrual cycle, polycystic ovarian disease (PCOD) and non-PCOD secondary amenorrhea. *J Clin Endocrinol Metab* 1985;61:1126–1132.

99. Christman GM, Randolph JF, Kelch RP, Marshall JC. Reduction of gonadotropin-releasing hormone pulse frequency is associated with subsequent selective follicle-stimulating hormone secretion in women with polycystic ovarian disease. *J Clin Endocrinol Metab* 1991;72:1278–1285.

100. Lobo RA, Kletzky OA, Campeau JD, diZerega GS. Elevated bioactive luteinizing hormone in women with the polycystic ovary syndrome. *Fertil Steril* 1983;39:674–678.

101. Lobo RA, Shoupe D, Chang SP, Campeau J. The control of bioactive luteinizing hormone secretion in women with polycystic ovary syndrome. *Am J Obstet Gynecol* 1984;148:423–428.

102. McClamrock HD, Bass KM, Adashi EY. Ovarian hyperandrogenism: the role of and sensitivity to gonadotropins. *Fertil Steril* 1991;55:73–79.

103. Mavroudis K, Evans A, Mamtora H, Anderson DC, Robertson WR. Bioactive LH in women with polycystic ovaries and the effect of gonadotropin suppression. *Clin Endocrinol (Oxf)* 1988;29:633–641.

104. Fauser BCJM, Pache TD, Lamberts SWJ, Hop WCJ, DeJong FH, Dahl KD. Serum bioactive and immunoreactive luteinizing hormone and follicle-stimulating hormone levels in women with cycle

abnormalities, with or without polycystic ovarian disease. *J Clin Endocrinol Metab* 1991;73:811–817.

105. Knobil E. The neuroendocrine control of the menstrual cycle. *Recent Prog Horm Res* 1980;36:53–88.

106. Tsai CC, Yen SSC. Acute effects of intravenous infusion of 17β-estradiol on gonadotropin release in pre- and post-menopausal women. *J Clin Endocrinol Metab* 1971;32:766–771.

107. Yen SSC, Tsai CC, Vandenberg G, Rebar R. Gonadotropin dynamics in patients with gonadal dysgenesis: model for the study of gonadotropin regulation. *J Clin Endocrinol Metab* 1972;35:897–904.

108. Lasley BL, Wang CW, Yen SSC. The effects of estrogen and progesterone on the functional capacity of the gonadotrophs. *J Clin Endocrinol* 1975;41:820–826.

109. Kazer RR, Kessel B, Yen SSC. Circulating LH pulse frequency in women with polycystic ovary syndrome. *J Clin Endocrinol Metab* 1987;65:233–236.

110. Venturoli S, Porcu E, Fabbri R, Magrini O, Gammi L, Paradisi R, Foccacci M, Bolzani R, Flamigni C. Episodic pulsatile secretion of FSH, LH, prolactin, oestradiol, oestrone, and LH circadian variations in polycystic ovary syndrome. *Clin Endocrinol (Oxf)* 1988;28:93–107.

111. Merriam GR. Neuroendocrine abnormalities in polycystic ovary syndrome: an overview. In: Dunaif A, Givens JR, Haseltine FP, Merriam GR, eds. *Polycystic ovary syndrome.* Cambridge, MA: Blackwell Scientific; 1992:51–56.

112. Heisenleder DJ, Khoury S, Zmeili SM, Papavasiliou S, Ortolano GA, Dee C, Duncan JA, Marshall JC. The frequency of gonadotropin-releasing hormone secretion regulates expression of α- and luteinizing hormone β-subunit messenger ribonucleic acids in male rats. *Mol Endocrinol* 1987;1:834–838.

113. Filicori M, Flamigni C, Campaniello E, Ferrari P, Meriggiola MC, Michelacci L, Pareschi A, Valdisirri A. Evidence for a specific role of GnRH pulse frequency in the control of the human menstrual cycle. *Am J Physiol* 1989;257:E930–936.

114. Soules MR, Clifton DK, Bremner WJ, Steiner RA. Corpus luteum insufficiency induced by a rapid gonadotropin-releasing hormone-induced gonadotropin secretion pattern in the follicular phase. *J Clin Endocrinol Metab* 1987;65:457–464.

115. Buckler HM, McLachlan RI, MacLachlan VB, Healy DL, Burger HG. Serum inhibin levels in polycystic ovary syndrome: basal levels and response to luteinizing hormone-releasing hormone agonist and exogenous gonadotropin administration. *J Clin Endocrinol Metab* 1988;66:798–803.

116. Kapen S, Boyar R, Hellman L, Weitzman ED. The relationship of luteinizing hormone secretion to sleep in women during the early follicular phase: effects of sleep reversal and a prolonged three-hour sleep-wake cycle. *J Clin Endocrinol Metab* 1976;42:1031–1040.

117. Wildt L, Marshall G, Hausler A, Plant TM, Belchetz PE, Knobil E. Amplitude of pulsatile GnRH input and pituitary gonadotropin secretion. *Fed Proc* 1979;38:978.

118. Spratt DI, Finkelstein JS, Butler JP, Badger TM, Crowley WF Jr. Effects of increasing the frequency of low doses of gonadotropinreleasing hormone (GnRH) on gonadotropin secretion in GnRH-deficient men. *J Clin Endocrinol Metab* 1987;64:1179–1186.

119. Hall JE, Whitcomb RW, Rivier JE, Vale WW, Crowley WF Jr. Differential regulation of luteinizing hormone, follicle-stimulating hormone, and free α-subunit secretion from the gonadotrope by gonadotropin-releasing hormone (GnRH): evidence from the use of two GnRH antagonists. *J Clin Endocrinol Metab* 1990;70:328–335.

120. Kourides IA, Re RN, Weintraub BD, Ridgway EC, Maloof F. Metabolic clearance and secretion rates of subunits of human thyrotropin. *J Clin Invest* 1977;59:508–516.

121. Hall JE, Taylor AE, Martin KA, Crowley WF Jr. New approaches to the study of the neuroendocrine abnormalities of women with the polycystic ovary syndrome. In: Tolis G, Bringer J, Chrousos GP, eds. *Intraovarian regulators and polycystic ovarian syndrome: recent progress on clinical and therapeutic aspects.* New York: Annals NY Academy of Sciences (Vol 687); 1993:182–192.

122. Berga SL, Guzick DS, Winters SJ. Increased luteinizing hormone and α-subunit secretion in women with hyperandrogenic anovulation. *J Clin Endocrinol Metab* 1993;77:182–192.

123. Bogovich K. Animal models for polycystic ovary syndrome. In: Dunaif A, Givens JR, Haseltine FP, Merriam GR, eds. *Polycystic ovary syndrome.* Cambridge, MA: Blackwell Scientific; 1992:129–140.

124. Poretsky L, Clemons J, Bogovich K. Hyperinsulinemia and human chorionic gonadotropin synergistically promote the growth of ovarian follicular cysts in rats. *Metabolism* 1992;41:903–910.

125. Zumoff B, Freeman R, Coupey S, Saenger P, Markowitz M, Kream J. A chronobiologic abnor-

mality in luteinizing hormone secretion in teenage girls with the polycystic-ovary syndrome. *N Engl J Med* 1983;309:1206–1209.

126. Porcu E, Venturoli S, Magrini O, Bolzani R, Gabbi D, Paradisi R, Fabbri R, Flamigni C. Circadian variations of luteinizing hormone can have two different profiles in adolescent anovulation. *J Clin Endocrinol Metab* 1987;65:488–493.

127. Geller S, Ayme Y, Lemasson C, Kandelman M, Grisoli F, Scholler R. Polykystose ovarienne; secretion inappropriee de LH "seule": microadenome hypophysaire a LH? *Nouv Presse Medicale* 1976;5:1492.

128. Soules MR, Steiner RA, Cohen NL, Bremner WJ, Clifton DK. Nocturnal slowing of pulsatile luteinizing hormone secretion in women during the follicular phase of the menstrual cycle. *J Clin Endocrinol Metab* 1985;61:43–49.

129. Futterweit W, Yeh HC, Mechanick JI. Ultrasonographic study of ovaries of 19 women with weight-loss related hypothalamic oligo-amenorrhea. *Biomed Pharmacother* 1988;42:279–284.

130. Fox R, Corrigan E, Thomas PG, Hull MGR. Oestrogen and androgen states in oligo-amenorrhoeic women with polycystic ovaries. *Br J Obstet Gynaecol* 1991;98:294–299.

131. Fox R, Hull M. Ultrasound diagnosis of polycystic ovaries. In: Tolis G, Bringer J, Chrousos GP, eds. *Intraovarian regulators and polycystic ovarian syndrome: recent progress on clinical and therapeutic aspects.* New York: Annals NY Academy of Sciences (Vol 687); 1993:217–223.

132. Jaffe RB, Keye WR Jr. Estradiol augmentation of pituitary responsiveness to gonadotropin-releasing hormone in women. *J Clin Endocrinol Metab* 1974;39:850–855.

133. Yen SSC, Lasley BL, Wang CF, Leblanc H, Siler TM. The operating characteristics of the hypothalamic–pituitary system during the menstrual cycle and observations of biological action of somatostatin. *Recent Prog Horm Res* 1975;31:321–363.

134. Katz M, Carr PJ. Abnormal luteinizing hormone response patterns to synthetic gonadotropin-releasing hormone in patients with polycystic ovarian syndrome. *J Endocrinol* 1976;70:163–171.

135. Patton WC, Berger MJ, Thompson IE, Chung AP, Grimes EM, Taymor ML. Pituitary gonadotropin responses to synthetic luteinizing hormone-releasing hormone in patients with typical and atypical polycystic ovary disease. *Am J Obstet Gynecol* 1975;121:382–386.

136. Zarate A, Canales ES, de la Cruz A, Soria A, Schally AV. Pituitary response to synthetic LH-RH in Stein-Leventhal syndrome and functional amenorrhea. *Obstet Gynecol* 1973;41:803–808.

137. Lobo RA, Granger L, Goebelsmann U, Mishell Jr DR. Elevations in unbound serum estradiol as a possible mechanism for inappropriate gonadotropin secretion in women with PCO. *J Clin Endocrinol Metab* 1981;52:156–158.

138. Dunaif A. Do androgens directly regulate gonadotropin secretion in the polycystic ovary syndrome? *J Clin Endocrinol Metab* 1986;63:215–221.

139. Yen SSC, Vandenberg G, Siler TM. Modulation of pituitary responsiveness to LRF by estrogen. *J Clin Endocrinol Metab* 1974;39:170–177.

140. Franks S, Hamilton-Fairley D, Sagle M, Polson D, Kiddy D, Watson H, White D. Low-dose gonadotropin therapy in polycystic ovary syndrome. In: Tolis G, Bringer J, Chrousos GP, eds. *Intraovarian regulators and polycystic ovarian syndrome: recent progress on clinical and therapeutic aspects.* New York: Annals NY Academy of Sciences (Vol 687); 1993:301–304.

141. Kamrava MM, Seibel MM, Berger MJ, Thompson I, Taymor ML: Reversal of persistent anovulation in polycystic ovarian disease by administration of chronic low-dose follicle-stimulating hormone. *Fertil Steril* 1982;37:520–523.

142. Schoemaker J, Wentz AC, Jones GS, Dubin NH. Stimulation of follicular growth with "pure" FSH in patients with anovulation and elevated LH levels. *Obstet Gynecol* 1978;51:270–277.

143. Fauser BCJM, De Jong FH. Gonadotropins in polycystic ovarian syndrome. In: Tolis G, Bringer J, Chrousos GP, eds. *Intraovarian regulators and polycystic ovarian syndrome: recent progress on clinical and therapeutic aspects.* New York: Annals NY Academy of Sciences (Vol 687); 1993:150–161.

144. Carmina E, Rosato F, Maggiore M, Gagliano AM, Indovina D, Janni A. Prolactin secretion in polycystic ovary syndrome (PCO): correlation with steroid pattern. *Acta Endocrinol (Copenh)* 1984;105:99–104.

145. Falaschi P, del Pozo E, Rocco A, Toscano V, Petrangeli E, Pompei P, Frajese G. Prolactin release in polycystic ovary. *Obstet Gynecol* 1980;55:579–582.

146. Wortsman J, Hirschowitz JF. Galactorrhea and hyperprolactinemia during treatment of polycystic ovarian syndrome. *Obstet Gynecol* 1980;55:460–463.

147. White MC, Ginsberg J. The hirsute female. In: Crosignani PG, Rubin BL, eds. *Endocrinology of human infertility: new aspects.* London: Academic Press; 1981:307–325.

148. Shoupe D, Lobo RA. Prolactin response after gonadotropin-releasing hormone in the polycystic ovary syndrome. *Fertil Steril* 1985;43:549–553.

149. Corenblum B, Taylor PJ. The hyperprolactinemic polycystic ovary syndrome may not be a distinct clinical entity. *Fertil Steril* 1982;38:549–552.

150. Quigley ME, Rakoff JS, Yen SSC. Increased luteinizing hormone sensitivity to dopamine inhibition in polycystic ovary syndrome. *J Clin Endocrinol Metab* 1981;52:231–234.

151. Ferrari C, Rampini P, Malinverni A, Scarduelli C, Benco R, Caldara R, Barbieri C, Testori G, Crosignani PG. Inhibition of luteinizing hormone release by dopamine infusion in healthy women and in various pathophysiological conditions. *Acta Endocrinol (Copenh)* 1981;97:436–440.

152. Shoupe D, Lobo RA. Evidence for altered catecholamine metabolism in polycystic ovary syndrome. *Am J Obstet Gynecol* 1984;150:566–571.

153. Lachelin GCL, Leblanc H, Yen SSC. The inhibitory effect of dopamine agonists on LH release in women. *J Clin Endocrinol Metab* 1977;44:728–732.

154. Judd SJ, Rakoff JS, Yen SSC. Inhibition of gonadotropin and prolactin release by dopamine: effect of endogenous estradiol levels. *J Clin Endocrinol Metab* 1978;47:494–498.

155. Seibel M. Toward understanding the pathophysiology and treatment of polycystic ovary disease. *Semin Reprod Endocrinol* 1984;2:297–304.

156. Falaschi P, Rocco A, Del Pozo E. Inhibitory effect of bromocriptine treatment on luteinizing hormone secretion in polycystic ovary syndrome. *J Clin Endocrinol Metab* 1986;62:348–351.

157. Spruce BA, Kendall-Taylor P, Dunlap W, Anderson AJ, Watson MJ, Cook DB, Gray C. The effect of bromocriptine in the polycystic ovary syndrome. *Clin Endocrinol (Oxf)* 1984;20:481–488.

158. Rosen GF, Lobo RA. Further evidence against dopamine deficiency as the cause of inappropriate gonadotropin secretion in patients with polycystic ovary syndrome. *J Clin Endocrinol Metab* 1987; 65:891–895.

159. Barnes RB, Mileikowsky GN, Cha KY, Spencer CA, Lobo RA. Effects of dopamine and metoclopramide in polycystic ovary syndrome. *J Clin Endocrinol Metab* 1986;63:506–509.

160. Barnes RB, Cha KY, Lee DG, Lobo RA. Modulation of luteinizing hormone immunoreactivity and bioactivity by dopamine but not norepinephrine in women. *Am J Obstet Gynecol* 1986;154; 445–450.

161. Steingold KA, Lobo RA, Judd HL, Lu JKH, Chang RJ. The effect of bromocriptine on gonadotropin and steroid secretion in polycystic ovarian disease. *J Clin Endocrinol Metab* 1986;62:1048–1051.

162. Murdoch AP, McClean KG, Watson MJ, Dunlop W, Taylor PK. Treatment of hirsutism in polycystic ovary syndrome with bromocriptine. *Br J Obstet Gynaecol* 1987;94:358–365.

163. Buvat J, Buvat-Herbaut M, Marcolin G, Racadot A, Fourlinnie JC, Beuscart R, Fossati P. A double-blind controlled study of the hormonal and clinical effects of bromocriptine in the polycystic ovary syndrome. *J Clin Endocrinol Metab* 1986;63:119–124.

164. Harrison RF, Synnott M, O'Moore R, O'Moore M. Can women with gonadotropin levels diagnostic of polycystic ovarian syndrome benefit from therapy with dopamine agonists? In: Tolis G, Bringer J, Chrousos GP, eds. *Intraovarian regulators and polycystic ovarian syndrome: recent progress on clinical and therapeutic aspects.* New York: Annals NY Academy of Sciences (Vol 687); 1993:272–279.

165. Futterweit W, Krieger DT. Pituitary tumors associated with hyperprolactinemia and polycystic ovarian disease. *Fertil Steril* 1979;31:608–613.

166. Futterweit W. Pituitary tumors and polycystic ovarian disease. *Obstet Gynecol* 1983;62:S74–S79.

167. Lunde O. Hyperprolactinemia in polycystic ovary syndrome. *Ann Chir Gynaecol* 1981;70:197–201.

168. Haesslein HC, Lamb EJ. Pituitary tumors in patients with secondary amenorrhea. *Am J Obstet Gynecol* 1976;125:759–767.

169. Shapiro AG. Pituitary adenoma, menstrual disturbance, hirsutism and abnormal glucose tolerance. *Fertil Steril* 1981;35:226–229.

170. Schlechte J, Sherman B, Halmi N, VanGilder J, Chapler F, Dolan K, Granner D, Duella T, Harris C. Prolactin-secreting pituitary tumors in amenorrheic women: a comprehensive study. *Endocr Rev* 1980;1:295–308.

171. Falcone T, Billiar R, Morris D. Serum inhibin levels in polycystic ovary syndrome: effect of insulin resistance and insulin secretion. *Obstet Gynecol* 1991;78:171–178.

172. McNatty KP, Smith DM, Makris A, Osathanondh R, Ryan KJ. The microenvironment of the human antral follicle: interrelationships among the steroid levels in antral fluid, the population of

granulosa cells, and the status of the oocyte in vivo and in vitro. *J Clin Endocrinol Metab* 1979;49: 851–860.

173. Hillier SG, Wickings EJ, Illingworth PI, Yong EL, Reichert LE Jr, Baird DT, McNeilly AS. Control of immunoreactive inhibin production by human granulosa cells. *Clin Endocrinol (Oxf)* 1991;35:71–78.

174. Yamoto M, Minami S, Nakano R, Kobayashi M. Immunohistochemical localization of inhibin/ activin subunits in human ovarian follicles during the menstrual cycle. *J Clin Endocrinol Metab* 1992;74:989–993.

175. Yamato M, Minami S, Nakano R. Immunohistochemical localization of inhibin subunits in polycystic ovary. *J Clin Endocrinol Metab* 1993;77:859–862.

176. Erickson GF, Hsueh AJW, Quigley ME, Rebar RW, Yen SSC. Functional studies of aromatase activity in human granulosa cells from normal and polycystic ovaries. *J Clin Endocrinol Metab* 1979;49:514–519.

177. Aleem FA, McIntosh T. Elevated plasma levels of β-endorphin in a group of women with polycystic ovarian disease. *Fertil Steril* 1984;42:686–689.

178. Jewelewicz R. The role of endogenous opioid peptides in control of the menstrual cycle. *Fertil Steril* 1984;42:683–685.

179. Giugliano D. Morphine, opioid peptides and pancreatic islet function. *Diabetes Care* 1984;7:92–98.

180. Giugliano D, Salvatore T, Cozzolino D, Ceriello A, Torella R, D'Onofrio F. Sensitivity to β-endorphins as a cause of human obesity. *Metabolism* 1987;36:974–978.

181. Barnes RB, Lobo RA. Central opioid activity in polycystic ovary syndrome with and without dopaminergic modulation. *J Clin Endocrinol Metab* 1985;61:779–782.

182. Aleem FA, Elbabbakh GH, Omar RA, Southren AL. Ovarian fluid β-endorphin levels in normal and polycystic ovaries. *Am J Obstet Gynecol* 1987;156:1197–1200.

183. Cumming DC, Reid RL, Quigley ME, Rebar RW, Yen SSC. Evidence for decreased endogenous dopamine and opioid inhibitory influences of LH secretion in polycystic ovary syndrome. *Clin Endocrinol (Oxf)* 1984;20:643–648.

184. Lanzone A, Cutillo G, Apa R, Caruso A, Fulghesu AM, Mancuso S. Long-term naltrexone treatment normalizes the pituitary response to gonadotropin-releasing hormone in polycystic ovarian syndrome. *Fertil Steril* 1993;59:734–737.

185. Petraglia F, D'Ambrigio G, Comitini G, Facchinetti F, Volpe A, Genazzani AR. Impairment of opioid control of luteinizing hormone secretion in menstrual disorders. *Fertil Steril* 1985;43:534–540.

186. Lobo RA, Granger LR, Paul WL, Goebelsmann U, Mishell DR. Psychological stress and increases in urinary norepinephrine metabolites, platelet serotonin, and adrenal androgens in women with polycystic ovary syndrome. *Am J Obstet Gynecol* 1983;145:496–503.

187. Paradisi R, Venturoli S, Capelli M, Spada M, Giambasi ME, Magrini O, Porcu E, Fabbri R, Flamigni C. Effects of a_1-adrenergic blockade on pulsatile luteinizing hormone, follicle-stimulating hormone, and prolactin secretion in polycystic ovary syndrome. *J Clin Endocrinol Metab* 1987; 65:841–846.

188. Siiteri PK, MacDonald PC: Role of extraglandular estrogen in human endocrinology. In: Greep RO, Astwood EB, eds. *Handbook of physiology Vol II, Section 7,* Washington, DC: American Physiological Society;1973:615–629.

189. Clarke IJ, Cummins JT. The temporal relationship between gonadotropin releasing hormone (GnRH) and luteinizing hormone (LH) secretion in ovariectomized ewes. *Endocrinology* 1982;111: 1737–1739.

190. Serafini P, Silva PD, Paulsen RJ, Elkind-Hirsch K, Hernandez M, Lobo RA. Acute modulation of the hypothalamic–pituitary axis by intravenous testosterone in normal women. *Am J Obstet Gynecol* 1986;155:1288–1292.

191. Nagamani M, Lingold JC, Gomez LG, Garza JR. Clinical and hormonal studies in hyperthecosis of the ovaries. *Fertil Steril* 1981;36:326–332.

192. Dunaif A, Scully RE, Andersen RN, Chapin DS, Crowley WF Jr. The effects of continuous androgen secretion on the hypothalamic–pituitary axis in woman: evidence from a luteinized ovarian thecoma. *J Clin Endocrinol Metab* 1984;59:389–393.

193. Givens JR, Andersen RN, Wiser WL, Donalson AJ, Coleman SA. A testosterone-secreting gonadotropin-responsive pure thecoma and polycystic ovarian disease. *J Clin Endocrinol Metab* 1975; 41:845–853.

194. Shelley D, Dobrjansky A, Futterweit W, Dunaif A. Ontogeny, mechanisms, and heterogeneity of androgen action on the hypothalamic–pituitary axis of women. *72nd Annual Meeting of Endocrine Society.* Atlanta, 1990: Abstract 1366.

195. Billiar RB, Richardson D, Anderson E, Mahajan D, Little B. The effect of chronic and acyclic elevation of circulating androstenedione or estrone concentrations on ovarian function in rhesus monkeys. *Endocrinology* 1985;116:2209–2220.

196. Scheele F, Hompes PGA, Gooren LJG, Spijkstra JJ, Spindra T. The effect of 6 weeks of testosterone treatment on pulsatile luteinizing hormone secretion in eugonadal female-to-male transsexuals. *Fertil Steril* 1991;55:608–611.

197. Goldzieher JW, Axelrod LR. Clinical and biochemical features of polycystic ovarian disease. *Fertil Steril* 1963;14:631–653.

198. Lobo RA, Goebelsmann U. Evidence for reduced 3β-ol-hydroxysteroid dehydrogenase activity in some hirsute women thought to have polycystic ovary syndrome. *J Clin Endocrinol Metab* 1981; 53:394–400.

199. Yen SSC. The polycystic ovary syndrome. *Clin Endocrinol (Oxf)* 1980;12:177–207.

200. Nestler JE, Clore JN, Blackard WG. The central role of obesity (hyperinsulinemia) in the pathogenesis of the polycystic ovary syndrome. *Am J Obstet Gynecol* 1989;161:1095–1097.

201. Siegel SF, Finegold DN, Lanes R, Lee PA. ACTH stimulation tests and plasma dehydroepiandrosterone sulfate levels in women with hirsutism. *N Engl J Med* 1990;323:849–854.

202. Eldar-Geva T, Hurwitz A, Vecsei P, Palti Z, Milwidsky A, Rosler A. Secondary biosynthetic defects in women with late-onset congenital adrenal hyperplasia. *N Engl J Med* 1990;323:855–863.

203. Chang RJ, Laufer LR, Meldrum DR, DeFazio J, Lu JKH, Vale WW, Rivier JE, Judd HL. Steroid secretion in polycystic ovarian disease after ovarian suppression by a long-acting gonadotropin-releasing hormone agonist. *J Clin Endocrinol Metab* 1983;56:897–903.

204. Geffner ME, Kaplan SA, Bersch N, Golde DW, Landaw EM, Chang RJ. Persistence of insulin resistance in polycystic ovarian disease after inhibition of ovarian steroid secretion. *Fertil Steril* 1986;45:327–333.

205. Dunaif A, Green G, Futterweit W, Dobrjansky A. Suppression of hyperandrogenism does not improve peripheral or hepatic insulin resistance in the polycystic ovary syndrome. *J Clin Endocrinol Metab* 1990;70:699–704.

206. Rosenfield RL, Ehrlich EN, Cleary RE. Adrenal and ovarian contributions to the elevated free plasma androgens in hirsute women. *J Clin Endocrinol Metab* 1972;34:92–98.

207. Kirschner MA, Jacobs JB. Combined ovarian and adrenal vein catheterization to determine the site(s) of androgen over-production in hirsute women. *J Clin Endocrinol Metab* 1971;33:199–209.

208. Rosenfield RL. Plasma free androgen patterns in hirsute women and their diagnostic implications. *Am J Med* 1979;66:417–421.

209. Barbieri RL. Hyperandrogenic disorders. *Clin Obstet Gynecol* 1990;33:640–654.

210. Poretsky L. On the paradox of insulin-induced hyperandrogenism in insulin-resistant states. *Endocr Rev* 1991;12:3–13.

211. Poretsky L, Glover B, Laumas V, Kalin M, Dunaif A. The effects of experimental hyperinsulinemia on steroid secretion, ovarian I-125 insulin binding and ovarian I-125 insulin-like growth factor-I binding in the rat. *Endocrinology* 1988;122:581–585.

212. Mechanick JI, Futterweit W. The aberrant puberty hypothesis of polycystic ovarian disease. *Mt Sinai J Med* 1986;53:311–314.

213. Mechanick JI, Futterweit W. Hypothesis: aberrant puberty and the Stein-Leventhal syndrome. *Int J Fertil* 1984;29:35–38.

214. Kase N, Kowal J, Perloff W, Soffer LJ. In vitro production of androgens by a virilizing adenoma and associated polycystic ovaries. *Acta Endocrinol (Copenh)* 1963;44:15–19.

215. Chrousos GP, Loriaux DL, Mann DL, Cutler GB Jr. Late-onset 21-hydroxylase deficiency mimicking idiopathic hirsutism or polycystic ovarian disease. *Ann Intern Med* 1982;96:143–148.

216. Scherzer WJ, Adashi EY. Adrenal hyperandrogenism. *Infertil Reprod Med Clin North Am* 1991;2: 479–494.

217. Hague WM, Adams J, Rodda C, Brook J, deBruyn R, Grant DB, Jacobs HS. The prevalence of polycystic ovaries in patients with congenital adrenal hyperplasia and their close relatives. *Clin Endocrinol (Oxf)* 1990;33:501–510.

218. Barnes RB, Rosenfield RL, Burstein S, Ehrmann DA. Pituitary–ovarian responses to nafarelin testing in the polycystic ovary syndrome. *N Engl J Med* 1989;320:559–565.

219. Dunaif A, Futterweit W. Polycystic ovary syndrome [Letter]. *N Engl J Med* 1988;319:584.
220. Kirschner MA, Zucker IR, Jespersen D. Idiopathic hirsutism: an ovarian abnormality. *N Engl J Med* 1976;294:637–640.
221. Lobo RA. The role of the adrenal in polycystic ovary syndrome. *Semin Reprod Endocrinol* 1984; 2:251–262.
222. Cedars MI, Chang RJ. Functional ovarian causes of hyperandrogenism. *Semin Reprod Endocrinol* 1986;4:143–153.
223. Gross MD, Wortsman J, Shapiro B, Mayers LC, Woodbury MC, Ayers JWP. Scintigraphic evidence of adrenal corticoid dysfunction in the polycystic ovary syndrome. *J Clin Endocrinol Metab* 1986;62:197–201.
224. Abraham GE, Chakmakjian ZH, Buster JE, Marshall JR. Ovarian and adrenal contributions to peripheral androgens in hirsute women. *Obstet Gynecol* 1975;46:169–173.
225. Horton R, Neisler J. Plasma androgens in patients with polycystic ovary syndrome. *J Clin Endocrinol Metab* 1968;28:479–484.
226. Melis GB, Mais V, Gambacciani M, Paolette AM, Antinori D, Fioretti P. Dexamethasone reduces the postcastration gonadotropin rise in women. *J Clin Endocrinol Metab* 1987;65:237–241.
227. Wilson EA, Erickson GF, Zarutski P, Finn AE, Tulchinsky D, Ryan KJ. Endocrine studies of normal and polycystic ovarian tissue in vitro. *Am J Obstet Gynecol* 1979;134:56–63.
228. Givens JR, Andersen RN, Ragland JB, Miser WL, Umstot ES. Adrenal function in hirsutism. I. Diurnal change and response of plasma androstenedione, 17-hydroxyprogesterone, cortisol, LH and FSH to dexamethasone and 1/2 unit of ACTH. *J Clin Endocrinol Metab* 1975;40:988–1000.
229. Lachelin GCL, Barnett M, Hopper BR, Brink G, Yen SSC. Adrenal function in normal women and women with polycystic ovary syndrome. *J Clin Endocrinol Metab* 1979;49:892–898.
230. Pang SY, Lerner AJ, Stoner E, Levine LS, Oberfield SE, Engel I, New MI. Late-onset adrenal steroid 3β-hydroxysteroid deficiency. I. A cause of hirsutism in pubertal and postpubertal women. *J Clin Endocrinol Metab* 1985;60:428–439.
231. Lucky AW, Rosenfield RL, McGuire J, Rudy S, Helke J. Adrenal androgen hyperresponsiveness to adrenocorticotropin in women with acne and/or hirsutism: adrenal enzyme defects and exaggerated adrenarche. *J Clin Endocrinol Metab* 1986;62:840–848.
232. Rich BH, Rosenfield RL, Lucky AW, Helke JC, Otto P. Adrenarche: changing adrenal response to adrenocorticotropin. *J Clin Endocrinol Metab* 1981;52:1129–1136.
233. Parker LN, Odell WD. Evidence for existence of cortical-androgen stimulating hormone. *Am J Physiol* 1979;236:E616–E620.
234. Parker LN, Lifrak ET, Odell WD. A 60,000 molecular weight human pituitary glycopeptide stimulates adrenal androgen secretion. *Endocrinology* 1983;113:2092–2096.
235. Chang RJ, Mandel FP, Wolfsen AR, Judd HL. Circulating levels of plasma adrenocorticotropin in polycystic ovary disease. *J Clin Endocrinol Metab* 1982;54:1265–1267.
236. Wajchenberg BL, Achando SS, Okada H, Czeresnia CE, Peixoto S, Lima SS, Goldman J. Determination of the source(s) of androgen overproduction in hirsutism associated with polycystic ovary syndrome by simultaneous adrenal and ovarian venous catherization. Comparison with the dexamethasone suppression test. *J Clin Endocrinol Metab* 1986;63:1204–1210.
237. Azziz R. The role of the ovary in the genesis of hyperandrogenism. In: Adashi EY, Leung PCK, eds. *The ovary*. New York: Raven Press; 1993:581–605.
238. Ettinger B, von Werder K, Thenaers GC, Forsham PH. Plasma testosterone stimulation–suppression dynamics in hirsute women. *Am J Med* 1971;51:170–175.
239. Lachelin GCL, Judd HL, Swanson SC, Hauck ME, Parker DC, Yen SSC. Long term effects of nightly dexamethasone suppression in patients with polycystic ovarian disease. *J Clin Endocrinol Metab* 1982;55:768–773.
240. Steinberger E, Smith KD, Rodriguez-Rigau LJ. Testosterone, dehydroepiandrosterone, and dehydroepiandrosterone sulfate in hyperandrogenic women. *J Clin Endocrinol Metab* 1984;59:471–477.
241. Karpas AE, Rodriguez-Rigau LJ, Smith KD, Steinberger E. Effect of acute and chronic androgen suppression by glucocorticoids on gonadotropin levels in hirsute women. *J Clin Endocrinol Metab* 1984;59:780–784.
242. McKenna TJ, Cunningham SK. Adrenal abnormalities in polycystic ovary syndrome and the impact of their correction. In: Dunaif A, Givens JR, Haseltine FP, Merriam GR, eds. *Polycystic ovary syndrome*. Cambridge, MA: Blackwell Scientific; 1992:183–193.
243. Janata J, Starka L. Effect of cortisol on the production of ovarian androgens. *J Endocrinol* 1964;29: 93–94.

244. Moltz L, Schwartz U, Sorensen R, Pickartz H, Hammerstein J. Ovarian and adrenal vein steroids in patients with nonneoplastic hyperandrogenism: selective catherization findings. *Fertil Steril* 1984;42:69–75.
245. Northrop G, Archie JT, Patel SK, Wilbanks GD. Adrenal and ovarian vein androgen levels and laparoscopic findings in hirsute women. *Am J Obstet Gynecol* 1975;122:192–198.
246. Laatikainen T, Apter D, Andersson B, Wahlstrom T. Follicular fluid steroid levels and ovarian steroid secretion in polycystic ovarian disease. *Eur J Obstet Gynaecol Reprod Biol* 1983;16:283–291.
247. Stahl NL, Teeslink CR, Greenblatt RB. Ovarian, adrenal, and peripheral testosterone levels in the polycystic ovary syndrome. *Am J Obstet Gynecol* 1973;117:194–200.
248. Wentz AC, White RI Jr, Migeon CJ, Hsu TH, Barnes HV, Jones GS. Differential ovarian and adrenal vein catheterization. *Am J Obstet Gynecol* 1976;125:1000–1007.
249. Bayliss RIS, Edwards OM, Starer E. Complications of adrenal venography. *Br J Radiol* 1970;43:531–533.
250. Judd HL, Rigg LA, Anderson DC, Yen SSC. The effects of ovarian wedge resection on circulating gonadotropin and ovarian steroid levels in patients with polycystic ovary syndrome. *J Clin Endocrinol Metab* 1976;43:347–355.
251. Katz M, Carr PJ, Cohen BM, Millar RP. Hormonal effects of wedge resection of polycystic ovaries. *Obstet Gynecol* 1978;52:437–443.
252. Greenblatt E, Casper RF. Endocrine changes after laparoscopic ovarian cautery in polycystic ovarian syndrome. *Am J Obstet Gynecol* 1987;156:279–285.
253. Kim MH, Rosenfield RL, Hosseinian AH, Schneier HG. Ovarian hyperandrogenism with normal and abnormal histologic findings of the ovaries. *Am J Obstet Gynecol* 1979;134:445–452.
254. Spratt DI, O'Dea LS, Schoenfeld D, Butler J, Rao PN, Crowley WF Jr. Neuroendocrine–gonadal axis in men: frequent sampling of LH, FSH, and testosterone. *Am J Physiol* 1987;254:E658–666.
255. Carr BR, Parker CR Jr, Madden JD, MacDonald PC, Porter JC. Plasma levels of adrenocorticotropin and cortisol in women receiving oral contraceptive steroid treatment. *J Clin Endocrinol Metab* 1979;49:346–349.
256. Wild RA, Umstot ES, Andersen RN, Givens JR. Adrenal function in hirsutism. II. Effect of an oral contraceptive. *J Clin Endocrinol Metab* 1982;54:676–681.
257. Fern M, Rose DP, Fern EB. Effect of oral contraceptives on plasma androgenic steroids and their precursors. *Obstet Gynecol* 1978;51:541–544.
258. Bardin CW, Lipsett MB. Testosterone and androstenedione blood production rates in normal women and women with idiopathic hirsutism or polycystic ovaries. *J Clin Invest* 1967;46:891–902.
259. Rosenfield RL, Rich BH, Wolsdorf JI, Cassorla F, Parks JS, Bongiovanni AM, Wu CH, Shackleton CHL. Pubertal presentation of congenital delta5-3 beta-hydroxysteroid dehydrogenase deficiency. *J Clin Endocrinol Metab* 1980;51:345–353.
260. Axelrod LR, Goldzieher JW. Steroid biosynthesis in normal and polycystic ovarian tissue. *J Clin Endocrinol Metab* 1962;22:431–440.
261. Pang SY, Softness B, Sweeney WJ III, New MI. Hirsutism, polycystic ovarian disease, and ovarian 17-ketosteroid reductase deficiency. *N Engl J Med* 1987;316:1295–1301.
262. Toscano V, Balducci R, Bianchi P, Mangiantini A, Sciarra F. Ovarian 17-ketosteroid reductase deficiency as a possible cause of polycystic ovarian disease. *J Clin Endocrinol Metab* 1990;71:288–292.
263. McNatty KP, Smith DM, Makris A, DeGrazia C, Tulchinsky D, Osathanondh R, Schiff I, Ryan KJ. The intraovarian sites of androgen and estrogen formation in women with normal and hyperandrogenic ovaries as judged by in vitro experiments. *J Clin Endocrinol Metab* 1980;50:755–763.
264. McNatty KP, Makris A, Reinhold VN, DeGrazia C, Osathanondh R, Ryan KJ. Metabolism of androstenedione by human ovarian tissues in vitro with particular reference to reductase and aromatase activity. *Steroids* 1979;34:429–443.
265. Rosenfield RL, Ehrmann DA, Barnes RB, Brigell DF, Chandler DW. Ovarian steroidogenic abnormalities in polycystic ovary syndrome: evidence for abnormal coordinate regulation of androgen and estrogen secretion. In: Dunaif A, Givens JR, Haseltine FP, Merriam GR, eds. *Polycystic ovary syndrome*. Cambridge, MA: Blackwell Scientific; 1992:83–110.
266. Dewailly D, Gillot-Longelin C, Cortet-Rudelli C, Fossati P. Clinical aspects of late onset 21-hydroxylase deficiency. *Semin Reprod Endocrinol* 1993;11:341–346.
267. Futterweit W, Deligdisch L. Histopathological effects of exogenously administered testosterone in 19 female-to-male transsexuals. *J Clin Endocrinol Metab* 1986;62:16–21.

268. Amirikia H, Savoy-Moore RT, Sundareson AS, Moghissi KS. The effect of long-term androgen treatment on the ovary. *Fertil Steril* 1986;45:202–208.
269. Futterweit W. The pathologic anatomy of polycystic ovarian disease. In: *Polycystic ovarian disease*. New York: Springer-Verlag; 1984:41–48.
270. Rosenfield RL, Ehrmann DA, Barnes RB, Sheikh Z. Gonadotropin-releasing agonist as a probe for the pathogenesis and diagnosis of ovarian hyperandrogenism. In: Tolis G, Bringer J, Chrousos GP, eds. *Intraovarian regulators and polycystic ovarian syndrome: recent progress on clinical and therapeutic aspects*. New York: Annals NY Academy of Sciences (Vol 687); 1993:162–181.
271. Futterweit W, Gabrilove JL, Smith H Jr. Testicular steroidogenic response to human chorionic gonadotropin of fifteen male transsexuals on chronic estrogen treatment. *Metabolism* 1984;33:936–942.
272. Ehrmann DA, Rosenfield RL, Barnes RB, Brigell DF, Sheikh Z. Detection of functional hyperandrogenism in women with androgen excess. *N Engl J Med* 1992;327:157–162.
273. Gibson M, Lackritz R, Schiff I, Tulchinsky D. Abnormal adrenal responses to adrenocorticotropic hormone in hyperandrogenic women. *Fertil Steril* 1980;33:43–48.
274. Nobels F, DeWailly D. Puberty and polycystic ovarian syndrome: the insulin/insulin-like growth factor I hypothesis. *Fertil Steril* 1992;58:655–666.
275. Schiebinger RJ, Albertson BD, Cassorla FG, Bowyer DW, Geelhoed GW, Cutler GB Jr. The developmental changes in plasma adrenal androgens during infancy and adrenarche are associated with changing activities of adrenal microsomal 17-hydroxylase and 17, 20-desmolase. *J Clin Invest* 1981;67:1177–1182.
276. Dickerman Z, Grant DR, Faiman C, Winter SDS. Intraadrenal steroid concentrations in man: zonal differences and developmental changes. *J Clin Endocrinol Metab* 1984;59:1031–1036.
277. Kennerson AR, McDonald DA, Adams JB. Dehydroepiandrosterone sulfotransferase localization in human adrenal glands: a light and electron microscopic study. *J Clin Endocrinol Metab* 1983; 56:786–790.
278. Erickson GF, Magoffin DA, Dyer CA, Hofeditz C. The ovarian androgen producing cells: a review of structure/function relationships. *Endocr Rev* 1985;6:371–399.
279. Hillier SG. Paracrine control of follicular estrogen synthesis. *Semin Reprod Endocrinol* 1991;9: 332–340.
280. Poretsky L, Grigorescu F, Seibel M, Moses AC, Flier JS. Distribution and characterization of insulin and insulin-like growth factor I receptors in normal human ovary. *J Clin Endocrinol Metab* 1985;61:728–734.
281. Cara JF, Rosenfield RL. Insulin-like growth factor I and insulin potentiate luteinizing hormone-induced androgen synthesis by rat ovarian thecal–interstitial cells. *Endocrinology* 1988;123:733–739.
282. Cara JF, Fan J, Azzarello J, Rosenfield RL. Insulin-like factor-I enhances luteinizing hormone binding to rat ovarian theca-interstitial cells. *J Clin Invest* 1990;86:560–565.
283. Eden JA, Jones J, Carter GD, Aldghband-Zadeh J. Follicular fluid concentrations of insulin-like growth factor I, epidermal growth factor, transforming growth factor-alpha and sex steroids in volume matched normal and polycystic human follicles. *Clin Endocrinol (Oxf)* 1990;32:395–405.
284. Erickson GF, Garzo VG, Magoffin DA. Insulin-like growth factor-I regulates aromatase activity in human granulosa and granulosa luteal cells. *J Clin Endocrinol Metab* 1989;69:716–724.
285. Steinkampf MP, Mendelson CR, Simpson ER. Effects of epidermal growth factor and insulin-like growth factor I on the levels of mRNA encoding aromatase cytochrome P-450 of human ovarian granulosa cells. *Mol Cell Endocrinol* 1988;59:93–99.
286. Adashi EY. The potential relevance of cytokines to ovarian physiology: the emerging role of resident ovarian cells of the white blood cell series. *Endocr Rev* 1990;11:454–464.
287. Erickson GF. An analysis of follicle development and ovum maturation. *Semin Reprod Endocrinol* 1986;4:233–254.
288. Erickson GF, Yen SSC. New data on follicle cells in polycystic ovaries: a proposed mechanism for the genesis of cystic ovaries. *Semin Reprod Endocrinol* 1984;2:231–243.
289. Adashi EY, Resnick CE, Hurwitz A, Ricciarelli E, Hernandez ER, Roberts CT, Leroith D, Rosenfeld R. Insulin-like growth factors: the ovarian connection. *Hum Reprod* 1991;6;1213–1219.
290. Erickson GF, Magoffin DA, Garzo VG, Cheung AP, Chang RJ. Granulosa cells of polycystic ovaries: are they normal or abnormal? *Hum Reprod* 1992;7:293–299.
291. Gospodarowicz D, Bialecki H. Fibroblast and epidermal growth factors are mitogenic agents for cultured granulosa cells of rodent, porcine, and human origin. *Endocrinology* 1979;104:757–764.

292. Delforge JP, Thomas K, Roux F, Carneiro de Siqueira J, Ferin J. Time relationships between granulosa cell growth and luteinization, and plasma luteinizing hormone discharge in humans. I. A morphometric analysis. *Fertil Steril* 1972;23:1–11.
293. Yong EL, Baird DT, Yates R, Reichert LE Jr, Hillier SG. Hormonal regulation of the growth and steroidogenic function of human granulosa cells. *J Clin Endocrinol Metab* 1992;74:842–849.
294. Erickson GF, Magoffin DA, Cragun JR, Chang RJ. The effects of insulin and insulin-like growth factors-I and-II on estradiol production by granulosa cells of polycystic ovaries. *J Clin Endocrinol Metab* 1990;70:894–902.
295. Brailly S, Gougeon A, Milgrom E, Bomsel-Helmreich O, Papiernik E. Androgens and progestins in the human ovarian follicle: differences in the evolution of preovulatory, healthy nonovulatory, and atretic follicles. *J Clin Endocrinol Metab* 1981;53:128–134.
296. Eden JA, Jones J, Carter GD, Alaghband-Zadeh J. A comparison of follicular fluid levels of insulin-like growth factor-I in normal dominant and cohort follicles, polycystic and multicystic ovaries. *Clin Endocrinol (Oxf)* 1988;29:327–336.
297. McNatty KP, Hunter WM, McNeilly AS, Sawers RS. Changes in the concentration of pituitary and steroid hormones in the follicular fluid of human Graafian follicles throughout the menstrual cycle. *J Endocrinol* 1975;64:555–571.
298. Lee DW, Shelden RM, Reichert LE Jr. Identification of low and high molecular weight follicle-stimulating hormone receptor-binding inhibitors in human follicular fluid. *Fertil Steril* 1990;53:830–835.
299. Ui M, Shimonaka M, Shimasaki S, Ling N. An insulin-like growth factor-binding protein in ovarian follicular fluid blocks follicle-stimulating hormone-stimulated steroid production by ovarian granulosa cells. *Endocrinology* 1989;125:912–916.
300. Shimasaki S, Shimonaka M, Ui M, Inoye S, Shibata F, Ling N. Structural characterization of a follicle-stimulating hormone action inhibitor in porcine ovarian follicular fluid. *J Biol Chem* 1990;265:2198–2202.
301. Vale WW, Rivier J, Vaughan J, McClintock R, Corrigan A, Woo W, Kan D, Spiess J. Purification and characterization of an FSH releasing protein from porcine ovarian follicular fluid. *Nature* 1986;321:776–779.
302. Ling N, Ying SY, Ueno N, Shimasani S, Eseh F, Hotia M, Guillemin R. A homodimer of the β-subunits of inhibin A stimulates the secretion of pituitary follicle stimulating hormone. *Biochem Biophys Res Commun* 1986;138:1129–1137.
303. Hsueh AJW, Dahl KD, Vaughan J, Tucker E, Rivier J, Bardin CW, Vale W. Heterodimers and homodimers of inhibin subunits have different paracrine action in the modulation of luteinizing hormone-stimulated androgen biosynthesis. *Proc Natl Acad Sci USA* 1987;84:5082–5086.
304. Cohick WS, Clemmons. OR. The insulin-like growth factors. *Ann Rev Physiol* 1993;55:131–153.
305. Adashi EY, Resnick CE, D'Ercole AJ, Svoboda ME, Van Wyk JJ. Insulin-like growth factors as intraovarian regulators of granulosa cell growth and function. *Endocr Rev* 1985;6:400–420.
306. Knecht M, Feng P, Catt KJ. Transforming growth factor-beta: autocrine, paracrine and endocrine effects in ovarian cells. *Semin Reprod Endocrinol* 1989;7:12–20.
307. May JV, Schomberg DW. The potential relevance of epidermal growth factor and transforming growth factor-alpha to ovarian physiology. *Semin Reprod Endocrinol* 1989;7:1–11.
308. Gospodarowicz D, Ferrara N, Schweigerer L, Neufeld G. Structural characterization and biological functions of fibroblast growth factor. *Endocr Rev* 1987;8:95–114.
309. Rosenfeld RG, Lamson GL, Oh Y, Conover C, DeLeon DD, Donovan S, Derant I, Giudice L. Insulin-like growth factor binding protein. *Recent Prog Horm Res* 1990;46:99–159.
310. Koistinen R, Suikkari AM, Tiifinen A, Kountula K. Human granulosa cells contain insulin-like growth factor binding protein (IGF-BP-1) mRNA. *Clin Endocrinol (Oxf)* 1990;32:635–640.
311. Suikkari A-M, Koivisto VA, Rutanen E-M, Yki-Jarvinen H, Karonen S-L, Seppala M. Insulin regulates the serum levels of low-molecular weight insulin-like growth factor-binding protein. *J Clin Endocrinol Metab* 1988;66:266–272.
312. Clemmons DR, Camacho-Hubner C, Jones JI, McCusker RH, Busby WH Jr. Insulin-like growth factor binding proteins: mechanisms of action at the cellular level. In: Spencer EM, ed. *Modern concepts of insulin-like growth factors.* New York: Elsevier Science; 1991:475–486.
313. Carlsson B, Carlsson L, Billig H. Estrus cycle-dependent covariation of insulin-like growth factor I (IGF-I) messenger ribonucleic acid and protein in the rat ovary. *Mol Cell Endocrinol* 1989;64:271–275.
314. Jesionowska H, Hemmings R, Guyda HJ, Posner BI. Determination of insulin and insulin-like growth factors in the ovarian circulation. *Fertil Steril* 1990;53:88–91.

315. Conover CA, Butler PC, Wang M, Rizza RA, Lee PDK. Lack of growth hormone effect on insulin-associated suppression of insulin-like growth factor binding protein 1 in humans. *Diabetes* 1990;39:1251–1256.

316. Cotterill AM, Cowell CT, Baxter RC, McNeil D, Silinik M. Regulation of the growth-hormone independent growth factor-binding protein in children. *J Clin Endocrinol Metab* 1988;67:882–887.

317. Baxter RC, Cowell CT. Diurnal rhythm of growth hormone-independent binding protein for insulin-like growth factors in human plasma. *J Clin Endocrinol Metab* 1987;65:432–440.

318. Adashi EY, Resnick CE, Rosenfeld RG. Insulin-like growth factor-I (IGF-I) and IGF-II hormonal action in cultured rat granulosa cells: mediation via type I but not type II IGF receptors. *Endocrinology* 1990;126:216–222.

319. Hsu C-J, Hammond JM. Gonadotropins and estradiol stimulate immunoreactive insulin-life growth factor-I production by porcine granulosa cells in vitro. *Endocrinology* 1987;120:198–207.

320. Adashi EY, Resnick CE, Brodie AMH, Svoboda ME, Van Wyk JJ. Somatomedin-C enhances induction of luteinizing hormone receptors by follicle stimulating hormone in cultured rat granulosa cells. *Endocrinology* 1985;116:2369–2375.

321. Homburg R, Eshel A, Abdalla HI, Jacobs HS. Growth hormone facilitates ovulation induction by gonadotropins. *Clin Endocrinol (Oxf)* 1988;29:113–117.

322. Adashi EY, Resnick CE, Brodie AMH, Svoboda ME, Van Wyk JJ. Somatomedin-C-mediated potentiation of follicle-stimulating hormone-induced aromatase activity of cultured rat granulosa cells. *Endocrinology* 1985;117:1313–1320.

323. Davoren JB, Hsueh AJW, Li CH. Somatomedin C augments FSH-induced differentiation of cultured rat granulosa cells. *Am J Physiol* 1985;249:E26–E33.

324. Adashi EY, Resnick CE, Hernandez ER, Hurwitz A, Rosenfeld RG. Follicle-stimulating hormone inhibits the constitutive release of insulin-like growth factor binding proteins by cultured rat ovarian granulosa cells. *Endocrinology* 1990;126:1305–1307.

325. Seppala M, Wahlstrom T, Koskimies AI, Tenhunen A, Rutanen EM, Koistinen R, Huhtaniemi I, Bohn H, Stenman UH. Human preovulatory follicular fluid, luteinized cells of hyperstimulated preovulatory follicles, and corpus luteum contain placental protein 12. *J Clin Endocrinol Metab* 1984;58:505–510.

326. Rutanen EM, Pekonen F, Makinen T. Soluble 34K binding protein inhibits the binding of insulin-like growth factor I to its cell receptors in human secretory phase endometrium: evidence for autocrine/paracrine regulation of growth factor action. *J Clin Endocrinol Metab* 1988;66:173–180.

327. Giudice LC, Milki AA, Milkowski DA, El-Danasouri I. Human granulosa cells contain messenger ribonucleic acids (mRNAs) encoding insulin-like growth factor binding proteins (IGFBPs) and secrete IGFBPs in culture. *Fertil Steril* 1991;56:475–480.

328. Pekonen F, Laatikainen T, Buyalos R, Rutanen EV. Decreased 34K insulin-like growth factor binding protein in polycystic ovarian disease. *Fertil Steril* 1989;51:972–975.

329. Suikkari AM, Ruutiainen K, Erkkola R, Seppala M. Low levels of low molecular weight insulin-like growth factor-binding protein in patients with polycystic ovarian disease. *Hum Reprod* 1989; 4:136–139.

330. Holly JMP, Eden JA, Alaghband-Zadeh J, Carter GD, Jemmott RC, Cianfarani S, Chard T, Wass JAH. Insulin-like growth factor binding proteins in follicular fluid from normal dominant and cohort follicles, polycystic and multicystic ovaries. *Clin Endocrinol (Oxf)* 1990;33:53–64.

331. Van Wyk JJ, Graves DC, Casella SJ, Jacobs S. Evidence from monoclonal antibody studies that insulin stimulates deoxyribonucleic acid synthesis through the type I somatomedin receptor. *J Clin Endocrinol Metab* 1985;61:639–643.

332. Cataldo NA, Giudice LC: Insulin-like growth factor binding profiles in human ovarian follicular fluid correlate with follicular functional status. *J Clin Endocrinol Metab* 1992;74:821–829.

333. Cataldo NA, Giudice LC. Follicular fluid insulin-like growth factor binding profiles in polycystic ovary syndrome. *J Clin Endocrinol Metab* 1992;74:695–697.

334. Bicsak TA, Shimonaka M, Malkowski M, Ling N. Insulin-like growth factor-binding protein (IGF-BP) inhibition of granulosa cell function: effect of cyclic adenosine 3′,5′-monophosphate, deoxyribonucleic acid synthesis, and comparison with the effect of an IGF-I antibody. *Endocrinology* 1990;126:2184–2189.

335. Hernandez ER, Hurwitz A, Vera A, Pellicel A, Adashi EY, LeRoith D, Roberts CT Jr. Expression of the genes encoding the insulin-like growth factors and their receptors in the human ovary. *J Clin Endocrinol Metab* 1992;74:419–425.

336. Gates GS, Bayer S, Seibel M, Poretsky L, Flier JS, Moses AC. Characterization of insulin-like

growth factor binding to human granulosa cells obtained during in vitro fertilization. *J Recept Res* 1987;7:885–902.

337. Hernandez ER, Resnick CE, Svoboda ME, Van Wyk JJ, Payne DW, Adashi EY. Somatomedin-C/insulin-like growth factor-I as an enhancer of androgen biosynthesis by cultured rat ovarian cells. *Endocrinology* 1988;122:1603–1612.

338. Garzo VG, Dorrington JH. Aromatase activity in human granulosa cells during follicular development and the modulation of follicle-stimulating hormone and insulin. *Am J Obstet Gynecol* 1984; 148:657–662.

339. Suikkari AM, Koivisto VA, Koistinen R, Seppala M, Yki-Jarvineng H. Dose-response characteristics for suppression of low molecular weight plasma insulin-like growth factor-binding protein by insulin. *J Clin Endocrinol Metab* 1989;68:135–140.

340. Conover CA, Lee PDK, Kanaley JA, Clarkson JT, Jensen MD. Insulin regulation of insulin-like growth factor binding protein-1 in obese and nonobese humans. *J Clin Endocrinol Metab* 1992;74: 1355–1360.

341. Urdl W. Polycystic ovarian disease: endocrinological parameters with special reference to growth hormone and somatomedin-C. *Arch Gynecol Obstet* 1988;243:13–36.

342. Rosenfeld RG, Ceda DM, Wilson M, Dollar LA, Hoffman AR. Characterization of high affinity receptors for insulin-like growth factor I and II on rat anterior pituitary cells. *Endocrinology* 1984; 114:1571–1575.

343. Holly JMP, Smith CP, Dunger DB, Howell RJS, Chard T, Perry LA, Savage MO, Cianfarani S, Rees LH, Wass JAH. Relationship between the pubertal fall in sex hormone binding globulin and insulin-like growth factor binding protein-I. A synchronized approach to pubertal development? *Clin Endocrinol (Oxf)* 1989;31:277–284.

344. Franks S. Growth factors: an overview. In: Dunaif A, Givens JR, Haseltine FP, Merriam GR, eds. *Polycystic ovary syndrome.* Cambridge, MA: Blackwell Scientific; 1992:223–227.

345. Ramashara K, Li CH. Human pituitary and placental hormones control human insulin-like growth factor II secretion in human granulosa cells. *Proc Natl Acad Sci USA* 1987;84:2643–2647.

346. Barreca A, Minuto F, Volpe A, Cecchelli E, Cella F, Del Monte P, Artini P, Giordano G. Insulin growth factor-I (IGF-I) and IGF-I binding protein in the follicular fluids of growth hormone treated patients. *Clin Endocrinol (Oxf)* 1990;32:497–505.

347. Laatikainen T. How IGF-I and IGF-I binding protein can be modulated in polycystic ovarian syndrome. In: Tolis G, Bringer J, Chrousos GP, eds. *Intraovarian regulators and polycystic ovarian syndrome: recent progress on clinical and therapeutic aspects.* New York: Annals NY Academy of Sciences (Vol 687); 1993:90–97.

348. Kazer RR, Unterman TG, Glick RL. An abnormality of the growth hormone/insulin-like growth factor-I axis in women with polycystic ovary syndrome. *J Clin Endocrinol Metab* 1990;71:958–962.

349. Kiddy DS, Hamilton-Fairley D, Seppala M, Koistinen R, James VHT, Reed MJ, Franks S. Diet-induced changes in sex hormone binding globulin and free testosterone in women with normal and polycystic ovaries: correlation with insulin and insulin-like growth factor-I. *Clin Endocrinol (Oxf)* 1989;31:757–763.

350. Lanzone A, Fulghesu AM, Pappalardo S, Proto C, Le Donne M, Andreani CL, Muscatello R, Caruso A, Mancuso S. Growth hormone and somatomedin-C secretion in patients with polycystic ovarian disease: their relationships with hyperinsulinism and hyperandrogenism. *Gynecol Obstet Invest* 1990;29:149–153.

351. Yamashita S, Melmed S. Effects of insulin on rat anterior pituitary cells: inhibition of growth hormone secretion and mRNA levels. *Diabetes* 1986;35:440–447.

352. Caufriez A, Goldstein J, Lebrun P, Herschuelz A, Furlanetto R, Copinschi G. Relations between immunoreactive somatomedin C, insulin and T3 patterns during fasting obese subjects. *Clin Endocrinol (Oxf)* 1984;20:65–70.

353. Bar RS, Harrison LC, Muggeo M, Gordon P, Kahn CR, Roth J. Regulation of insulin receptors in normal and abnormal physiology in humans. *Adv Intern Med* 1979;24:23–52.

354. Conway GS, Agrawal R, Betteridge DJ, Jacobs HS. Risk factors for coronary heart disease in lean and obese women with the polycystic ovary syndrome. *Clin Endocrinol (Oxf)* 1992;36:1–7.

355. Siiteri PK. Extraglandular estrogen formation and serum binding of oestradiol: relationship to cancer. *J Endocrinol* 1981;89:119P–129P.

356. McDonald PC, Edman CD, Hemsell DL, Porter JC, Siiteri PK. Effect of obesity on conversion of plasma androstenedione to estrone in post menopausal women with and without endometrial cancer. *Am J Obstet Gynecol* 1978;130:448–455.

357. Kirschner MA, Schneider G, Ertel NH, Worton E. Obesity, androgens, estrogens and cancer risk. *Cancer Res* 1982;42(Suppl):3281s–3285s.

358. Lobo RA, March CM, Goebelsmann U, Mishell Jr RD. The modulating role of obesity and 17β-estradiol (E2) on bound and unbound E2 and adrenal androgens in oophorectomized women. *J Clin Endocrinol Metab* 1982;54:320–324.

359. Jasonni VM, Bulletti C, Ferraretti AP, Franceschetti F, Bolelli GF, Bonavia M, Flamigni C. Metabolic aspects of estrone sulphate in postmenopausal women. In: Jasonni VM, Nenci I, Flamigni C, eds. *Steroids and endometrial cancer*. New York: Raven Press; 1983:157–165.

360. Longcope C. The metabolism of estrone sulfate in normal males. *J Clin Endocrinol Metab* 1972; 34:113–122.

361. Fishman J, Hellman L. Comparative fate of estrone and estrone sulfate in man. *J Clin Endocrinol Metab* 1973;36:160–164.

362. Grodin JM, Siiteri PK, McDonald PC. Source of estrogen production in postmenopausal women. *J Clin Endocrinol Metab* 1973;36:207–214.

363. Deslypere JP, Verdonck L, Vermeulen A. Fat tissue: a steroid reservoir and site of steroid metabolism. *J Clin Endocrinol Metab* 1985;61:564–570.

364. Perel E, Killinger DW. The interconversion and aromatization of androgens by human adipose tissue. *J Steroid Biochem* 1979;10:623–627.

365. Facchinetti F, Livieri L, Petraglia F, Cortona L, Severi F, Genazzani AR. Dexamethasone fails to suppress hyperendorphinemia of obese children. *Acta Endocrinol (Copenh)* 1987;116:90–94.

366. Glass AR, Burman KD, Dahms WT, Boehm TM. Endocrine function in human obesity. *Metabolism* 1981;30:89–104.

367. Grulet H, Hecart AC, Delemer B, Gross A, Sulmont V, Leutenegger M, Caron J. Roles of LH and insulin resistance in lean and obese polycystic ovary syndrome. *Clin Endocrinol (Oxf)* 1993;38: 621–626.

368. Kopelman PG, Pilkington TRE, White N, Jeffcoate SL. Abnormal sex steroid secretion and binding in massively obese women. *Clin Endocrinol (Oxf)* 1980;14:113–116.

369. Pasquali R, Antenucci D, Melchionda N, Fabbri R, Venturoli S, Patrono D, Capelli M. Sex hormones in obese premenopausal women and their relationship to body fat mass and distribution, β-cell function and diet composition. *J Endocrinol Invest* 1987;10:345–350.

370. Plymate SR, Matej LA, Jones RE, Friedl KE. Inhibition of sex hormone-binding globulin production in the human hepatoma (Hep G2) cell line by insulin and prolactin. *J Clin Endocrinol Metab* 1988;67:460–464.

371. Singh A, Hamilton-Fairley D, Koistinen R, Seppala M, James VHT, Franks S, Reed MJ. Effect of insulin-like growth-factor type I (IGF-I) and insulin on the secretion of sex hormone binding globulin and IGF-I binding protein (IBP-I) by human hepatoma cells. *J Endocrinol* 1990;124:R1–R3.

372. Apter D, Bolton NJ, Hammond GL, Vihko R. Serum sex hormone-binding globulin during puberty in girls and in different types of adolescent menstrual cycles. *Acta Endocrinol (Copenh)* 1984;107: 413–418.

373. Evans DJ, Hoffmann RG, Kalkhoff RK, Kissebah AH. Relationship of androgenic activity to body fat topography, fat cell morphology and metabolic aberrations in premenopausal women. *J Clin Endocrinol Metab* 1983;57:304–310.

374. Lapidus L, Bengtsonn C, Larsson B, Penert K, Rybo E, Sjostrom L. Distribution of adipose tissue and risk of cardiovascular disease and death: a twelve year follow up of participants in the population study of women in Gothenburg, Sweden. *Br Med J* 1984;289:1257–1261.

375. Wild R. Consequences and treatment of polycystic ovary syndrome. In: Dunaif A, Givens JR, Haseltine FP, Merriam GR, eds. *Polycystic ovary syndrome*. Cambridge, MA: Blackwell Scientific; 1992:311–317.

376. Kissebah AH, Peiris AN. Biology of regional body fat distribution: relationship to non-insulin dependent diabetes mellitus. *Diabetes Metab Rev* 1988;2:83–109.

377. Kissebah AH, Vydelingum N, Murray R, Evans DJ, Hartz AJ, Kalkhoff RK, Adams PW. Relation of body fat distribution to metabolic complications of obesity. *J Clin Endocrinol Metab* 1982;54: 254–260.

378. Kitabchi AE, Buffington CK, Givens JR, Inouye H. The role of testosterone and dehydroepiandrosterone on insulin resistance and sensitivity in hyperandrogenic females: use of activated T-lymphocytes as an in vitro study model and its correlation to in vivo studies. In: Dunaif A, Givens JR, Haseltine FP, Merriam GR, eds. *Polycystic ovary syndrome*. Cambridge, MA: Blackwell Scientific; 1992:289–305.

379. Freedman DS, Jacobsen SJ, Barboriak JJ, Sobocinski KA, Anderson AJ, Kissebah AH, Sasse EA, Gruchow HW. Body fat distribution and male/female differences in lipids and lipoproteins. *Circulation* 1990;81:1498–1506.
380. Kirschner MA, Bardin CW. Androgen production and metabolism in normal and virilized women. *Metabolism* 1972;21:667–686.
381. Stein IF, Leventhal ML. Amenorrhea associated with bilateral polycystic ovaries. *Am J Obstet Gynecol* 1935;29:181–191.
382. Rogers J, Mitchell GW. The relation of obesity to menstrual disturbances. *N Engl J Med* 1952;247: 53–55.
383. Hartz AJ, Barboriak PN, Wong A, Katayama KP, Rimm AA. The association of obesity with infertility and related menstrual abnormalities in women. *Int J Obes* 1979;3:57–73.
384. Pasquali R, Casamirri F, Antenucci D, Melchionda N, Colombi C, Gaddi D. Relationship between onset of obesity and onset of oligomenorrhea in females with obesity and polycystic ovaries. In: Flamigni C, Venturoli S, Givens JR, eds. *Adolescence in females.* Chicago: Year Book Medical; 1985:363–365.
385. Venturoli S, Porcu E, Fabbri R, Paradisi R, Gammi I, Passarini M, Orsini LF, Flamigni C. Ovarian multifollicularity, high LH and androgen plasma levels, and anovulation are frequent and strongly linked in adolescent irregular cycles. *Acta Endocrinol (Copenh)* 1986;111:368–374.
386. Apter D, Vihko R. Endocrine determinants of fertility: serum androgen concentration during follow-up of adolescence into the third decade of life. *J Clin Endocrinol Metab* 1990;71:970–974.
387. Dunaif A, Graf M, Mandeli J, Laumas U, Dobrjansky A. Characterization of groups of hyperandrogenic women with acanthosis nigricans, impaired glucose tolerance, and/or hyperinsulinemia. *J Clin Endocrinol Metab* 1987;65:499–507.
388. Graf MJ, Richards CJ, Brown V, Meisner L, Dunaif A. The independent effect of hyperandrogenemia, hyperinsulinemia, and obesity on lipid and lipoprotein profiles in women. *Clin Endocrinol (Oxf)* 1990;33:119–131.
389. Kiddy DS, Sharp PS, White DM, Scanlon MF, Mason HD, Bray CS, Polson DW, Reed MJ, Franks S. Differences in clinical and endocrine features between obese and non-obese subjects with polycystic ovary syndrome: an analysis of 263 consecutive cases. *Clin Endocrinol (Oxf)* 1990;32: 213–220.
390. Dunaif A, Mandeli J, Fluhr H, Dobrjansky A. The impact of obesity and chronic hyperinsulinemia on gonadotropin release and gonadal steroid secretion in the polycystic ovary syndrome. *J Clin Endocrinol Metab* 1988;66:131–139.
391. Laatikainen T, Tulenheimo A, Anderson B, Karkkainen A. Obesity, serum steroid levels and pulsatile gonadotropin secretion in polycystic ovary disease. *Eur J Obstet Gynaecol Reprod Biol* 1983;15:45–50.
392. Combes R, Altomare E, Tramoni M, Vague J. Obesity and menstrual disorders. In Mancini M, Lewis B, Contaldo F, eds. *Medical complications of obesity.* London: Academic Press; 1979:285–288.
393. Reshef E, Wild RA. Hyperandrogenic effects on lipid metabolism. *Infertil Reprod Med Clin North Am* 1991;2:599–610.
394. Wild RA, Painter PC, Coulsen RB, Carruth KB, Ranney GB. Lipoprotein lipid concentrations and cardiovascular risk in women with polycystic ovary syndrome. *J Clin Endocrinol Metab* 1985;61: 946–951.
395. Dunaif A, Shelley D, Green G, Dobrjansky A, Licholai T. Evidence for distinctive and intrinsic defects in insulin action in the polycystic ovary syndrome. *Diabetes* 1992;41:1257–1266.
396. Stern MP. Type II diabetes mellitus interface between clinical and epidemiological investigation. *Diabetes Care* 1988;11:119–126.
397. Burghen GA, Givens JR, Kitabchi AE. Correlation of hyperandrogenism with hyperinsulinism in polycystic ovarian disease. *J Clin Endocrinol Metab* 1980;50:113–116.
398. Marshall S, Olefsky JM. Effects of insulin on insulin binding, glucose transport, and insulin degradation by isolated rat adipocytes: evidence for hormone-induced desensitization at the receptor and postreceptor level. *J Clin Invest* 1980;66:763–772.
399. Moller DE, Flier JS. Insulin resistance: mechanisms, syndromes and implications. *N Engl J Med* 1991;325:938–949.
400. Dahlgren E, Johansson S, Linstedt G, Knuttson F, Oden A, Janson PO, Mattson LA, Crona N, Lunberg PE. Women with polycystic ovary syndrome wedge resected in 1956 to 1965: a long-term followup focusing on natural history and circulating hormones. *Fertil Steril* 1992;57:505–513.

401. Conway GS, Clark PM, Wong D, Hales CN. Hyperinsulinaemia in the polycystic ovary syndrome (PCOS) confirmed with specific immunoradiometric (IRMA) assays for insulin, proinsulin and 32–33 split proinsulin. *J Endocrinol* 1991;131(abst 30).
402. Barbieri RL, Hornstein MD. Hyperinsulinemia and ovarian hyperandrogenism. *Endocrinol Metab Clin North Am* 1988;17:685–703.
403. Barbieri RL, Ryan KJ. Hyperandrogenism, insulin resistance, and acanthosis syndrome: a common endocrinopathy with distinct pathophysiological features. *Am J Obstet Gynecol* 1983;147:90–101.
404. Flier JS. Metabolic importance of acanthosis nigricans. *Arch Dermatol* 1985;121:193–194.
405. Stuart CA, Pate CJ, Peters EJ. Prevalence of acanthosis nigricans in an unselected population. *Am J Med* 1989;87:269–272.
406. Stuart CA, Peters EJ, Prince MJ, Richards G, Cavallo A, Meyer WJ. Insulin resistance with acanthosis nigricans: the roles of obesity and androgen excess. *Metabolism* 1986;35:197–205.
407. Flier JS, Eastman RC, Minaker KL, Matteson D, Rowe JW. Acanthosis nigricans in obese women with hyperandrogenism: characterization of an insulin resistant state distinct from the type A and B syndromes. *Diabetes* 1985;34:101–107.
408. Dunaif A, Green G, Phelps RG, Lebwohl M, Futterweit W, Lewy L. Acanthosis nigricans, insulin action and hyperandrogenism: clinical, histological and biochemical findings. *J Clin Endocrinol Metab* 1991;73:590–595.
409. Peters EJ, Stuart CA, Prince MJ. Acanthosis nigricans and obesity: acquired and intrinsic defect in insulin action. *Metabolism* 1986;35:807–813.
410. Cohen P, Harel C, Bergman R, Daoud D, Pam Z, Barzilai N, Armoni M, Karnieli E. Insulin resistance and acanthosis nigricans: evidence for a postbinding defect in vivo. *Metabolism* 1990;39: 1006–1011.
411. Chang RJ, Nakamura RM, Judd HL, Kaplan SA. Insulin resistance in nonobese patients with polycystic ovarian disease. *J Clin Endocrinol Metab* 1983;57:356–359.
412. Smith S, Ravnikar VA, Barbieri RL. Androgen and insulin response to an oral glucose challenge in hyperandrogenic women. *Fertil Steril* 1987;48:72–77.
413. Shoupe D, Kumar DD, Lobo RA. Insulin resistance in polycystic ovary syndrome. *Am J Obstet Gynecol* 1983;147:588–592.
414. Pasquali R, Casimirri F, Venturoli S, Paradisi R, Mattioli L, Capelli M, Melchionda N, Labo G. Insulin resistance in patients with polycystic ovaries: its relationship to body weight and androgen levels. *Acta Endocrinol (Copenh)* 1983;104:110–116.
415. Pasquali R, Fabbri R, Venturoli S, Paradisi R, Antenucci D, Melchionda N. Effect of weight loss and antiandrogenic therapy on sex-hormone blood levels and insulin resistance in obese patients with polycystic ovaries. *Am J Obstet Gynecol* 1986;154:139–144.
416. Bruno B, Poccia G, Fabbrini A. Insulin resistance and secretion in polycystic ovarian disease. *J Endocrinol Invest* 1986;8:443–448.
417. Attila L, Ding YQ, Ruutiainen K, Erkkola R, Irjala K, Huhtaniemie I. Clinical features and circulating gonadotrophin, insulin, and androgen interactions in women and polycystic ovarian disease. *Fertil Steril* 1991;55:1057–1061.
418. Jialal I, Naiker P, Reddi K, Moodley J, Joubert SM. Evidence for insulin resistance in nonobese patients with polycystic ovarian disease. *J Clin Endocrinol Metab* 1987;64:1066–1069.
419. Buyalos RP, Geffner ME, Bersch N, Judd HL, Watanabe RM, Bergman RN, Golde DW. Insulin and insulin-like growth factor-I responsiveness in polycystic ovarian syndrome. *Fertil Steril* 1992; 57:796–803.
420. Tiitinen A, Pekonen F, Stenman UH, Laatikainen T. Plasma androgens and oestradiol during oral glucose tolerance test in patients with polycystic ovaries. *Hum Reprod* 1990;5:242–245.
421. Kinoshita T, Kato J. Impaired glucose tolerance test in patients with polycystic ovary syndrome (PCOS). *Horm Res* 1990;33(Suppl 2):18–20.
422. Sharp PS, Kiddy DS, Reed MJ, Anyaoku V, Johnston DG, Franks S. Correlation of plasma insulin and insulin like growth factor-I with indices of androgen transport and metabolism in women with polycystic ovary syndrome. *Clin Endocrinol (Oxf)* 1991;35:253–257.
423. Kiddy DS, Hamilton-Fairley D, Bush A, Short F, Anyaoku V, Reed MJ, Franks S. Improvement in endocrine and ovarian function during dietary treatment of obese women with polycystic ovary syndrome. *Clin Endocrinol (Oxf)* 1992;36:105–111.
424. Robinson S, Kiddy D, Gelding SV, Willis D, Niththyanananthan R, Bush A, Johnston DG, Franks S. The relationship of insulin insensitivity to menstrual pattern in women with hyperandrogenism and polycystic ovaries. *Clin Endocrinol (Oxf)* 1993;39:351–355.

425. Peiris AN, Aiman EJ, Drucker WD, Kissebah AH. The relative contributions of hepatic and peripheral tissues to insulin resistance in hyperandrogenic women. *J Clin Endocrinol Metab* 1989;68: 715–720.
426. Poretsky L, Grigorescu F, Seibel M, Pazianos A, Moses AC, Flier JS. Specific insulin binding sites in human ovary. *J Clin Endocrinol Metab* 1984;59:809–811.
427. Poretsky L. Role of insulin resistance in the pathogenesis of polycystic ovary syndrome. In: Schoemaker J, Schats R, eds. *Ovarian Endocrinopathies*. London: Parthenon; 1994;169–176.
428. Kopelman PG, White N, Pilkington TRE, Jeffcoate SL. The effect of weight loss on sex steroid secretion and binding in massively obese women. *Clin Endocrinol (Oxf)* 1981;14:133–166.
429. Harlass FE, Plymate SR, Fariss BL, Belts RP. Weight loss is associated with correction of gonadotropin and sex steroid abnormalities in the obese anovulatory female. *Fertil Steril* 1984;42: 649–652.
430. Pasquali R, Antenucci D, Casamirri F, Venturoli S, Paradisi R, Fabbri R, Balestra V, Melchionda N, Barbara L. Clinical and hormonal characteristics of obese amenorrheic hyperandrogenic women before and after weight loss. *J Clin Endocrinol Metab* 1989;68:173–179.
431. Bates GW, Whitworth NS. Effect of body weight reduction on plasma androgens in obese, infertile women. *Fertil Steril* 1982;38:406–409.
432. Grenman S, Ronnemaa T, Irjala K, Kaihola HL, Gronross M. Sex steroid, gonadotropin, cortisol, and prolactin levels in healthy, massively obese women: correlation with abdominal fat cell size and effect of weight reduction. *J Clin Endocrinol Metab* 1986;63:1257–1261.
433. Hamilton-Fairley D, Kiddy D, Anyaoku V, Koistinen R, Seppala M, Franks S. Response of sex hormone binding globulin and insulin-like growth factor binding protein-1 to an oral glucose tolerance test in obese women with polycystic ovary syndrome before and after calorie restriction. *Clin Endocrinol (Oxf)* 1993;39:363–367.
434. Weaver JU, Holly JMP, Kopelman PG, Noonan K, Giadom CG, White N, Virdee S, Wass JAH. Decreased sex hormone-binding globulin (SHBG) and insulin-like growth factor binding protein-1 (IGFBP-1) in extreme obesity. *Clin Endocrinol (Oxf)* 1990;33:415–422.
435. Smith CP, Archibald HR, Thomas JM, Tarn AC, Williams AJK, Gale EAM, Savage MO. Basal and stimulated insulin levels rise with advancing puberty. *Clin Endocrinol (Oxf)* 1988;28:7–14.
436. Dunaif A. Diabetes mellitus and polycystic ovary syndrome. In: Dunaif A, Givens JR, Haseltine FP, Merriam GR, eds. *Polycystic ovary syndrome*. Cambridge, MA: Blackwell Scientific; 1992: 347–358.
437. Dunaif A. Insulin resistance in polycystic ovary syndrome. In: Tolis G, Bringer J, Chrousos GP, eds. *Intraovarian regulators and polycystic ovarian syndrome: recent progress on clinical and therapeutic aspects*. New York: Annals NY Academy of Sciences (Vol 687); 1993:60–64.
438. Dunaif A, Graf M. Insulin administration alters gonadal steroid metabolism independent of changes in gonadotropin secretion in insulin resistant women with the polycystic ovary syndrome. *J Clin Invest* 1989;83:23–29.
439. Ciaraldi TP, El-Roeiy A, Madar Z, Reichart D, Olefsky JM, Yen SSC. Cellular mechanisms of insulin resistance in polycystic ovarian syndrome. *J Clin Endocrinol Metab* 1992;75:577–583.
440. Schwartz LB, Diamond MP. The coexistence of hyperandrogenism and hyperinsulinemia: a relationship between reproductive function and carbohydrate metabolism. *Infertil Reprod Med Clin North Am* 1991;2:611–635.
441. Cole C, Kitabchi AE. Remission of insulin resistance with Orthonovum in a patient with polycystic ovarian disease and acanthosis nigricans. *Clin Res* 1978;26:412A.
442. Woodard TL, Burghen GA, Kitabchi AE, Wilimas JA. Glucose intolerance and insulin resistance in aplastic anemia treated with oxymetholone. *J Clin Endocrinol Metab* 1981;53:905–908.
443. Cohen JC. Hickman R. Insulin resistance and diminished glucose tolerance in powerlifters ingesting anabolic steroids. *J Clin Endocrinol Metab* 1987;64:960–963.
444. Shoupe D, Lobo RA. The influence of androgens on insulin resistance. *Fertil Steril* 1984;41:385–388.
445. Elkind-Hirsch KE, Valdes CT, Malinak LR. Insulin resistance improves in hyperandrogenic women treated with Lupron. *Fertil Steril* 1993;60:634–641.
446. Amiel SA, Sherwin RS, Simonson DC, Lauritano AA, Tamborlane WV. Impaired insulin action in puberty: a contributing factor to poor glycemic control in adolescents with diabetes. *N Engl J Med* 1986;315:215–219.
447. Amiel SA, Caprio S, Sherwin RS, Plewe G, Haymond MW, Tamborlane WV. Insulin resistance of puberty: a defect restricted to peripheral glucose metabolism. *J Clin Endocrinol Metab* 1991;72: 277–282.

448. Kahn CR, Flier JS, Bar RS, Archer JA, Gorden P, Martin MM, Roth J. The syndromes of insulin resistance and acanthosis nigricans: insulin receptor disorders in man. *N Engl J Med* 1976;294: 739–745.

449. Taylor SI, Dons RF, Hernandez E, Roth J, Gorden P. Insulin resistance associated with androgen excess in women with autoantibodies to the insulin receptor. *Ann Intern Med* 1982;97:851–855.

450. Barbieri RL. Effects of insulin on ovarian steroidogenesis. In: Dunaif A, Givens JR, Haseltine FP, Merriam GR, eds. *Polycystic ovary syndrome*. Cambridge, MA: Blackwell Scientific; 1992:249–263.

451. Moller DE, Flier JS. Detection of an alteration in the insulin-receptor gene in a patient with insulin resistance, acanthosis nigricans, and the polycystic ovary syndrome (Type A insulin resistance). *N Engl J Med* 1988;319:1526–1529.

452. Yoshimasa S, Seino S, Whittaker D, Kakehi T, Kosaki A, Kuzuha H, Imura H, Bell GI, Steiner DF. Insulin resistant diabetes due to a point-mutation that prevents insulin proreceptor processing. *Science* 1988;240:784–787.

453. Annos T, Taymor ML. Ovarian pathology associated with insulin resistance and acanthosis nigricans. *Obstet Gynecol* 1981;58:662–664.

454. Nagamani M, Dinh TV, Kelver ME. Hyperinsulinemia in hyperthecosis of the ovaries. *Am J Obstet Gynecol* 1986;154:384–389.

455. Billiar RB, Richardson D, Schwartz R, Posner B, Little B. Effect of chronically elevated androgen or estrogen on the glucose tolerance test and insulin response in female rhesus monkeys. *Am J Obstet Gynecol* 1987;157:1297–1302.

456. Singer F, Bhargava G, Poretsky L. Persistent insulin resistance after normalization of androgen levels in a woman with congenital adrenal hyperplasia: a case report. *J Reprod Med* 1989;34:921–922.

457. Friedl KE, Jones RE, Hannan CJ Jr, Plymate SR. The administration of pharmacological doses of testosterone or 19-testosterone to normal men is not associated with increased insulin secretion or impaired glucose tolerance. *J Clin Endocrinol Metab* 1989;68:971–975.

458. Kaplowitz PB, D'Ercole AJ. Fibroblasts from a patient with leprechaunism are resistant to insulin, epidermal growth factor, and somatomedin C. *J Clin Endocrinol Metab* 1982;55:741–748.

459. Nestler JE, Clore JN, Strauss JF III, Blackard WG. The effects of hyperinsulinemia on serum testosterone, progesterone, dehydroepiandrosterone sulfate and cortisol levels in normal women and in a woman with hyperandrogenism, insulin resistance and acanthosis nigricans. *J Clin Endocrinol Metab* 1987;64:180–184.

460. Declue TJ, Shah SC, Marchese M, Malone JI. Insulin resistance and hyperinsulinemia induce hyperandrogenism in a young type B insulin-resistant female. *J Clin Endocrinol Metab* 1991;72: 1308–1311.

461. Stuart CA, Prince MJ, Peters EJ, Mayer WJ. Hyperinsulinemia and hyperandrogenemia: in vivo responses to insulin infusion. *Obstet and Gynecology* 1987;69:921–925.

462. Micic D, Popovic V, Nesovic M, Sumarac M, Dragasevic M, Kendereski A, Markovic D, Djordjevic P, Manojlovic D, Micic J. Androgen levels during sequential insulin euglycemic clamp studies in patients with polycystic ovary disease. *J Steroid Biochem* 1988;31:995–999.

463. Fox JH, Licholai T, Green G, Dunaif A. Differential effects of oral-glucose mediated intravenous hyperinsulinemia on circulating androgen levels in women. *Fertil Steril* 1993;60:994–1000.

464. Hubert GD, Schriok ED, Givens JR, Buster JE. Suppression of circulating delta-4-androstenedione and dehydroepiandosterone sulfate during oral glucose tolerance test in normal females. *J Clin Endocrinol Metab* 1991;73:781–784.

465. Bonora E, Moghetti P, Zancanano C, Cigolini M, Querena M, Cacciatori V, Corgnati A, Muggeo M. Estimates of in vivo insulin action in man: comparison of insulin tolerance tests with euglycemic and hyperglycemic glucose clamp studies. *J Clin Endocrinol Metab* 1989;68:374–378.

466. Falcone T, Finegood DT, Fantus IG, Morris D. Androgen response to endogenous insulin secretion during the frequently sampled intravenous glucose tolerance test in normal and hyperandrogenic women. *J Clin Endocrinol Metab* 1990;71:1653–1657.

467. Diamond MP, Grainger DK, Landano AJ, Starick-Zydr K, DeFaonzo C. Effect of acute physiological elevations of insulin on circulating androgen levels in nonobese women. *J Clin Endocrinol Metab* 1991;72:883–887.

468. Nestler JE, Clore JN, Blackard WG. Effects of insulin on steroidogenesis in vivo. In: Dunaif A, Givens JR, Haseltine FP, Merriam GR, eds. *Polycystic ovary syndrome*. Cambridge, MA: Blackwell Scientific; 1992:265–278.

469. Schriock ED, Buffington CK, Hubert GD, Kurtz BR, Kitabchi AE, Buster JE, Givens JR. Divergent correlations of circulating dehydroepiandrosterone sulfate and testosterone with insulin levels and insulin receptor binding. *J Clin Endocrinol Metab* 1988;66:1329–1331.
470. Farah MJ, Givens JR, Kitabchi AE. Bimodal correlation between the circulating insulin level and the production rate of dehydroepiandrosterone: positive correlation in controls and negative correlation in the polycystic ovary syndrome with acanthosis nigricans. *J Clin Endocrinol Metab* 1990;70:1075–1081.
471. Nestler JE, Usiskin KS, Barlascini CO, Welty DF, Clore JN, Blackard WG. Suppression of serum dehydroepiandrosterone sulfate levels by insulin: an evaluation of possible mechanisms. *J Clin Endocrinol Metab* 1989;69:1040–1046.
472. Jarrett JC, Ballejo G, Tsibris JCM, Spellacy WN. Insulin binding to human ovaries. *J Clin Endocrinol Metab* 1985;60:460–463.
473. Poretsky L, Bhargava G, Kalin MF, Wolf SA. Regulation of insulin receptors in the human ovary: in vitro studies. *J Clin Endocrinol Metab* 1988;67:774–778.
474. Hernandez ER, Resnick ER, Holtzclaw DW, Payne DW, Adashi EY. Insulin as a regulator of androgen biosynthesis by cultured rat ovarian cells: cellular mechanism(s) underlying physiological and pharmacological hormonal actions. *Endocrinology* 1988;122:2034–2043.
475. Nestler JE, Powers LP, Matt DW, Steingold KA, Plymate SR, Rittmaster RS, Clore JN, Blackard WG. A direct effect of hyperinsulinemia on serum sex hormone-binding globulin levels in obese women with polycystic ovary syndrome. *J Clin Endocrinol Metab* 1991;72:83–89.
476. Glickman SP, Rosenfield RL, Bergenstal RM, Helke J. Multiple androgenic abnormalities, including elevated free testosterone, in hyperprolactinemic women. *J Clin Endocrinol Metab* 1982;55: 251–257.
477. Moll GW Jr, Rosenfield RL, Helke JH. Estradiol–testosterone binding interactions and free plasma estradiol under physiological conditions. *J Clin Endocrinol Metab* 1981;52:868–874.
478. Rosenfield RL, Fang VS, Dupon C, Kim MH, Refetoff S. The effects of low doses of depot estradiol and testosterone in teenagers with ovarian failure and Turner's syndrome. *J Clin Endocrinol Metab* 1973;37:574–580.
479. Hall K, Brismar K, Grissom F, Lindgren B, Povoa G. IGF BP-1: production and control mechanism. *Acta Endocrinol (Copenh)* 1991;124:48–54.
480. Holly JMP. The physiological role of IGFBP-1. *Acta Endocrinol (Copenh)* 1991;124:55–62.
481. Conway GS, Jacobs HS, Holly JMP, Wass JAH. Effects of luteinizing hormone, insulin, insulin-like growth factor-I and insulin like growth factor small binding protein I in the polycystic ovary syndrome. *Clin Endocrinol (Oxf)* 1990;33:593–603.
482. Hammond JM, Baranao JLS, Skaleris D, Knight AB, Romanus JA, Rechler MM. Production of insulin-like growth factors by ovarian granulosa cells. *Endocrinology* 1985;117:2553–2555.
483. Veldhuis JD, Rodgers RR, Furdanetto RW, Azimi P, Juckter D, Garmey J. Synergistic actions on estradiol and the insulin-like growth factor/somatomedin-C on swine ovarian granulosa cells. *Endocrinology* 1986;119:530–538.
484. Adashi EY, Resnick CE, Svoboda ME, Van Wyk JJ, Hascall VC, Masaki Y. Independent and synergistic actions of somatomedin-C in the stimulation of proteoglycan biosysnthesis by cultured rat granulosa cells. *Endocrinology* 1986;118:456–458.
485. Fradkin JE, Eastman RC, Lesniak MA, Roth J. Specificity spillover at the hormone receptor: exploring its role in human disease. *N Engl J Med* 1989;320:640–645.
486. Soos MA, Siddle K. Immunological relationships between receptors for insulin and insulin-like growth factor I. Evidence for structural heterogeneity of insulin-like growth factor I receptor involving hybrids with insulin receptors. *Biochem J* 1989;263:553–563.
487. Treadway JL, Morrison BD, Goldfine ID, Pessin JE: Assembly of insulin/insulin-like growth factor-I hybrid receptors in vitro. *J Biol Chem* 1989;264:21450–21453.
488. Poretsky L, Bhargava G, Saketos M, Dunaif A. Regulation of human ovarian insulin receptors in-vivo. *Metabolism* 1990;39:161–166.
489. Adashi EY, Hsueh A, Yen SSC. Insulin enhancement of luteinizing hormone and follicle-stimulating hormone release by cultured pituitary cells. *Endocrinology* 1981;108:1441–1449.
490. Adashi EY, Resnick CE, Hernandez ER, Svoboda ME, Van Wyk JJ. Potential relevance of insulin-like growth factor I to ovarian physiology: from basic science to clinical application. *Semin Reprod Endocrinol* 1989;7:94–103.
491. Futterweit W. Genetics of polycystic ovarian disease. In: *Polycystic ovarian disease*. New York: Springer-Verlag; 1984:47–48.

492. Wilroy RS, Givens JR, Wiser WL, Coleman SA, Andersen RN, Summitt RL. Hyperthecosis: an inheritable form of polycystic ovarian disease. *Birth Defects (Series XI)* 1975:81–85.
493. Cohen PN, Givens JR, Wiser WL, Wilroy RS, Summitt RL, Coleman SA, Andersen RN. Polycystic ovarian disease, maturation arrest of spermiogenesis and Klinefelter's syndrome in siblings of a family with familial hirsutism. *Fertil Steril* 1975;26:1228–1238.
494. Ferriman D, Purdie AW. The inheritance of PCO and possible relationship to premature balding. *Clin Endocrinol (Oxf)* 1979;11:291–300.
495. Parker R, Ming PLL, Rajan R, Goodner DM, Reme A. Clinical and cytogenetic studies of patients with polycystic ovary disease. *Am J Obstet Gynecol* 1980;137:656–659.
496. Hague WM, Adams J, Reeders ST, Peto TEA, Jacobs HS. Familial polycystic ovaries: a genetic disease? *Clin Endocrinol (Oxf)* 1988;29:593–605.
497. Lunde O, Magnus P, Sandvik L, Hoglo S. Familial clustering in the polycystic ovarian syndrome. *Gynecol Obstet Invest* 1989;28:23–30.
498. Friedman CI, Richards S, Kim MH. Familial acanthosis nigricans: a longitudinal study. *J Reprod Med* 1987;32:531–536.
499. Sagle M, Bishop K, Ridley N, Alexander FM, Michel M, Bonney RC, Beard RW, Franks S. Recurrent early miscarriage and polycystic ovaries. *Br Med J* 1989;297:1027–1028.
500. Franks S. The ubiquitous polycystic ovary. *J Endocrinol* 1991;129:317–319.
501. Bouchard C. Genetic aspects of human obesity. In: Bjorntorp P, Brodoff BN, eds. *Obesity.* Philadelphia: JB Lippincott; 1992:343–351.

Androgenic Disorders,
edited by G. P. Redmond.
Raven Press, Ltd., New York © 1995.

7

Ovarian Pathology in Androgenic Disorders

Shu-Yuan Liao

*Department of Medicine, College of Medicine, University of California,
Irvine, California 92717.*

One of two major functions of the ovary is the secretion of the steroid hormones estrogen, progesterone, and androgen. The theca cell and stroma, including the hilar cells, are the main sources of androgen secretion in the normal ovary. Not all the factors that influence androgen secretion are fully understood, but it is at least in part regulated or enhanced by the anterior pituitary gonadotropin, luteinizing hormone (LH), and human chorionic gonadotropin (hCG). Recent data suggest that insulin and insulin-like growth factor I are also engaged in the regulation of ovarian androgen production (1,2).

The principal ovarian androgens are testosterone and androstenedione, but dehydroepiandrosterone and other weaker androgens are also secreted in small quantities by the ovary. In premenopausal women, the estrogen is primarily derived from the theca cell as androstenedione and then converted to estradiol by the granulosa cell. Only small amounts of ovarian androgen are secreted into the circulation. After menopause the ovary continues to produce testosterone and, to a lesser degree, androstenedione. Ovarian androgen secretion combines with adrenal secretion to make up the total circulatory pool of androgen in normal women. After cessation of follicular activity, the cellular sources of these hormones are uncertain, but in vitro and in vivo studies indicate that the ovarian stroma retains its steroidogenic potential and gonadotropin responsiveness in postmenopausal subjects (3,4,5). Therefore, it can be concluded that the ovarian stroma is responsible for androgen production. In fact, stromal hyperplasia is not an uncommon phenomenon observed in normal postmenopausal women.

Under certain circumstances, when there is abnormal proliferation, either reactive or neoplastic, of lutein cells, stromal cells, or hilar cells (pure or varied in combination), an excess amount of androgen is secreted. The term ovarian hyperandrogenism is applied to this condition. Patients with very severe ovarian hyperandrogenism usually present with a history of rapid or progressive onset of virilization of varying degrees with an accompanying palpable or nonpalpable ovarian mass. The first clinical sign of androgenic syndrome is usually oligomenorrhea, followed by amenorrhea, defeminization, atrophy of the breasts, loss of body con-

TABLE 1. *Ovarian pathology in androgenic disorders*

Nontumorous lesions in nonpregnant women
  Polycystic ovary disease
  Stromal hyperthecosis
  Massive ovarian edema
Nontumorous lesions in pregnant women
  Luteoma of pregnancy
  Hyperreactio luteinalis
Androgen-producing tumors
  Sertoli-Leydig cell tumor (androblastoma)
  Steroid cell tumors
    Stromal luteoma
    Leydig cell tumors (hilar, nonhilar types)
    Steroid cell tumor, not otherwise specified
Ovarian tumors with functional stroma
  Germ cell tumors containing syncytiotrophoblast
  Tumors in pregnant women
  Idiopathic group

tours, acne, and hirsutism. Later, deepening of the voice, clitoral enlargement, and recession of the hair line occur. In most cases, ovarian hyperandrogenism produces more moderate changes, as discussed elsewhere in this book.

The plasma testosterone level in ovarian hyperandrogenism is typically elevated, but urinary 17-ketosteroid is normal or slightly elevated. In adrenal disorders, the adrenal cortex often secretes mainly weak androgens: androstenedione, dehydro-epiandrosterone, and urinary 17-kestosteroid levels are high. In other instances of adrenal androgen excess, testosterone may be elevated.

Ovarian pathology in androgenic disorders can generally be divided into four major groups: nontumorous lesions in nonpregnant women, nontumorous lesions in pregnant women, androgen-producing tumors, and ovarian tumors with functional stroma. Several subtypes are encountered in each major group (Table 1). The clinicopathology and pathophysiology of these groups of lesions have been described in detail elsewhere (6,7,8). Only the most common salient clinicopathologic features will be discussed in this chapter.

NONTUMOROUS LESIONS IN NONPREGNANT WOMEN WITH HYPERANDROGENISM

Polycystic Ovary Disease (PCO)

This is a common idiopathic disorder and most likely reflects a spectrum of related disorders that is considerably broader than the syndrome initially defined by Stein and Leventhal in 1935 (9). The disorder is clinicopathologically characterized by chronic anovulation, sclerocystic ovaries, associated inappropriate gonadotropin secretion, and increased peripheral conversion of androgen to estrogen (7,9,10). Affected patients often present in their third decade with a history of premenarchal obesity, oligomenorrhea, infertility, and hirsutism, often with onset in adolescence. Virilization is rare. The pathophysiology of PCO is complex and poorly understood,

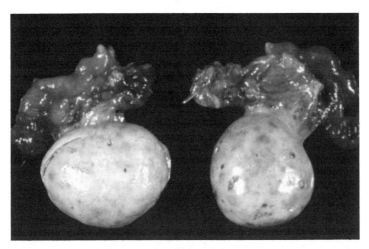

FIG. 1. Polycystic ovary. Follicle cysts are visible through the smooth surface of the enlarged, rounded ovaries.

but at least it is known that the luteinized theca cells and stromal cells induced by abnormal levels of plasma LH are a source of excess androgen (11).

Pathologic features. Both ovaries are typically rounded and two to five times normal size, but on rare occasions their size may be normal (Fig. 1). The cut surfaces reveal multiple follicle cysts in the outer cortex beneath a thickened, white, superficial zone associated with a central mass of stroma, with a few or no stigmata of ovulation (corpora lutea or albicantia) (Fig. 2). Three major changes are observed microscopically: (a) collagenization of the outer cortex; (b) cystic or atretic follicles

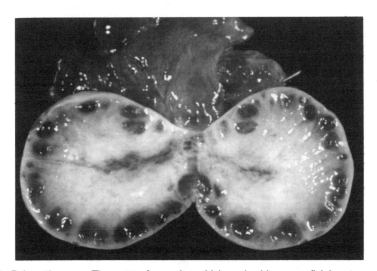

FIG. 2. Polycystic ovary. The cut surfaces show thickened, white, superficial cortex, adjacent multiple follicle cysts, and a central mass of stroma.

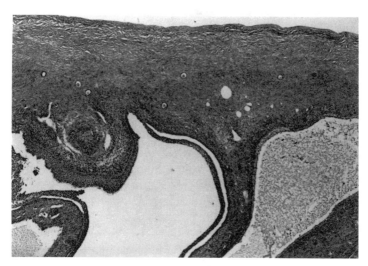

FIG. 3. Polycystic ovary. Follicle cysts are situated beneath a zone of fibrotic superficial cortex. (H&E stain, ×40.)

with a thickened layer of luteinized theca interna cells (follicular hyperthecosis); (c) varying degrees of proliferation of the medullary stromal cells, which occasionally contain foci of lutein cells (7,11) (Figs. 3,4). However, sclerocystic ovaries similar to PCO may also represent a nonspecific morphologic expression of chronic anovulation resulting in other disorders (i.e., adrenal, pituitary, or ovarian lesions). On rare occasions, adrenal disorders can give rise to classic clinicopathologic find-

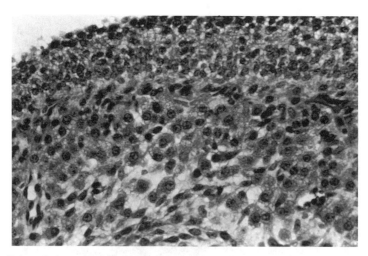

FIG. 4. Polycystic ovary. The cystic follicle is lined by an inner layer of nonluteinized granulosa cells and an outer thicker layer of luteinized theca interna cells. (H&E stain, ×400.)

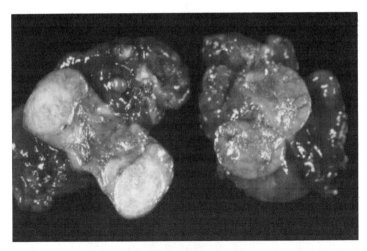

FIG. 5. Stromal hyperplasia and stromal hyperthecosis. The cut surfaces of both ovaries are solid, homogenous, and have white to yellow color in the unfixed state.

ings of PCO as well (12,13). It should also be noted that most normal prepubertal ovaries have a sclerocystic appearance (14). Treatment of PCO is complex and is discussed in detail in Chapter 14. The associated infertility has been treated with wedge resection of the ovary (now rarely used) or clomiphene citrate or gonadotropin administration.

Stromal Hyperplasia (SH) and Hyperthecosis (SHT)

This is a condition in which both ovaries are enlarged due to varying degrees of nonneoplastic proliferation of stromal cells. The term stromal hyperthecosis refers to the finding of accompanying focal luteinization of the stromal cells. Both SH and SHT are most commonly encountered in postmenopausal women who are over the sixth decade of life. Varying degrees of virilization have also been observed (15). However, florid examples of SHT are more common in patients in a younger reproductive age group. These patients characteristically exhibit marked virilization, obesity, hypertension, a disturbed glucose tolerance and, less commonly, clinical findings more characteristic of PCO (16). The serum levels of testosterone and androstenedione are usually markedly elevated, but, unlike PCO, the gonadotropin levels are normal.

Pathologic features. Both ovaries are enlarged, and sometimes the size can be up to 7 cm in diameter. The cut surfaces are homogeneous, firm, and white to yellow (Fig. 5). Microscopically, the cortex and medulla are replaced by proliferated stromal cells arranged in nodular or diffuse patterns (Fig. 6). Clusters of luteinized stromal cells are typically found in SHT (Fig. 7). Immunohistochemical studies have also demonstrated the presence of testosterone, estradiol, and follicle stimulating hormone (FSH), but not LH in the luteinized stromal cells (17).

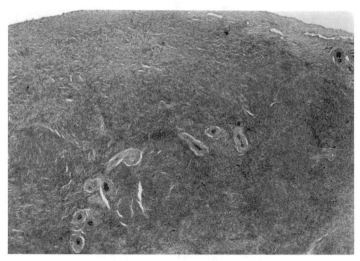

FIG. 6. Stromal hyperplasia. The cortex and medulla are replaced by hyperplastic stromal cells in a diffuse pattern. (H&E stain, × 40.)

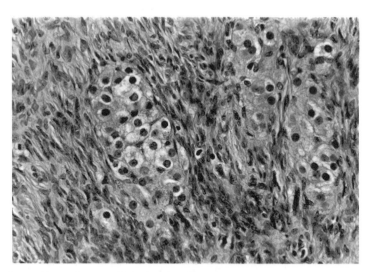

FIG. 7. Stromal hyperthecosis. Clusters of luteinized stromal cells are seen within the hyperplastic ovarian stroma. (H&E stain, × 400.)

Clinicopathologically there is an overlap between SHT and PCO, but the former has little or no response to wedge resection of the ovary or clomiphene treatment. Patients with SH or SHT usually require bilateral oophorectomy to halt progressive virilization.

Massive Ovarian Edema

Approximately 20% of patients with massive ovarian edema exhibit clinical signs and symptoms of hirsutism or virilization (18,19). The lesion typically occurs in young patients ranging in age from 6 to 33 years. The pathogenesis of the disorder is not fully understood. It is most likely related to interference of the blood circulation by intermittent partial torsion of the mesovarium, resulting in accumulation of edema fluid in the ovarian stroma. Stromal lutein cells are observed in 40% of cases and are the source of androgen. The luteinization probably represents either a secondary phenomenon, due to stimulation by the edema fluid containing possible LH-like substance, or a pre-existing stromal hyperthecosis (19,20,21).

Pathologic features. The enlarged ovary is soft and fluctuant. The size ranges from 5 cm to 35 cm and the cut surfaces are white, gelatinous, and sometimes hemorrhagic (Fig. 8). Bilateral involvement is occasionally encountered. The striking histologic finding is a marked diffuse stromal edema that usually spares the superficial cortex. Luteinized stromal cells are observed scattered throughout the stroma (Figs. 9,10).

Most of the reported patients with massive ovarian edema have been treated with

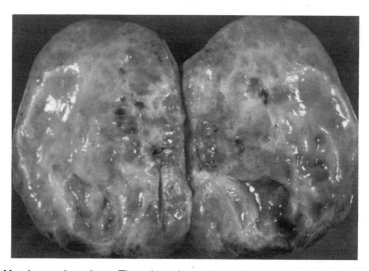

FIG. 8. Massive ovarian edema. The enlarged ovary has solid, edematous cut surfaces.

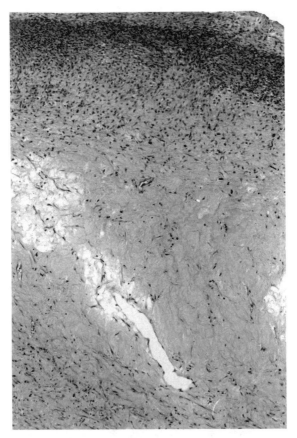

FIG. 9. Massive ovarian edema. The ovarian stromal cells are widely separated by edematous fluid, but the superficial cortex is not involved. (H&E stain, ×40.)

oophorectomy, but there are a small number in which the enlarged ovary returns to normal size simply by wedge resection. Therefore, intraoperative recognition of the disorder is important in order to avoid unnecessary surgery.

NONTUMOROUS LESIONS IN PREGNANT WOMEN WITH HYPERANDROGENISM

Pregnancy Luteoma

This lesion represents nonneoplastic, solid proliferation of luteinized cells. The pathogenesis is not completely clear, but the condition appears dependent on hCG for its structural and functional integrity. A pre-existing endocrinopathy (such as stromal hyperthecosis or PCO) may predispose to the development of the lesion in some patients (7). The patients are usually in their third or fourth decade and are

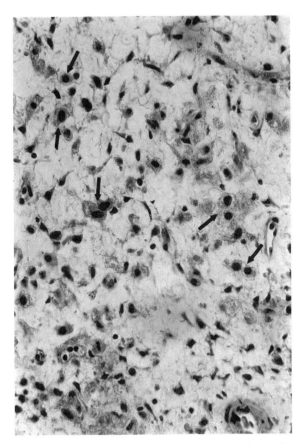

FIG. 10. Massive ovarian edema. Luteinized stromal cells (*arrow*) are dispersed within the edematous stroma. (H&E stain, × 400.)

black in 80% of cases; multiparity is seen in 80% of cases. The enlarged ovary is incidentally discovered at the time of cesarean section or tubal ligation during the third trimester of pregnancy. Approximately 100 cases have been reported and in one-quarter of the cases the patient has become hirsute or virilized. At least two-thirds of the offspring also show masculinization (6,7).

Pathologic features. The size of pregnancy luteoma varies from microscopic to over 20 cm in diameter. Both ovaries are involved in one-third of cases, and half present as multiple nodules. The nodules are well-circumscribed and have solid, yellow to red to brown cut surfaces. Microscopically, the nodule is composed of luteinized cells which have abundant eosinophilic cytoplasm, with little or nonstainable lipid (Figs. 11,12). Mitotic activity is usually present.

There are numbers of benign or malignant conditions such as thecomas, steroid cell tumors, or metastatic carcinomas which may also occur during pregnancy and have a gross appearance similar to pregnancy luteomas. The differential diagnosis

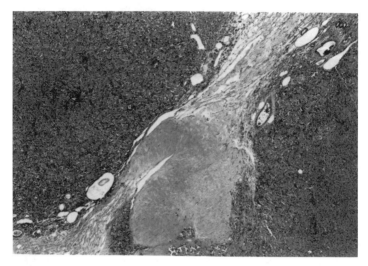

FIG. 11. Pregnancy luteoma. Two solid nodules of luteinized cells are seen in the ovarian stroma. (H&E stain, × 40.)

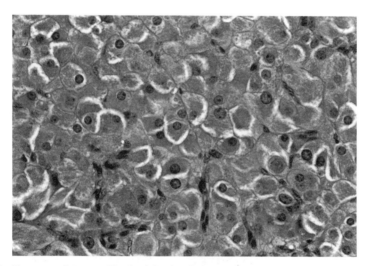

FIG. 12. Pregnancy luteoma. The luteinized cells have abundant eosinophilic cytoplasm with slight variation in nuclear size. (H&E stain, × 400.)

can usually be made by excisional biopsy of one nodule. Therefore, frozen section of the nodule during surgery is necessary in order to establish the diagnosis and preserve the remaining ovarian tissue. The lesions always spontaneously regress and the ovary returns to normal size within several weeks after delivery.

Hyperreactio Luteinalis (HL)

This condition is most commonly associated with a high level of circulating hCG resulting from intrinsic disorders such as molar pregnancy, choriocarcinoma, Rh sensitization with fetal hydrops, and multiple gestation (6,22), but 60% of cases of HL unassociated with gestational trophoblastic disease have accompanied a single normal pregnancy (23). Occasionally the lesion is produced by extrinsic factors such as the administration of ovulation-inducing drugs (Clomid or some form of FSH followed by hCG) (24). The latter is referred to as ovarian hyperstimulation syndrome (an iatrogenic form of HL).

Pathologic features. There is usually moderate to massive enlargement of both ovaries due to the presence of numerous luteinized follicle cysts and/or corpora lutea with marked edema of the stroma. The cysts may be filled with clear or hemorrhagic fluid (Fig. 13). Microscopically, there is striking luteinization of the theca interna layer, and sometimes of granulosa cells, in and around the follicle cysts (Fig. 14). Stromal luteinization sometimes can be prominent. The luteinized theca cells or stromal cells are most likely responsible for the elevation of plasma testosterone and signs of virilization which are observed in 25% of cases unassociated with trophoblastic disease. However, the offspring are not affected (25).

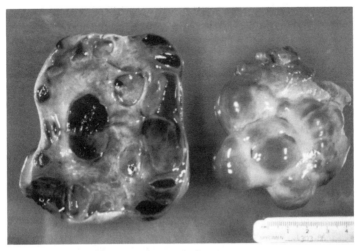

FIG. 13. Hyperreactio luteinalis. The enlarged cystic ovaries have multiple thin-walled follicle cysts within the cortex (*left*). Some of the cysts are hemorrhagic.

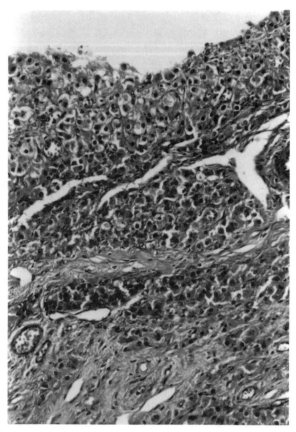

FIG. 14. Hyperreactio luteinalis. The cyst lining consists of luteinized granulosa cells (*top*), surrounded by a thicker layer of luteinized theca cells. Note: lutein cells are also present in the ovarian stroma (*bottom*). (H&E stain, ×100.)

Clinically, the symptoms may occur during any of the three trimesters, or after ovulation when it is induced by drugs. The lesion usually regresses during puerperium, or within a few weeks after conservative therapy in an iatrogenic form of HL. Surgical intervention is necessary only in rare patient with torsion or rupture of the cyst, or to diminish androgen production in virilized patients.

ANDROGEN-PRODUCING TUMORS

Almost all of the androgenic tumors are composed of theca cells and their luteinized derivatives: Sertoli cells, Leydig cells, and fibroblasts of gonadostromal origin, as pure cell type or in various combinations. There are two major categories: Sertoli-Leydig cell tumors and steroid cell tumors.

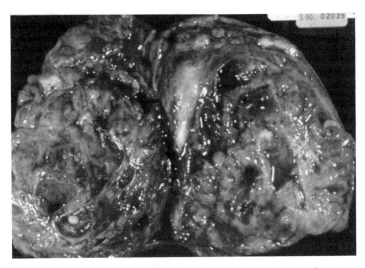

FIG. 15. Sertoli-Leydig cell tumor. The enlarged ovary has lobulated yellow-brown cut surfaces in the unfixed state, in which small cystic areas are present.

Sertoli-Leydig Cell Tumors (SLCTs)

These tumors account for less than 0.2% of ovarian neoplasms. Greater than 75% of patients are in the reproductive age group with the average age at diagnosis being 25 to 30 years. Only 10% of cases are encountered in patients over 50 years of age (26). Clinically, the patients usually present with a palpable pelvic mass and typical androgenic syndrome, which is observed in approximately 50% of cases.

Pathologic features. The enlarged ovary commonly has solid, yellow-brown cut surfaces with occasional blood-filled cyst formations (Fig. 15). The unilocular, thin-walled cyst has never been described. The histology of the tumors is divided into five categories in the new World Health Organization classification: well-differentiated (Fig. 16), intermediate differentiation (Fig. 17), poorly differentiated (Fig. 18), retiform (Fig. 19), and mixed. The well-differentiated lesion is composed of hollow or solid tubules lined by, or filled with, benign-appearing Sertoli cells and separated by variable numbers of Leydig cells. The poorly differentiated SLCTs in general resemble an unclassified sarcoma with focal Sertoli or Leydig cell differentiation. Tumors with glandular formation simulating the rete of the testis are designated as SLCTs with retiform pattern and are almost always accompanied by an otherwise typical intermediate or poorly-differentiated group. The lesions are commonly encountered in a younger age group than other subtypes (27,28). In approximately 20% of the cases, the tumors may contain heterologous elements. Mucinous epithelium of the gastrointestinal type is most commonly encountered (Fig. 20), but mesenchymal components such as skeletal muscle, cartilage, etc., mature or immature, have also been described. Most of the tumors with heterologous elements are

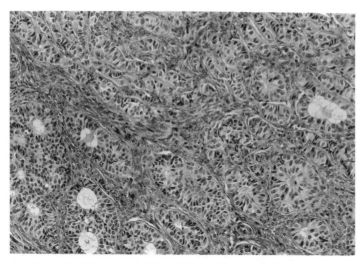

FIG. 16. Sertoli-Leydig cell tumor, well differentiated. Hollow or solid tubules are lined by Sertoli cells and separated by ovarian stroma in which Leydig cells are seen (*arrow*). (H&E stain, ×100.)

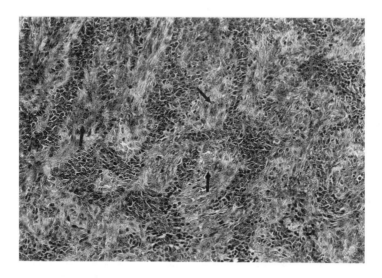

FIG. 17. Sertoli-Leydig cell tumor of intermediate differentiation. Anastomosing columns of immature Sertoli cells and clusters of Leydig cells in the intervening stroma are present. (H&E stain, ×100.)

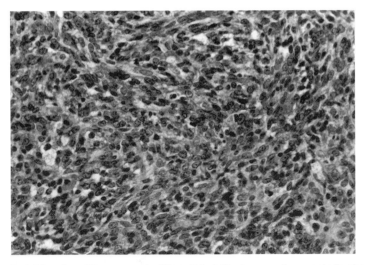

FIG. 18. Sertoli-Leydig cell tumor, poorly differentiated. The tumor cells are spindle-shaped and exhibit nuclear atypia and mitotic activity. (H&E stain, × 400.)

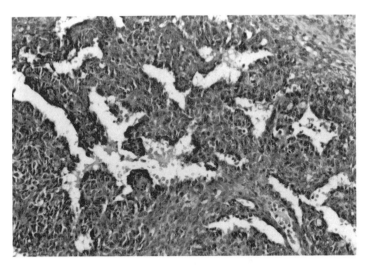

FIG. 19. Sertoli-Leydig cell tumor with retiform pattern. The retiform tubules are lined by epithelial cells and surrounded by immature mesenchymal tissue. (H&E stain, × 200.)

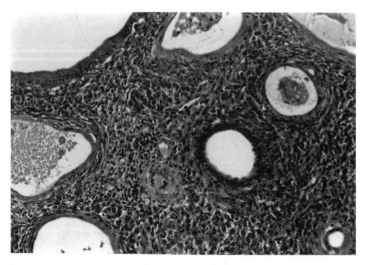

FIG. 20. Sertoli-Leydig cell tumor with heterologous elements. The mucinous glands are separated by ill-defined aggregates of Sertoli cells with intermediate differentiation. (H&E stain, ×200.)

of intermediate differentiation, but some are poorly differentiated with a retiform pattern, or are mixed (29,30).

In general, SLCTs are of low-grade malignancy. The prognosis is closely related to the clinical stage and degree of differentiation. No well-differentiated SLCTs have been reported as clinically malignant. The majority of recurrent or fatal tumors have been observed in one of three categories: poorly-differentiated tumor, those with mesenchymal heterologous elements, and those with a predominant retiform component (31). Overall, the incidence of malignancy is 13% and five-year survival rates reported in the literature have ranged from under 70% to over 90% (7,8). These tumors occur predominantly in young women and are bilateral in fewer than 1.5% of cases. Unilateral salpingo-oophorectomy can be offered for clinical stage Ia disease (7,26).

Steroid Cell Tumors

The designation of steroid cell tumors has been recently proposed to apply to the group of tumors formerly known as lipid or lipoid cell tumors. The tumors are composed exclusively of cells resembling steroid hormone-secreting cells: lutein cells, Leydig cells, and adrenal cortical cells. Depending on the presumed cell of origin, the tumors are subclassified into three major categories: stromal luteoma, Leydig cell tumors (hilar and nonhilar types), and steroid cell tumors not otherwise specified (NOS) (7,32–34). Clinically, virilization has been found in 10% of stromal luteoma, 80% of Leydig cell tumors, and 50% of steroid cell tumors NOS. The

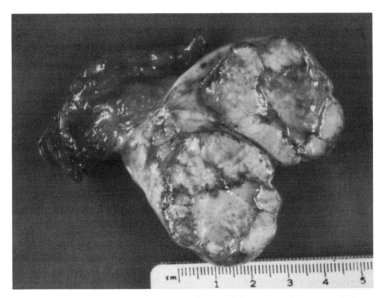

FIG. 21. Steroid cell tumor. The sectioned surfaces of the ovary show a well-circumscribed mass with an area of degeneration. The color is golden yellow to brown in the unfixed state.

former two categories tend to occur in postmenopausal women, but the steroid cell tumors NOS usually affect younger patients (mean age 43 years) (34) and occasionally occur in children. The plasma testosterone level is typically elevated and the urine 17-ketosteroid level is usually normal or slightly elevated. Occasionally, some steroid cell tumors NOS may functionally resemble adrenal cortical tumors with clinical manifestation of adrenogenital syndrome or Cushing's syndrome (35).

Pathologic features. In general, these tumors are rarely bilateral, and the gross appearance is almost always solid, with the color ranging from golden yellow to dark brown (Fig. 21). Microscopically the steroid cell tumors of all types disclose generally similar features. The neoplastic cells have abundant cytoplasm which is pink and granular in luteoma (Fig. 22) and Leydig cell tumors (Fig. 23), but is more foamy due to the content of lipid in steroid cell tumor NOS (Fig. 24). Leydig cell tumors are diagnosed only when the pathognomonic Reinke crystals are identified in the cytoplasm of neoplastic cells (Fig. 23). The majority of Leydig cell tumors are localized in the hilus of the ovary. The nonhilar type is extremely rare and is thought to directly derive from the ovarian stromal cells (36).

There are no convincing examples of malignant stromal luteoma or Leydig cell tumors (hilar type). However, approximately 25% to 40% of steroid cell tumors in the NOS category are clinically malignant, and are more frequently encountered in older patients. Most malignant tumors are larger than 7 cm and tend to show hemorrhage, necrosis, nuclear atypia, and increased mitotic activity (>2/10 HPFS) (34). Because of the rare bilaterality, conservative treatment is usually applied for benign lesions.

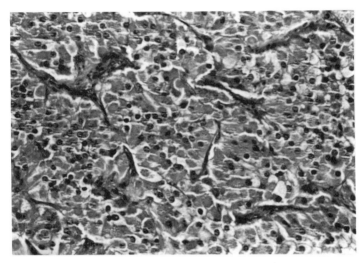

FIG. 22. Stromal luteoma. Nests of polygonal eosinophilic tumor cells are separated by a thin fibrovascular network. (H&E stain, ×200.)

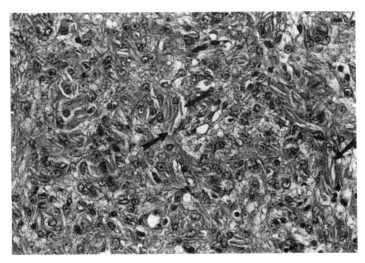

FIG. 23. Leydig cell tumor. Solid sheets of polygonal eosinophilic cells in which pathognomonic crystals of Reinke are identified (*arrow*). (H&E stain, ×200.)

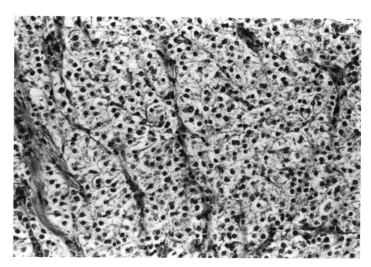

FIG. 24. Steroid cell tumor NOS. The lipid-rich steroid type cells with clear cytoplasm are arranged diffusely. (H&E stain, ×200.)

OVARIAN TUMORS WITH FUNCTIONAL STROMA ASSOCIATED WITH HYPERANDROGENISM

There are a number of nonfunctional ovarian tumors associated with hirsutism or virilization due to an excess of androgen produced by luteinized stromal cells, so-called functional stroma. The mechanisms which regulate why some neoplasms, and not others, may cause virilization, are unknown. Several hypotheses have been proposed: (a) Certain tumors induce mitotic activity in stromal cells, and post-mitotic cells are highly responsive to various stimuli such as luteinizing hormone (37); (b) The expanding tumor exerts pressure on the stroma and induces a reaction similar to theca cell formation surrounding a developing follicle (38,39); and (c) The neoplastic cells produce hCG which induces luteinized stromal cells. By immunohistochemical studies, hCG has been identified in tumor cells of 6% to 42% of common epithelial tumors of the ovary (40,41,42).

This group of tumors can basically be divided into three major categories (43): (a) germ cell tumors containing syncytiotrophoblast cells that produce hCG, (b) tumors in pregnant patients, and (c) an idiopathic group. The last group accounts for the majority of cases with hyperandrogenism. Although most tumors with functional stroma are estrogenic, in a study of 24 functioning ovarian tumors with peripheral steroid cell proliferation, androgenic manifestations were found in 42% of the patients (44). Almost all types of common epithelial ovarian tumors may be associated with stromal activation, but endocrine manifestations are seen with significant frequency only in patients with mucinous tumors. In rare instances, struma ovarii,

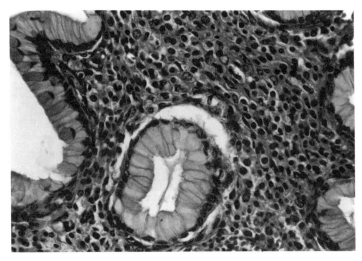

FIG. 25. Mucinous cystadenoma with functional stroma. The mucinous glands are separated by masses of luteinized stromal cells. (H&E stain, ×400.)

stromal carcinoid, dermoid cyst, Brenner tumor, and cyst of rete ovary origin have been reported (44). In metastatic carcinoma with virilization, the most common type of tumor is Krukenberg's tumor of gastric origin, although cases of breast, appendix, and colon have also been reported.

Pathologic features. The ovary reveals varying degrees of stromal cell proliferation accompanying epithelial tumors. The stromal cells typically have abundant

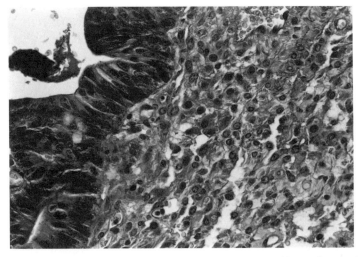

FIG. 26. Metastatic colonic adenocarcinoma with functional stroma. The malignant glands are surrounded by a band of luteinized stromal cells. (H&E stain, ×400.)

eosinophilic cytoplasm, which resembles lutein or Leydig cells. Sometimes Reinke crystals characteristic of Leydig cells are found. These cells are almost always distributed within the tumor singly, diffusely, or in clusters (Figs. 25,26). On rare occasions, these luteinized stromal cells may form a peripheral band outside the tumor mass (44). However, it is worthwhile to mention that the presence of steroid-type cells is not always associated with hormone overproduction and steroid type cells may not be prominent in tumors with functional stroma.

Clinical management of these tumors with functional stroma is the same as that of tumors without functional stroma. Abnormal endocrine manifestations usually disappear after the ovarian tumor is removed.

CONCLUSIONS

The pathologies mentioned above are the most commonly encountered lesions associated with hyperandrogenism. However, on occasion, other tumors that usually secrete estrogens may be androgen-secreting, and vice versa. Among these estrogenic tumors, granulosa cell tumors and thecomas with androgenic manifestations have been described.

As noted previously, lutein cells and luteinized stromal cells, including Leydig cells and hilar cells of the ovary, are the cellular sources of excess androgen, in which the main components are testosterone and small quantities of androstenedione. Therefore, accurate measurement of testosterone and urinary 17-ketosteroids usually will aid in the correct diagnosis of androgen-secreting lesions or tumors. However, some patients may have hirsutism or virilization with normal levels of plasma testosterone. Thus, virilization in any woman, especially with a rapid onset history, warrants further investigation either by vaginal ultrasound, CT scan, or other methods.

It must be emphasized that not all virilized women have associated ovarian tumors. Many functional states such as PCO, stromal hyperthecosis, pregnant luteoma, or hyperreactio luteinalis, may mimic a neoplasm. Frozen section of the removed tissues during surgical exploration is essential to achieve accurate diagnosis and appropriate therapy.

REFERENCES

1. Barbieri RL, Makris A, Randall RW, et al. Insulin stimulates androgen accumulation in incubation of ovarian stroma obtained from women with hyperandrogenism. *J Clin Endocrinol Metab* 1986; 62:904.
2. Hagamani M, Stuart CA. Specific binding sites for insulin-like growth factor I in the ovarian stroma of women with polycystic ovarian disease and stromal hyperthecosis. *Am J Obstet Gynecol* 1990; 163:1992.
3. Clement PB. Anatomy and histology of the ovary. In: Kurman RJ, ed. *Pathology of the female genital tract, Blaustein A*. 4th ed. New York: Springer-Verlag; 1994: chap 15.
4. Longcope C, Hunter R, Franz C. Steroid secretion by the postmenopausal ovary. *Am J Obstet Gynecol* 1980;138:564–568.
5. Dennefors BL, Janson PO, Knutsson F, Hamberger L. Steroid production and responsiveness to

gonadotropin in isolated stromal tissue of human postmenopausal ovaries. *Am J Obstet Gynecol* 1980;136:997–1002

6. Clement PB. Nonneoplastic lesions of the ovary. In: Kurman RJ, ed. *Pathology of the female genital tract, Blaustein A*, 4th ed. New York: Springer-Verlag; 1994: chap 16.

7. Scully RE. Tumors of the ovary and maldeveloped gonads. In: *Atlas of tumor pathology,* second series, Fascicle 16. Washington, DC, Armed Forces Institute of Pathology; 1979.

8. Young RH, Scully RE. Sex cord–stromal and steroid cell ovarian tumors. In: Kurman RJ, ed. *Pathology of the female genital tract, Blaustein A*, 4th ed. New York: Springer-Verlag; 1994: chap 19.

9. Coney P. Polycystic ovarian disease: current concepts of pathophysiology and therapy. *Fertil Steril* 1984;42:667–682.

10. Biggs JSG. Polycystic ovarian disease: Current concepts. Aust NZ. *J Obstet Gynecol* 1981;21:26–36.

11. Biggs JSG, Thomas FJ. Sites of steroid production in the polycystic ovary. *Br J Obstet Gynaecol* 1981;88:42–46.

12. Erickson, GF, Magoffin DA, Jones KL. Theca function in polycystic ovaries of a patient with virilizing congenital adrenal hyperplasia. *Fertil Steril* 1989;51:173.

13. Lobo RA. Ovarian hyperandrogenism and androgen-producing tumors. *Endocrinol Metab Clin North Am* 1991;20:773–805.

14. Merrill JA. The morphology of the prepubertal ovary: relationship to the polycystic ovary syndrome. *South Med J* 1963;56:225–231.

15. Boss JH, Scully RE, Wegner KH, Cohen RB. Structural variations in the adult ovary: clinical significance. *Obstet Gynecol* 1965;25:747–763.

16. Wentz AC, Gutai JP, Jones GS, Migeon CJ. Ovarian hyperthecosis in an adolescent patient. *J Pediatr* 1976;88:488–493.

17. Madeido G, Tieu TM, Aiman J. Atypical ovarian hyperthecosis in a virilized post menopausal women. *Am J Clin Pathol* 1985;83:101–107.

18. Vasquez SB, Sotos JF, Kim MH. Massive edema of the ovary and virilization. *Obstet Gynecol* 1982;59:95S–99S.

19. Young RH, Scully RE. Fibromatosis and massive edema of the ovary, possibly related entities: A report of 14 cases of fibromatosis and 11 cases of massive edema. *Int J Gynecol Pathol* 1984;3:153–178.

20. Kalstone CE, Jaffe RB, Abell MR. Massive edema of the ovary simulating fibroma. *Obstet Gynecol* 1969;34:564–571.

21. Sternberg WH, Dhurandhar HN. Functional ovarian tumors of stromal and sex cord origin. *Hum Pathol* 1977;8:565–582.

22. Girouard DP, Barclay DL, Collins CG. Hyperreactio luteinalis: review of the literature and report of 2 cases. *Obstet Gynecol* 1964;23:513–525.

23. Clement PB. Tumor-like ovarian lesions in pregnancy. *Int J Gynecol Pathol* 1993;12:108–115.

24. Haning RV Jr, Strawn EY, Nolten WE. Pathophysiology of the ovarian hyperstimulation syndrome. *Obstet Gynecol* 1985;66:220–224.

25. Hensleigh PA, Woodruff JD. Differential maternal–fetal response to androgenizing luteoma or hyperreactio luteinalis. *Obstet Gynecol Surv* 1978;33:262–271.

26. Young RH, Scully RE. Ovarian Sertoli-Leydig cell tumors: a clinicopathological analysis of 207 cases. *Am J Surg Pathol* 1985;9:543–569.

27. Young RH, Scully RE. Ovarian Sertoli-Leydig cell tumors with a retiform pattern: a problem in histopathologic diagnosis. A report of 25 cases. *Am J Surg Pathol* 1983;7:755–771.

28. Roth LM, Slayton RR, Brady LW, et al. Retiform differentiation in ovarian Sertoli-Leydig cell tumors: a clinicopathologic study of six cases from a gynecologic oncology study group. *Cancer* 1985;55:1093–1098.

29. Young RH, Prat J, Scully RE. Ovarian Sertoli-Leydig cell tumors with heterologous elements. (i)Gastrointestinal epithelium and carcinoid: a clinicopathologic analysis of thirty-six cases. *Cancer* 1982;50:2448–2456.

30. Prat J, Young RH, Scully RE. Ovarian Sertoli-Leydig cell tumors with heterologous elements. (ii)Cartilage and skeletal muscle: a clinicopathologic analysis of twelve cases. *Cancer* 1982;50: 2465–2475.

31. Zaloudek C, Norris HJ. Sertoli-Leydig tumors of the ovary: a clinicopathologic study of 64 intermediate and poorly differentiated neoplasms. *Am J Surg Pathol* 1984;8:405–418.

32. Hayes MC, Scully RE. Stromal luteoma of the ovary; a clinicopathologic analysis of 25 cases. *Int J Gynecol Pathol* 1987;6:313–321.

33. Paraskevas M, Scully RE. Hilus cell tumor of the ovary: clinicopathological analysis of 12 Reinke-crystal-positive and 9 crystal negative cases. *Int J Gynecol Pathol* 1989;8:299–310.

34. Hayes MC, Scully RE. Ovarian steroid cell tumor (not otherwise specified): a clinicopathological analysis of 63 cases. *Am J Surg Pathol* 1987;11:835–845.

35. Young RH, Scully RE. Ovarian steroid cell tumors associated with Cushing's syndrome: a report of three cases. *Int J Gynecol Pathol* 1987;6;40.

36. Roth LM, Sternberg WH. Ovarian stromal tumors containing Leydig cells. II: Pure Leydig cell tumor, nonhilar type. *Cancer* 1973;32;952.

37. Talerman A. Ovarian Sertoli-Leydig cell tumor (androblastoma) with retiform pattern: a clinico-pathologic study. *Cancer* 1987;60:3056–3064.

38. Woodruff JD, Williams TJ, Goldberg B. Hormone activity of the common ovarian neoplasm. *Am J Obstet Gynecol* 1963;87:679–698.

39. Scott JS, Lumsden CE, Levell MJ. Ovarian endocrine activity in association with hormonally inactive neoplasia. *Am J Obstet Gynecol* 1967;97:161–70.

40. Connor TB, Ganis FM, Levin HS, Migeon CJ, Martin LG. Gonadotropin-dependent Krukenberg tumor causing virilization during pregnancy. *J Clin Endocrinol* 1968;28:198–214.

41. Mohabeer J, Buckley CH, Fox H. An immunohistochemical study of the incidence and significance of human chorionic gonadotropin synthesis by epithelial ovarian neoplasms. *Gynecol Oncol* 1983;16:74–84.

42. Casper S, van Nagell JR, Powell DF, et al. Immunohistochemical localization of tumor markers in epithelial ovarian cancer. *Am J Obstet Gynecol* 1984;149:154–158.

43. Scully RE. Ovarian tumors with functioning stroma. In: Fox H, ed. *Hains and Taylor's gynecological and obstetrical pathology,* 3rd ed. Edinburgh: Churchill-Livingstone; 1987.

44. Rutgers JL, Scully RE. Functioning ovarian tumors with peripheral steroid cell proliferation: a report of twenty-four cases. *Int J Gynecol Pathol.* 1986;5:319–337.

Androgenic Disorders,
edited by G. P. Redmond.
Raven Press, Ltd., New York © 1995.

8

Adrenal Hyperplasia

Sandro Loche and *Maria I. New

*Pediatric Endocrinology Service, Ospedale Regionale per le Microcitemie,
Cagliari, 09121 Italy; *Department of Pediatrics, Division of Endocrinology,
The New York Hospital–Cornell Medical Center, New York, New York 10021.*

Congenital adrenal hyperplasia (CAH) is the result of reduced enzymatic activity at any of the biosynthetic steps in the production of cortisol (Fig. 1,2) (1). The synthesis of cortisol takes place in the zona fasciculata of the adrenal cortex and is regulated by pituitary pulsatile release of adrenocorticotropin hormone (ACTH), which is, in turn, inhibited by cortisol at the pituitary and hypothalamic level. Impaired synthesis of cortisol via feedback mechanism induces oversecretion of ACTH, hyperplasia of the adrenal cortical tissue, and overproduction of precursor steroids proximal to the site of the enzymatic defect. The different abnormal secretion patterns of glucocorticoid, mineralocorticoid, and sex steroids produce the clinical syndromes of genital ambiguity (hyperandrogenemia) and imbalance in sodium metabolism, hypertension, and hypoandrogenemia. Somatic growth and fertility also are affected. Patients with CAH can conduct relatively normal lives with hormonal treatment and corrective surgery of the genitalia.

In overview there are two degrees of severity of CAH. Classical CAH involves near-total block of an enzyme activity while nonclassical CAH is milder than the classical form and is usually diagnosed later in life. While they are distinguished clinically, these two forms, classical and nonclassical, show surprisngly wide ranges of hormonal values, and cannot always be classified based on the genetic mutation.

The following enzymatic defects of adrenal steroidogenesis will be discussed:

1. 21-Hydroxylase deficiency: classical (salt-wasting and simple virilizing) and nonclassical;
2. 11β-Hydroxylase deficiency (hypertensive CAH) with corticosterone methyl oxidase types I and II (salt-wasting) deficiencies;
3. 3β-hydroxysteroid dehydrogenase deficiency;
4. 17α-hydroxylase deficiency with or without 17,20-lyase deficiency;
5. Cholesterol desmolase deficiency (lipoid hyperplasia).

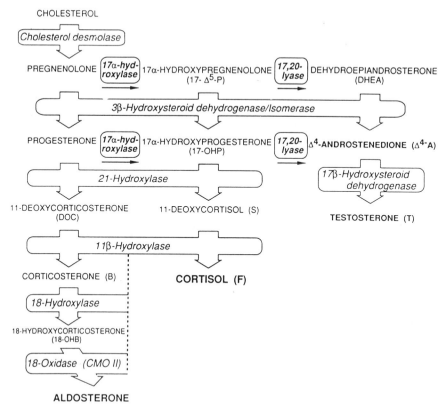

FIG. 1. General schema of steroidogenesis. Minor pathways in the adrenal (such as DHEA to androstenediol to testosterone), steroid sulfation, and aromatization are not shown.

21-HYDROXYLASE DEFICIENCY

Steroid 21-hydroxylase deficiency accounts for most cases of CAH (2). The enzyme is a cytochrome P450 expressed in the adrenal cortex (CYP21). According to international newborn screening, the classical form is found to occur at a frequency of 1 in 15,000 births (3). In 21-hydroxylase deficiency, 17-hydroxyprogesterone (17-OHP) is not converted to 11-deoxycortisol in the cortisol synthetic pathway. Secretion of ACTH is increased owing to the cortisol deficiency via the negative feedback system. ACTH stimulation of the adrenal cortex leads to accumulation of precursors proximal to the 21-hydroxylation step (Fig. 2). The 17-hydroxylated precursors are metabolized to androgens. The abnormally high levels of circulating androgens result postnatally in progressive virilism and advanced somatic development. Prenatally, the excess androgens masculinize the external genitalia of the genetic female.

CAH due to 21-hydroxylase deficiency is the most common cause of ambiguous genitalia in females. Females with classical 21-hydroxylase deficiency manifest varying degrees of genital ambiguity at birth, ranging from mild clitoral enlargement

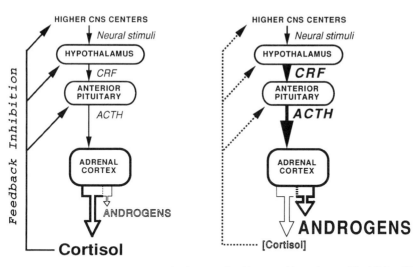

FIG. 2. The regulation of cortisol secretion in normal subjects and in patients with virilizing CAH (formerly andrenogenital syndrome [AGS], usually [90% of cases] due to 21-hydroxylase deficiency).

to the profound morphological anomaly of a penile urethra. The development of the internal genitalia is normal, and childbearing capacity exists. Therefore, it is important to recognize the disorder in newborns with ambiguous genitalia and make a female sex assignment. Postnatally, untreated children of either sex exhibit accelerated somatic growth with advanced bone maturation, early closure of the epiphyses, and final adult stature below that predicted on the basis of parental heights. Other symptoms of androgen excess include premature appearance of sexual hair, acne, adult body odor, and temporal balding. Females may develop polycystic ovarian syndrome and amenorrhea or irregular menses. Because genital formation in males at birth is normal, the syndrome often goes unrecognized until signs of androgen excess such as accelerated linear growth and precocious sexual hair appear later in childhood (4). In pubertal males, high levels of adrenal androgens may suppress gonadotropin secretion, resulting in reduced fertility.

In about 66% to 75% of classical cases of 21-hydroxylase deficiency, there is salt wasting from deficient aldosterone synthesis. It is manifested by hyponatremia and hyperkalemia, inappropriately high urinary sodium, and low serum and urinary aldosterone with high plasma renin activity (PRA). In severe cases, hypovolemia and shock may occur. Salt losing in infancy from an aldosterone biosynthetic defect may improve with age (5–7), and possible adjustments in sodium intake and mineralocorticoid replacement in patients labeled neonatally as salt wasters can be made on the basis of careful monitoring of PRA. Patients not demonstrating salt wasting are said to have simple virilizing disease. In the simple virilizing type there is measurable aldosterone and response to changes in PRA and salt status. The presence or absence of salt wasting in 21-hydroxylase deficiency may be seen consistently within families, and subsequently affecting offspring thus having the same form of the disease as the index case. Discordance for salt wasting and aldosterone synthetic capacity among affected siblings in several families (6). Distinct zonal defects in the two classical forms of 21-hydroxylase deficiency have been clinically investigated (9).

The nonclassical attenuated or late-onset form has been shown to have an extremely high frequency in the general population (1/100) with a remarkable increase in incidence among [1/27] Ashkenazi Jews, [1/53] in Hispanics and [1/63] in Yugoslavs (Croatians, Serbians, and other groups). An incidence of 1/333 was seen in Italians (10). The existence of this form of adrenal hyperplasia was first suspected in the early 1950s by gynecologists in clinical practice who used glucocorticoids for the treatment of women with physical signs of hyperandrogenism, including infertility (11,12). Females with nonclassical 21-hydroxylase deficiency who are not born with ambiguous genitalia, clinical features secondary to androgen excess that are variable and may present at any age (Fig. 3). Nonclassical 21-hydroxylase deficiency can result in premature development of pubic hair in children (13,14). High serum concentrations of adrenal androgens promote the early fusion of epiphyseal growth plates which results in final adult height less than predicted on the basis of parental heights (15). Severe cystic acne has been attributed to nonclassical 21-

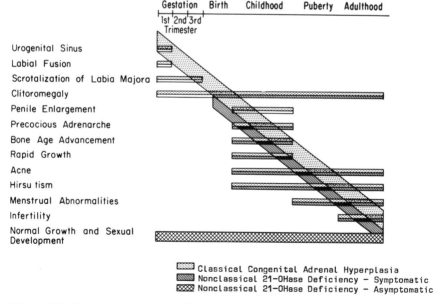

FIG. 3. Clinical spectrum of 21-OHD. There is a wide spectrum of clinical presentation in 21-OHD, ranging from prenatal virilization with labial fusion to precocious adrenarche to pubertal or postpubertal virilization. (From ref. 98, with permission.)

hydroxylase deficiency (16,17). Male-pattern baldness has been noted in other cases as the sole presenting symptom in young women with nonclassical 21-hydroxylase deficiency. Menarche in females may be normal or delayed, and secondary amenorrhea occurs frequently. Women with polycystic ovarian syndrome may in fact be patients with nonclassical 21-hydroxylase deficiency. Adrenal sex steroid excess may initially disrupt the normal cyclicity of gonadotropin release, leading to the formation of ovarian cysts, which then may continue to produce androgens autonomously. The prevalence of nonclassical 21-hydroxylase deficiency as an etiology of hirsutism and oligomenorrhea ranges from 1.2% to 30%. The wide range of frequencies reported may be related to differences in the ethnic composition of the groups studied, since the disease frequency varies in different ethnic groups (10). In women with polycystic ovaries, sonograms of the ovaries do not distinguish women with nonclassical 21-hydroxylase deficiency, and ACTH tests are required for differential diagnosis. Chronic hypersecretion of androgen precursors can induce a reduction in insulin sensitivity in female patients with nonclassical 21-hydroxylase deficiency (18).

In boys, early beard growth, acne, and a growth spurt may be the clinical signs. In adult men, androgen excess is difficult to identify, and its manifestations may be limited to short stature or to oligozoospermia and reduced fertility.

Some individuals with identical biochemical abnormalities (e.g., equally elevated serum 17-OHP after an intravenous injection of ACTH) remain entirely asymptomatic. Longitudinal follow-up of these patients often shows that signs of hyperandrogenism wax and wane.

HLA and 21-Hydroxylase Deficiency

The human major histocompatibility complex, or HLA, located on the short arm of chromosome 6, is an assembly of genes coding for cell surface antigens that are the major barriers for allogenic transplantation. The class I antigens, and others, the class II antigens, expressed on activated T lymphocytes, and provide a basis for recognition of non-self within the context of self and thus control the immune response. In addition, in the HLA region there are class III genes coding for expressed factors with functions outside the histocompatibility and immune responses, including adrenal cytochrome P450 specific for steroid 21-hydroxylation (CYP21).

Classic genetic analysis showed the HLA complex to span a recombinative distance of approximately 3 cM (centimorgans) (19). At the same time the gene for 21-hydroxylase deficiency was mapped between HLA-B and HLA-DR (a distance of 0.8 cM), segregating more frequently with HLA-B (20). Molecular genetic studies have led to the isolation and characterization of an increasing number of genes within this extended region (21–23), which by physical measure is approximately 3500–4000 kb (kilobase pairs) in length.

Linkage between HLA and 21-hydroxylase deficiency was first shown by Dupont et al. (24) and later confirmed by the same group (25) and by other groups (reviewed in ref. 20). Compiled data on intra-HLA recombinations strongly indicated a gene locus for 21-hydroxylase between HLA-B and HLA-DR (26). The more recent molecular studies have confirmed this location in class III. Steroid 21-hydroxylase deficiency is a monogenic trait, and the close genetic linkage of the 21-hydroxylase gene to HLA is utilized for genotyping siblings in pedigrees with an affected proband. Thus, with few exceptions (27), a sibling sharing both HLA haplotypes with the proband is predicted to be affected, one who shares a single haplotype is predicted to be heterozygote, and one who shares no HLA haplotype is predicted to be unaffected (Fig. 4). In the rare cases in which an HLA-identical sibling is not affected, a de novo pathological mutation has been described (28–31).

In addition to linkage of the 21-hydroxylase locus with the HLA-B and HLA-DR loci, 21-hydroxylase deficiency alleles are found in linkage disequilibrium (i.e., the nonrandom association of particular alleles of different genetic loci) with HLA antigen genes or haplotypic combinations that may include specific alleles of C4 of serum complement (32). The salt-wasting form of 21-hydroxylase deficiency shows increased association with the extended haplotype HLA-A3,Bw47,DR7, which also carries a null allele at C4B (33,34). Patients with nonclassical 21-hydroxylase deficiency may be genetic compounds carrying two recessive genetic defects; a severe 21-hydroxylase deficiency gene and a mild nonclassical 21-hydroxylase deficiency allele, or they can be homozygous for the mild 21-hydroxylase deficiency allele (35). Nonclassical disease is associated with the haplotype HLA-B14,DR1, which has been shown to have a duplicated C4A isotype (36–38). The association of nonclassical 21-hydroxylase deficiency with HLA-B14,DR1 has been observed in all ethnic groups examined (10) except the Yugoslav population (39). Negative association with 21-hydroxylase deficiency has been noted for the haplotype HLA-A1, B8,DR3 (37), which carries a null allele at C4A; this haplotype occurs with somewhat greater frequency in certain autoimmune disorders.

Molecular Genetics

The structural gene encoding the adrenal cytochrome P-450 specific for steroid 21-hydroxylation (P-450c21) is named CYP21 or CYP21B and contains 10 exons. This gene and a 98% identical pseudogene (CYP21P or CYP21A) are located in close proximity (30 kb) in the HLA complex adjacent to and alternating with the C4B and C4A genes encoding the fourth component of the serum complement (Fig. 5). The pseudogene CYP21P owing to several deleterious mutations does not give rise to an enzyme protein.

Mutations in CYP21 appear to be generated by either of two types of recombination mechanisms. Misalignment of the tandem C4A-CYP21P-C4B-CYP21 arrangement during meiosis leads to unequal crossing over, resulting in a complete deletion of a DNA segment, including C4B and CYP21. Alternatively, small deleterious mutations appear to be transferred from CYP21P to CYP21 in gene conversion events (40). The frequency of gene deletions in different ethnic groups ranges from

A. FAMILY Zurich-7 (Levine *et al.* 1978)

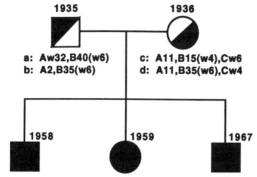

B. FAMILY NYC-16 (Levine *et al.* 1978)

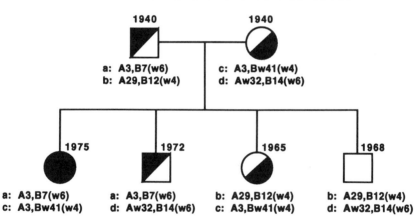

FIG. 4. Pedigrees for two families with classical 21-OHD. The HLA haplotypes for the HLA-A, HLA-B, and HLA-C alleles are given in each family. The paternal haplotypes are labeled a and b and the maternal haplotypes c and d. The parents are obligate heterozygous carriers for the 21-OHD gene (denoted by the half-black symbols). The affected children are denoted by black symbols. In A, three affected siblings are HLA genotypically identical. In B, one affected child is genotypically different from the three unaffected siblings. One sibling that carries the paternal a and d haplotypes is presumed to be a heterozygous carrier for 21-OHD because he shares the haplotype with the patient. Another sibling has the parental b and c haplotypes and shares the c haplotype with the patient, and should be a carrier of the classical 21-OHD gene. The child with the b and d haplotypes should be normal for the gene. (From ref. 25, with permission.)

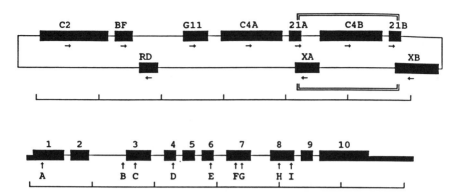

FIG. 5. *Top.* Diagram of the chromosomal region containing the CYP21 (21A and 21B) 21-hydroxylase genes. HLA-B is about 600 kb to the left and HLA-DR about 400 kb to the right of the diagrammed region. Other genes in this region are BF (properdin factor B), C2, C4A, and C4B (second and fourth serum complement components). These genes are all transcribed in the same direction. Additional genes of unknown function are transcribed from the opposite chromosomal strand: RD, XA, and XB. A scale is marked every 20 kb. The bracket indicates the region deleted in about 20% of classic 21-OHD alleles.

Bottom. A CYP21 gene is diagrammed. A scale is marked every 500 bp. Numbered bars represent exons which are sequences found in mRNA. Full bars are protein-coding sequences whereas half-height bars are untranslated sequences. Nine deleterious mutations normally found only in the CYP21A pseudogene are marked: A, mutation of codon 30 from CCG, encoding proline, to CTG, leucine; B, A or C to G mutation in intron 2 causing aberrant splicing; C, 8 base-pair deletion in codons 110-112; D, mutation of codon 172 from ATC, isoleucine, to AAC, asparagine; E, cluster of three mutations in codons 235-238 changing the amino acid sequence from isoleucine-valine-glutamate-methionine to asparagine-glutamate-glutamate-lysine; F, mutation of codon 281 from GTG, valine, to TTG, leucine; G, single-base insertion between codons 306-307; H, nonsense mutation, CAG to TAG, in codon 318; I, mutation of codon 356 from CGG, arginine, to TGG, tryptophan. (From ref. 99, with permission.)

11% to 35%, and in many cases are found to be associated with the haplotype HLA-B47,DR7 (41). Gene conversion events explain 65% to 90% of the disease haplotypes (that is, most of the haplotypes in which deletional mutations were not identified). Nine mutations in the CYP21 sequence having adverse effects at some stage of gene expression are normally present in the CYP21P pseudogene.

A nonsense mutation in codon 318 (C→T substitution) would result in an encoded translation product that would be truncated and completely inactive. This was seen in 4% to 7% of classical 21-hydroxylase deficiency haplotypes (42). The 8-bp deletion in exon 3 normally found in CYP21P shifts the reading frame and encodes a completely inactive enzyme. This mutation is found in 3% to 10% of disease haplotypes and is predicted to result in a salt-wasting phenotype (41). A cluster of mutations, Ile-Val-Glu-Met-236-239→Asn-Glu-Glu-Lys (43), and a single substitution, Arg-356→Trp (44), also have been described in patients with the salt-wasting disease.

A point mutation (A or C→G substitution) in the second intron introduces a new acceptor site to be recognized by the intron splicing mechanism. Mutation A/C to G constitutes the single most frequent nondeleted allele causing classical 21-hydroxylase deficiency and causes intron 2 to end prematurely so that 19 nucleotides normally spliced out of mRNA are retained (45). This leads to a shift in the translational reading frame, preventing synthesis of an active protein. Almost all of the mRNA is aberrantly spliced, but in vitro a small amount of normally spliced mRNA can be detected. If no other mutations are present, a small amount of normal enzyme might thus be synthesized. The presence of the aberrantly spliced mRNA in small amounts has been demonstrated in vitro after transfection of COS cells with the functional CYP21 gene. It is possible, therefore, that abnormal protein can be produced in the adrenal tissue of normal individuals. We do not know what proportion of mRNA is normally spliced in the adrenal glands of patients with this mutation. Most (but not all) patients who are homozygous or hemizygous for this mutation have the salt-wasting form of the disorder, indicating that they have insufficient enzymatic activity to permit adequate aldosterone synthesis (45). In addition, a Gly-291→Ser mutation (46), a T→C transition at base 398 (46), a G→C transition at the conserved, splice donor site of intron 7 (47), and a TGG→TAG (nonsense) mutation at Trp-406 in exon 9 (47), and two different mutations at position 483 of exon 10 [an Arg-483→Pro codon change and a frameshift mutation GG→C (46,48)] have been found in patients with the salt-wasting phenotype. A single base change in exon 4 isoleucine-172 to asparagine (polar to nonpolar substitution) (44,49) has been associated with the simple virilizing phenotype (49).

Associated with the HLA-B14,DR1 haplotype (the haplotype seen in 78% of patients with nonclassical CAH) is a change in codon 281 of CYP21 from GTC, valine, to TTG, leucine. It has been speculated that Val-281→Leu, which is a conservative amino acid substitution, increases the likelihood of an α-helix forming in a region that is normally not to be in a helical conformation (50), and that such a change in secondary structure accounts for the deleterious effect on activity is supported by recent studies correlating mutations at this site with reduced rates of heme insertion into the protein (51). In addition, a Pro-105→Leu, Pro-453→Ser, and C→T transition at 4 bases upstream of translation initiation were identified together in one allele producing the nonclassical phenotype (52,53).

Recently, a missense mutation at residue 30 in exon 1, changing proline to leucine, was revealed in 16% of haplotypes in patients with the less severe, nonclassical phenotype of the disease (52).

Correlation of Genotype with Phenotype

In general, mutant P450c21 enzymes carrying specific amino acid substitutions identified in patients with 21-hydroxylase deficiency display activities that correspond roughly to the clinical severity of the disease and to the associated biochemical abnormalities. Like homozygous deletion, which precludes the expression of any enzyme, deletion in conjunction with a stop mutation, or with the cluster of mutations at exon 6, which confers zero enzyme activity in vitro, would be predicted to result in 0% overall 21-hydroxylase activity in vivo and the severe salt-wasting phenotype. Homozygosity for the mutation Ile-172→Asn, which confers about 2% of normal activity on the gene product, usually results in the simple virilizing phenotype. However, the distinction between the two forms of classical 21-hydroxylase deficiency is not absolute. There are reports of HLA-identical sibling pairs in which one sibling demonstrates salt wasting whereas in the other there is adequate aldosterone synthesis (54,55). One patient with the Ile-172→Asn mutation has been shown to have mild salt wasting, and patients with identical mutations are reported to have variable amelioration of aldosterone deficiency with age.

As we mentioned above, homozygotes for milder mutations, such as Val-281→Leu and Pro-30→Leu, which have approximately 50% of wild type enzyme activity in vitro (56), usually manifest the phenotype of the nonclassical form of the disease (52,53).

Recently, Speiser et al. (55) classified 90 patients into three mutation groups based on the degree of predicted enzymatic compromise. Mutation group A (no enzymatic activity) consisted primarily of salt-wasting patients, group B (2% activity) of simple virilizing patients, and group C (10% to 20% activity) of nonclassical patients. Mutation groups were correlated with clinical diagnosis, but each group contained patients with phenotypes either more or less severe than predicted. The phenotype was accurately predicted in 87% (54/62) of group A, 72% (16/22) of group B, and 62.5% of group C. It is possible that individuals with phenotypes that are more severe than those predicted from the genotype and are discordant with sibs have additional, as yet unidentified, mutations within the CYP21 gene. It is also plausible that at least some differences in clinical disease expression are governed by factors remote from the CYP21 locus. Finally, one might postulate that phenotypic severity is influenced by parental imprinting or by negative allelic complementation, that is, exaggerated gene dosage effect (55).

Diagnosis and Treatment

Nomograms relating the baseline and ACTH-stimulated levels of 17-OHP, Δ^4-androstenedione, DHHEA, the DEA/Δ^4-androstenedione ratio, and testosterone (T) provide hormonal standards to use in the assignment of the 21-hydroxylase deficiency genotype; that is, patients whose hormonal values fall on the regression line within a defined groups are assigned to that group (Fig. 6) (57). Clinically symptomatic and asymptomatic cases of nonclassical 21-hydroxylase deficiency are found to be biochemically indistinguishable. Heterozygotes for classical and heterozygotes for nonclassical 21-hydroxylase deficiency demonstrate a similar 17-OHP response to ACTH stimulation. Baseline 17-OHP levels of nonclassical 21-hydroxylase deficiency subjects obtained at random times may be insufficiently elevated to identify affected status, but early morning (0800 h) measurements are informative.

The distribution of hormonal responses along a regression line suggests that there is a spectrum of enzymatic deficiency in these groups: patients with classical CAH have the most severe deficiency, patients with the nonclassical form have a less

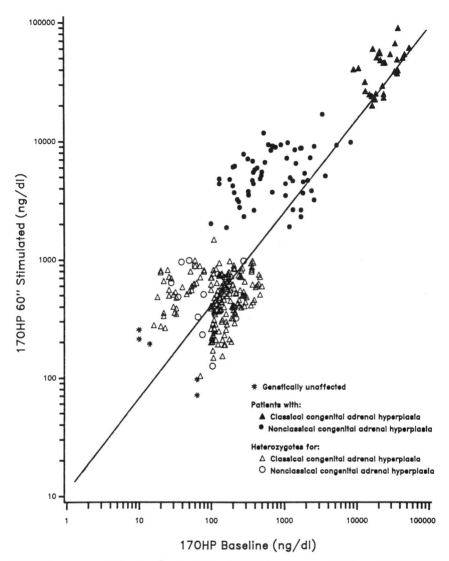

FIG. 6. Nomogram relating baseline to ACTH-stimulated serum concentrations of 17OHP. The scales are logarithmic. A regression line for all data points is shown. (Data for this nomogram was collected between 1982 and 1991 at the Department of Pediatrics, The New York Hospital–Cornell Medical Center, New York, New York 10021.)

severe deficiency, while heterozygotes have an even milder deficiency unmasked only upon ACTH stimulation. It should be stated that measurement of ACTH-stimulated 17-OHP levels is reflective solely of the 21-hydroxylase defect in the zona fasciculata.

With the demonstration of linkage between the genes for HLA and 21-hydroxylase deficiency, HLA genotyping makes it possible to predict which siblings are carriers and which siblings are genetically unaffected. The validity of the HLA prediction is supported by pedigree analysis and hormonal studies (58–61). The 21-hydroxylase deficiency remains the only adrenal cortical enzyme defect for which heterozygosity can be reliably demonstrated by means of hormonal response to ACTH stimulation and corroborated by genetic linkage marker analysis.

Hormone replacement of the essential gluco- and/or mineralocorticoids remains the principal therapy for 21-hydroxylase deficiency as well as for all the other forms of CAH. It corrects metabolism, lowers ACTH levels to normal, and reduces inappropriate adrenal steroid overproduction with remission of symptoms of virilization and/or hypertension. Steroids are administered in dosages approximating physiologic requirements according to potency. Hydrocortisone is preferred in childhood management as it directly replaces cortisol and reduces the possibility of cushingoid signs and slowed growth from overtreatment. Dosage is generally 10 to 15 mg/m^2/day. In cases of poor hormonal control and in adults, the more potent, longer-acting synthetic analogs prednisone and dexamethasone are often used. The synthetic steroid 9α-fluorocortisol is used for mineralocorticoid replacement in cases of salt wasting. The standard dosage range is 0.05 to 0.1 mg/day. 9α-Fluorocortisol has been found beneficial in correcting the renin–aldosterone axis in simple virilizing patients also, normalizing PRA and reducing the glucocorticoid requirement (62). In nonclassical patients, dexamethasone in low doses (0.25 to 0.5 mg) given at bedtime can be used. Given the 9-month life expectancy of established hair follicles, remission of hirsutism takes at least one or two years. Resumption of normal menstrual cycles is usually the first clinical sign of good hormonal treatment, followed by remission of acne.

Prenatal Diagnosis and Treatment

Hormonal therapy also is possible in prenatal life (63–65). Fetal adrenal suppression is achieved by administration to the mother of dexamethasone, which crosses the placenta without being metabolized appreciably and thus is able to suppress fetal adrenal steroid production. The current dosage is 20 μg/kg maternal–fetal weight per day. This greatly reduces masculinization of the external genitalia in utero in the female fetus with 21-hydroxylase deficiency. In a family at risk, treatment must begin before the 9th week of gestation and is continued to term in the affected female fetus. Prenatal diagnosis is made by chorionic villus sampling at 8 to 10 weeks gestational age, or by amniocentesis (at 15 to 18 weeks gestational age). Diagnosis has heretofore been accomplished by detection of restriction fragment polymorphism in the closely linked HLA loci, permitting the affected chromosomes to be identified in any family in which a index case (i.e., a prior affected offspring) is available for study (64,65). Use of HLA linkage is no longer in common use. The vast majority of mutations causing 21-hydroxylase deficiency can be directly identified using molecular genetic diagnostic techniques to detect deletions and point mutations in DNA (66–68). Treatment is discontinued if the fetus is a genetic male or an unaffected female (Fig. 7).

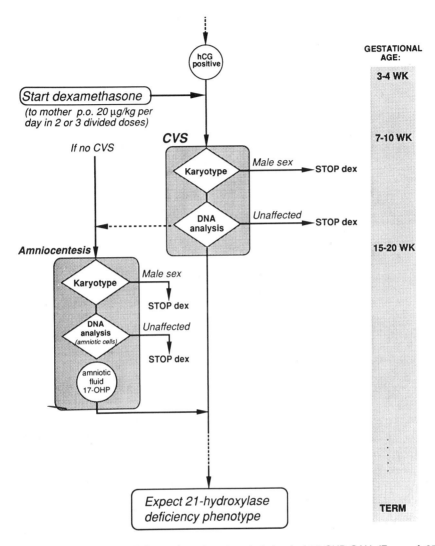

FIG. 7. Schedule of prenatal diagnosis and treatment of classical 21-OHD CAH. (From ref. 65, with permission.)

11β-HYDROXYLASE DEFICIENCY
(HYPERTENSIVE, VIRILIZING CAH)

11β-Hydroxylase deficiency (11β-OHD) is the second-most common form of CAH (5% to 8% of all cases in the general population). The classical form occurs in about 1 in 100,000 births in the general Caucasian population and in 1 in 5,000 to 1 in 7,000 births in Israel (69). This unexpected clustering of cases was traced to Jewish families of North African origin.

There is defective conversion of 11-deoxycortisol to cortisol and usually reduced or absent conversion of deoxycorticosterone (DOC) to corticosterone. Elevation of serum 11-deoxycortisol and DOC and marked urinary elevation of the corresponding tetrahydrometabolites is characteristic. Excess adrenal androgen production from shunted cortisol precursors, as in 21-hydroxylase deficiency, results in genital ambiguity of the affected female fetuses, with normal female internal reproductive organs.

Hypertension, with or without hypokalemic alkalosis, clinically distinguishes 11β-OHD. Two-thirds of the patients become hypertensive; the degree of hypertension does not correlate with the degree of virilization or with biochemical parameters (serum DOC, PRA). Hypertension is attributable to elevated DOC levels (70,71). DOC-induced sodium retention results in suppression of PRA and reduced secretion of aldosterone and 18-hydroxycorticosterone from the zona glomerulosa (72,73). Glucocorticoid administration results in reduction of DOC secretion and natriuresis; renin suppression ceases and PRA increases angiotensin II production, stimulating aldosterone secretion. Suppression of DOC may not lower blood pressure in hypertensive 11β-OHD patients, although this lack of response is a feature of long-standing hypertension of many causes. Mild, late onset, and even cryptic (detected by hormonal tests only) forms have been reported (74,75).

Molecular Genetics

Deficiency of 11β-hydroxylase activity is inherited in an autosomal recessive manner, but unlike 21-hydroxylase deficiency, it is not HLA linked. Distinct isoenzymes of the mitochondrial P450 enzyme P450c11 participate in cortisol and aldosterone synthesis in humans. These isoenzymes encoded by two genes, CYP11B1 and B2, are 93% identical and located on the long arm of chromosome 8 (76,77).

In the zona fasciculata, 11β-hydroxylation of 11-deoxycortisol yields cortisol in a single step. In the zona glomerulosa, P450c11 11β-hydroxylates DOC to corticosterone and has 18-hydroxylase and 18-oxidase activities converting corticosterone to 18-hydroxycorticosterone and then aldosterone (78). These steps are also called corticosterone methyl oxidase (CMO) type I and type II. In the zona fasciculata there is some 18-hydroxylation of DOC and corticosterone but no aldosterone synthesis.

Studies of patients with defective cortisol or aldosterone synthesis caused by respective deficiencies in 11β-hydroxylase and CMO type II activities confirmed the hypothesis that the isoenzyme encoded by CYP11B1 synthesizes cortisol in the zona fasciculata whereas the isoenzyme encoded by CYP11B2 synthesizes aldosterone in the zona glomerulosa (79,80).

Mutations in the zona fasciculata gene result in defective cortisol synthesis and hypertension from elevated levels of DOC, whereas mutations in the zona glomerulosa gene result in defective aldosterone synthesis and salt wasting. Many cases in the Moroccan–Israeli population share the same mutation, Arg-448→His in

CYP11B1, which encodes a defective enzyme (81). Most known mutations (81–84) are clustered in exons 6 to 8 (83). This clustering may reflect the location of functionally important amino acid residues within the enzyme or an increased tendency to develop mutations within this region of the gene. Prenatal diagnosis is now possible for this disease by polymerase chain reaction (PCR) amplification of exons and selective probing with allele-specific oligonucleotides or by direct sequencing (83).

3β-HYDROXYSTEROID DEHYDROGENASE DEFICIENCY

The exact frequency of 3β-hydroxysteroid dehydrogenase deficiency (3β-HSD) is unknown. The enzyme 3β-hydroxysteroid dehydrogenase has the compound function of 3β-hydroxysteroid dehydrogenation and 3-oxosteroid isomerization. This enzyme function is present in the adrenal cortex, gonads, and placenta, but also in the liver and many peripheral tissues.

In the classical form of 3β-HSD, there is poor or absent conversion to Δ^4-steroids, and overproduction of Δ^5-steroid precursors, which are relatively inactive, causing variable degrees of salt wasting and cortisol insufficiency (85). Gonadal androgen production also is deficient. Genetic males exhibit genital ambiguity at birth. In affected females, the elevated circulating levels of DHEA are converted to more potent androgens in the periphery that may produce a limited androgen effect (usually only clitoral enlargement). Deficient aldosterone production in cases of near-complete 3β-HSD enzyme block results in salt wasting (85), while in other cases the ability to conserve sodium has been intact (86–89).

In the nonclassical form, 3β-HSD deficiency is an attenuated enzyme defect with no major developmental abnormalities (90). The onset is peripubertal or postadrenarchal, and the zona glomerulosa is not involved, ensuring adequate aldosterone synthesis. The signs of virilization in females are similar to those in nonclassical 21-hydroxylase deficiency (premature adrenarche, irregular menses, infertility, severe acne, temporal balding, and hirsutism).

Biochemically, elevated serum levels of the Δ^5-steroids pregnenolone, 17-hydroxypregnenolone, and DHEA, and increased excretion of the Δ^5-metabolite pregnenetriol in the urine are diagnostic for this enzyme disorder.

Molecular Genetics

The 3β-HSD deficiency is inherited in an autosomal recessive manner. Two genes encoding 3β-HSD mapped to the 1p13 chromosome have been cloned to date: a skin-placental form (type I) and an adrenal–gonadal form (type II). Studies on the type II 3β-HSD gene from index cases revealed a number of mutations associated with different phenotypic forms of 3β-HSD deficiency (91). For example, insertion of a single C between codons 186 and 187 shifts the translation frame leading to premature termination. A stop codon introduced by virtue of G→A transition in codon 171 also would lead to a truncated protein product (mutation W171X). Other point mutations that have been identified include: T→A transversion converting Tyr-253→Asn, a G→A transition converting Glu-142→Lys, a missense mutation at codon 248 (Val→Asn) followed by a frameshift mutation at codon 248 (92), and a G→C change converting Ala-245→Pro. The last missense mutation was identified in a homozygote individual with classical 3β-HSD deficiency who was able to conserve salt. Although the activity of this mutant enzyme was found to be 12% of the activity endowed by the wild type II 3β-HSD, it was adequate to prevent salt wasting. Molecular analysis to date has not shown any DNA abnormality in patients with the nonclassical form of the disease (91) except a heterozygous mutation of the type II gene in one recent case (93).

17α-HYDROXYLASE/17,20-LYASE DEFICIENCY

The mitochondrial P450c17 enzyme can catalyze both the 17α-hydroxylase and 17,20-lyase reactions. Patients have been described with either combined 17α-hydroxylase and 17,20-lyase deficiency, or isolated 17,20-lyase deficiency. Defects on the single polypeptide P450c17 appear to be the molecular basis of both these deficiencies.

The enzyme is shared by the adrenals and the gonads, and defects result in reduced production of all androgens and estrogens. In the genetic male there is pseudohermaphroditism and gynecomastia (94), whereas in the female there are infantile genitalia. In both sexes, normal puberty fails to occur, even to the extent that the patients have no sexual hair. They also may develop hypokalemia and hypertension owing to elevated levels of DOC. They are less likely to suffer adrenal crisis than are individuals affected with other steroidogenic enzyme deficiencies that impair cortisol synthesis, as a result of the corticosterone they produce at high levels. There are at least 122 cases reported (95). The diagnosis is confirmed by marked elevations of serum DOC and corticosterone and the metabolites of these two hormones. Aldosterone is usually suppressed, although there are cases described with normal or elevated aldosterone levels. Gonadotropin production is extremely high in both sexes because of the absence of any sex steroid feedback.

Diagnosis is often made with the young female or apparent female presenting at pubertal age with primary amenorrhea or lack of development of secondary sex characteristics. The disorder may be revealed earlier in 46,XY karyotype cases presenting in infancy or childhood with inguinal hernia or mass. These patients are hypokalemic and hypertensive at the time of diagnosis. Alternately, hypokalemia and hypertension may be the first manifestations of the disorder. In long-standing cases that are untreated or undertreated, hypertension of considerable severity may develop. Treatment consists of glucocorticoid replacement in prepuberty, and sex steroid replacement as appropriate for the phenotypic sex starting at pubertal age. In 46,XY patients the testes may be abdominal, inguinal, or labial; if therapy is directed toward phenotypic development as a male, the gonads may be preserved by orchiopexy. Estrogen replacement induces the breasts to develop satisfactorily and menstrual cycles may be established in genetic females.

Molecular Genetics

The gene for the P450c17 enzyme has been located on chromosome 10. In all the studied patients, mutations in the structural gene (CYP17) were found (95). These include a stop codon introduced in the first exon by a single base substitution and a 7-bp (frameshift) duplication, both identified in patients who had complete combined 17α-hydroxylase and 17,20-lyase deficiency. Two additional patients had a 4-bp duplication late in the coding sequence encoding a protein that showed no enzyme activity in transfection studies. Other identified mutations include, again near the end of the coding sequence, a 3-bp deletion eliminating one of two adjacent phenylalanine residues, a stop codon introduced by a single base substitution, and a nonconservative Pro→Thr substitution.

CHOLESTEROL DESMOLASE DEFICIENCY (LIPOID ADRENAL HYPERPLASIA)

This is the most fundamental steroidogenic defect. It occurs rarely. The defective conversion of cholesterol to pregnenolone appears to involve the enzyme cytochrome P450scc. There is negligible reproduction of all steroids and the adrenal glands have a characteristic fatty appearance caused by massive accumulation of cholesterol. Affected individuals present with hypogonadism, severe fluid and electrolyte disturbances, addisonian pigmentation, and susceptibility to infection. They often do not survive infancy.

The gene for the P450scc enzyme has been localized on chromosome 15 (96). Mutation of the structural gene has not yet been identified (97).

SUMMARY

Congenital adrenal hyperplasia may present in the newborn period with either ambiguous or normal genitalia, depending on the type of steroidogenic enzyme defect responsible for the individual patient's disease. In the most commonly diagnosed form of CAH, the 21-hydroxylase enzyme is defective, resulting in insufficient cortisol production, lack of negative feedback inhibition to the hypothalamus and pituitary, and consequent overstimulation of the adrenal gland, resulting in excess secretion of androgens which do not require 21-hydroxylase for their synthesis. Thus, females undergo virilization in prenatal life and are born with a variable degree of genital ambiguity, while males have normal genitalia at birth. Two-thirds of patients with 21-hydroxylase deficiency have the salt-wasting trait, which may not be solely related to the severity of the mutation at the active HLA-linked 21-hydroxylase locus on chromosome 6.

Nonclassical forms of adrenal hyperplasia are recognized in which newborn females have normal genitalia and postnatally have variable clinical manifestations. The nonclassical 21-hydroxylase deficiency is an allelic variant of the classical disorder, with mild elevation of hormonal precursors and a phenotype which ranges from no apparent clinical abnormality, to precocious adrenarche, to hirsutism, oligomenorrhea and infertility. The frequency of the nonclassical disorder is approximately 100 times the frequency of the classical 21-hydroxylase deficiency in the general Caucasian population.

To date, the molecular basis of forms of CAH resulting from deficiencies in CYP21, CYP17, CYP11B, and 3β-HSD have been identified. The only gene in which a structural defect has not been identified is that encoding P450scc. Treatment of CAH involves replacement of cortisol and, if necessary, mineralocorticoids and/or salt. Proper longitudinal care of patients must include careful attention to adrenocortical hormone levels, growth, sexual maturation, and psychosexual status.

Prenatal diagnosis may be reliably performed by molecular genetic characterization of the defect after chorionic villus sampling. Prenatal therapy in at-risk pregnancies reduces in utero virilization of the female fetus.

REFERENCES

1. New MI. Congenital adrenal hyperplasia. In: Degroot LJ, Besser M, Burger HG et al., eds. *Endocrinology*. 3rd ed. Philadelphia: WB Saunders 1995;1813–1835.
2. New MI, White PC, Pang S, Dupont B, Speiser PW. The adrenal hyperplasias. In: Scriver CL, Beaudet AL, Sly WS, Valle D, eds. *The metabolic basis of inherited disease*. 6th ed. New York: McGraw-Hill, 1989:1881–1917.
3. Pang S and Clark A. Congenital adrenal hyperplasia due to 21-hydroxylase deficiency: Newborn screening and its relationship to the diagnosis and treatment of the disorder. *Screening* 1993;2:105–139.
4. Wilkins L. *The diagnosis and treatment of endocrine disorders in childhood and adolescence*. 3rd ed. Springfield, IL: Charles C. Thomas; 1965:410.
5. Luetscher JA. Studies of aldosterone in relation to water and electrolyte balance in man. *Recent Prog Horm Res* 1956;12:175–198.
6. Stoner E, DiMartino J, Kuhnle U, Levine LS, Oberfield SE, New MI. Is salt wasting in congenital adrenal hyperplasia genetic? *Clin Endocrinol (Oxf)* 1986;24:9–20.
7. Speiser PW, Adgere L, Ueshiba H, White PC, New MI. Aldosterone synthesis in salt-wasting congenital adrenal hyperplasia with complete absence of adrenal 21-hydroxylase. *N Engl J Med* 1991;324:145–149.
8. Rosenbloom AL, Smith DW. Varying expression for salt losing in related patients with congenital adrenal hyperplasia. *Pediatrics* 1966;38:215–219.
9. Kuhnle U, Chow D, Rapaport R, Pang S, Levine LS, New MI. The activity of the 21-hydroxylase (21-OH) enzyme in the glomerulosa and fasciculata of the adrenal cortex in congenital adrenal hyperplasia (CAH). *J Clin Endocrinol Metab* 1981;52:534–544.
10. Speiser PW, Dupont B, Rubinstein P, Piazza A, Kastelan A, New MI. High frequency of nonclassical adrenal steroid 21-hydroxylase deficiency. *Am J Hum Genet* 1985;37:650–657.
11. Jones HW, Jones GES. The gynecological aspects of adrenal hyperplasia and allied disorders. *Am J Obstet Gynecol* 1954;68:1330–1365.
12. Jeffries WM, Weir WC, Weir DR, Prouty RL. The use of cortisone and related steroids in infertility. *Fertil Steril* 1958;9:145–150.
13. Kohn B, Levine LS, Pollack MS, et al. Late onset steroid 21-hydroxylase deficiency: a variant of classical congenital adrenal hyperplasia. *J Clin Endocrinol Metab* 1982;55:817–827.
14. Temeck JW, Pang S, Nelson C, New MI. Genetic defects of steroidogenesis in premature pubarche. *J Clin Endocrinol Metab* 1987;64:609–617.
15. New MI, Gertner JM, Speiser PW, Del Balzo P. Growth and final height in classical and nonclassical 21-hydroxylase deficiency. *J Endocrinol Invest* 1989;12(S3):91–95.
16. Rose LI, Newmark SR, Strauss JS, Pochi PE. Adrenocortical hydroxylase deficiencies in acne vulgaris. *J Invest Dermatol* 1976;66:324–326.
17. Lucky AW, Rosenfield RL, McGuire J, Rudy S, Helke J. Adrenal androgen hyperresponsiveness to

adrenocorticotropin in women with acne and/or hirsutism: adrenal enzyme defects and exaggerated adrenarche. *J Clin Endocrinol Metab* 1986;62:840–848.

18. Speiser PW, Serrat J, New MI, Gertner JM. Insulin insensitivity in adrenal hyperplasia due to nonclassical steroid 21-hydroxylase deficiency. *J Clin Endocrinol Metab* 1992;75:1421–1424.

19. Baur MP, Sigmund S, Sigmund M, Rittner C. Analysis of MHC recombinant families. In: Albert ED, Baur MP, Mayr WR, eds. *Histocompatibility testing 1984*. Berlin: Springer-Verlag; 1984:324.

20. New MI. Congenital adrenal hyperplasia. In: Farid N, ed. *The immunogenetics of endocrine disorders*. 2nd ed. New York: Alan Liss; 1988:305

21. Moller G. Molecular genetics of class I and II MHC antigens. 1. *Immunol Rev* 1985;84:1–168.

22. Moller G. Molecular genetics of class I and II MHC antigens 2. *Immunol Rev* 1985;85:1–168.

23. Moller G. Molecular genetics of class III MHC antigens. *Immunol Rev* 1985;87:1–208.

24. Dupont B, Oberfield SE, Smithwick EM, Lee TD, Levine LS. Close genetic linkage between HLA and congenital adrenal hyperplasia (21-hydroxylase deficiency). *Lancet* 1977;2:1309–1312.

25. Levine LS, Zachmann M, New MI, et al. Genetic mapping of the 21-hydroxylase deficiency gene within the HLA linkage group. *N Engl J Med* 1978;299:911–915.

26. Dupont B, Pollack MS, Levine LS, O'Neill GJ, Hawkins B, New MI. Congenital adrenal hyperplasia and HLA: joint report from the eighth International Histocompatibility Workshop. In: Terasaki PI, ed. *Histocompatibility testing 1980*. Los Angeles: HLA Tissue Typing Laboratory; 1981:693–706.

27. Sinnott PJ, Dyer PA, Price DA, Harris R, Strachan T. 21-hydroxylase deficiency families with HLA-identical affected and unaffected sibs. *J Med Genet* 1989;28:10–17.

28. Sinnott P, Collier S, Costigan C, Dyer PA, Harris R, Strachan T. Genesis by meiotic unequal crossover of a de novo deletion that contributes to steroid 21-hydroxylase deficiency. *Proc Natl Acad Sci USA* 1990;87:2107–2111

29. Collier S, Tassabehji M, Strachan T. A de novo pathological point mutation at the 21-hydroxylase locus: implications for gene conversion in the human genome. *Nature Genet* 1993;3:260–265.

30. Hejtmancik JF, Black S, Harris S, et al. Congenital 21-hydroxylase deficiency as a new deletion mutation. *Hum Immunol* 1992;35:246–252.

31. Tajima T, Fujieda K, Fujii-Kuriyama Y. De novo mutation causes steroid 21-hydroxylase deficiency in one family of HLA-identical affected and unaffected siblings. *J Clin Endocrinol Metab* 1993;77:86–89.

32. Awdeh ZL, Raum D, Yunis EJ, Alper CA. Extended HLA complement allele haplotypes: evidence for T/t-like complex in man. *Proc Natl Acad Sci USA* 1983;80:259–263.

33. Klouda PT, Harris R, Price DA. Linkage and association between HLA and 21-hydroxylase deficiency. *J Med Genet* 1980;17:337–341.

34. Dupont B, Virdis R, Lerner AJ, Nelson C, Pollack MS, New MI. Distinct HLA-B antigen associations for the salt-wasting and simple virilizing forms of congenital adrenal hyperplasia due to 21-hydroxylase deficiency. In: Albert ED, Baur MP, Mayr WR, eds. *Histocompatibility testing 1984*. Berlin: Springer-Verlag; 1984:660.

35. New MI, Speiser P. Genetics of adrenal steroid 21-hydroxylase deficiency. *Endocr Rev* 1986;7:331–349.

36. O'Neill GJ, Dupont B, Pollack MS, Levine LS, New MI. Complement C4 allotypes in congenital adrenal hyperplasia due to 21-hydroxylase deficiency: further evidence for different allele variants at the 21-hydroxylase locus. *Clin Immunol Immunopathol* 1982;23:312–332.

37. Fleischnick E, Raum D, Alosco SM, et al. Extended MHC haplotypes in 21-hydroxylase deficiency congenital adrenal hyperplasia: shared genotypes in unrelated patients. *Lancet* 1983;1:152–156.

38. Raum DL, Awdeh ZL, Anderson J, et al. Human C4 haplotypes with duplicated C4A or C4B. *Am J Hum Genet* 1984;36:72–79.

39. Kastelan A, Brkljacic-Surkalovic LJ, Dumic M. The HLA associations in congenital adrenal hyperplasia due to 21-hydroxylase deficiency in a Yugoslav population. *Ann NY Acad Sci* 1985;458:41–45.

40. White PC, Vitek A, Dupont B, New MI. Characterization of frequent deletions causing steroid 21-hydroxylase deficiency. *Proc Natl Acad Sci USA* 1988;85:4436–4440.

41. White PC, New MI, Dupont B. HLA-linked congenital adrenal hyperplasia results from a defective gene encoding a cytochrome P450 specific for steroid 21-hydroxylation. *Proc Natl Acad Sci USA* 1984;81:7505–7509.

42. Globerman H, Amor M, Parker KL, New MI, White PC. A nonsense mutation causing steroid 21-hydroxylase deficiency. *J Clin Invest* 1988;82:139–144.

43. Higashi Y, Hiromasa T, Tanae A, et al. Effects of individual mutations in the P-450(C21) pseu-

dogene on the P-450(C21) activity and their distribution in the patient genomes of congenital steroid 21-hydroxylase deficiency. *J Biochem* 1991;109:638–644.

44. Chiou SH, Hu MC, Chung BC. A missense mutation at Ile[172]→Asn or Arg[356]Trp causes steroid 21-hydroxylase deficiency. *J Biol Chem* 1990;265:3549–3552.

45. Higashi Y, Tanae A, Inoue H, Hiromasa T, Fujii-Kuriyama Y. Aberrant splicing and missense mutations cause steroid 21-hydroxylase [P450c(21)] deficiency in humans. *Proc Natl Acad Sci USA* 1988;85:7486–7490.

46. Wedell A, Ritzén EM, Haglund-Stengler B, Luthman L. Steroid 21-hydroxylase deficiency: three additional mutated alleles and establishment of phenotype-genotype relationships of common mutations. *Proc Natl Acad Sci USA* 1992;89:7232–7236.

47. Wedell A, Luthman H. Steroid 21-hydroxylase deficiency: two additional mutations in salt-wasting disease and rapid screening of disease-causing mutations. *Hum Mol Genet* 1993;2:499–504.

48. Wedell A, Luthman H. Steroid 21-hydroxylase (P450c21): a new allele and spread of mutations through the pseudogene. *Hum Genet* 1993;91:236–240.

49. Amor M, Parker KL, Globerman H, New MI, White PC. Mutation in the CYP21B gene (Ile-172 to Asn) causes steroid 21-hydroxylase deficiency. *Proc Natl Acad Sci USA* 1988;85:1600–1604.

50. Speiser PW, New MI, White PC. Molecular genetic analysis of nonclassic steroid 21-hydroxylase deficiency associated with the HLA haplotype B14;DR1. *N Engl J Med* 1988;319:19–23.

51. Wu DA, Chung BC. Mutations of P450c21 (steroid 21-hydroxylase) at Cys428, Val281, and Ser268 result in complete, partial or no loss of enzymatic activity, respectively. *J Clin Invest* 1991;88:519–523.

52. Tusie-Luna MT, Speiser PW, Dumic M, New MI, White PC. A mutation (Pro-30 to Leu-30) in CYP21 represents a potential nonclassic steroid 21-hydroxylase deficiency allele. *Mol Endocrinol* 1991;5:685–692.

53. Owerbach D, Sherman L, Ballard A-L, Azziz R. Pro-453 to Ser mutation in CYP21 is associated with nonclassic steroid 21-hydroxylase deficiency. *Mol Endocrinol* 1992;6:1211–1215.

54. Morel Y, David M, Forest MG, et al. Gene conversions and rearrangements cause discordance between inheritance of forms of 21-hydroxylase deficiency and HLA types. *J Clin Endocrinol Metab* 1989;68:592–599.

55. Speiser PW, Dupont B, Zhu D, et al. Disease expression and molecular genotype in congenital adrenal hyperplasia due to 21-hydroxylase deficiency. *J Clin Invest* 1992;90:594–595.

56. Tusie-Luna MT, Traktman P, White PC. Determination of functional effects of mutations in the steroid 21-hydroxylase gene (CYP21) using recombinant vaccinia virus. *J Biol Chem* 1990;265:20,916–922.

57. New MI, Lorenzen F, Lerner AJ, et al. Genotyping steroid 21-hydroxylase deficiency: hormonal reference data. *J Clin Endocrinol Metab* 1983;57:320–326.

58. Gutai JP, Kowarski AA, Migeon CJ. The detection of the heterozygous carrier for congenital virilizing adrenal hyperplasia. *J Pediatr* 1977;90:924–929.

59. Lorenzen F, Pang S, New MI, et al. Studies on the C-21 and C-19 steroids and HLA genotyping in siblings and parents of patients with congenital adrenal hyperplasia due to 21-hydroxylase deficiency. *J Clin Endocrinol Metab* 1980;50:572–577.

60. Lorenzen F, Pang S, New MI, Dupont B, Pollack MS, Chow D, Levine LS. Hormonal phenotype and HLA-genotype in families of patients with congenital adrenal hyperplasia (21-hydroxylase deficiency). *Pediatr Res* 1979;13:1356–1360.

61. Grosse-Wilde H, Weil J, Albert E, Scholz S, Bidlingmaier F, Sippel WG, Knorr D. Genetic linkage studies between congenital adrenal hyperplasia and the HLA blood group system. *Immunogenetics* 1979;8:41–49.

62. Rosler A, Levine LS, Schneider B, Novogroder M, New MI. The interrelationship of sodium balance, plasma renin activity and ACTH in congenital adrenal hyperplasia. *J Clin Endocrinol Metab* 1977;45:500–512.

63. David M, Forest MG. Prenatal treatment of congenital adrenal hyperplasia resulting from 21-hydroxylase deficiency. *J Pediatr* 1984;105:799–803.

64. Karaviti LP, Mercado AB, Mercado MB, et al. Prenatal diagnosis/treatment in families at risk for infants with steroid 21-hydroxylase deficiency (congenital adrenal hyperplasia). *J Steroid Biochem Mol Biol* 1992;41:445–451.

65. Speiser PW, Laforgia N, Kato K, et al. First trimester prenatal treatment and molecular genetic diagnosis of congenital adrenal hyperplasia (21-hydroxylase deficiency). *J Clin Endocrinol Metab* 1990;70:838–848.

66. Owerbach D, Draznin MB, Carpenter RJ, Greenberg F. Prenatal diagnosis of 21-hydroxylase deficiency congenital adrenal hyperplasia using the polymerase chain reaction. *Hum Genet (Oxf)* 1992; 89:109–110.
67. Rumsby G, Honour JW, Rodeck C. Prenatal diagnosis of congenital adrenal hyperplasia by direct detection of mutations in the steroid 21-hydroxylase gene. *Clin Endocrinol* 1993;38:421–425.
68. Forest MG, David M, Morel Y. Prenatal diagnosis and treatment of 21-hydroxylase deficiency. *J Steroid Biochem Mol Biol* 1993;45:75–82.
69. Rosler A. Classic and nonclassic congenital adrenal hyperplasia among non-ashkenazi Jews. In: Bonne-Tamir B, ed. *New perspectives on genetic markers and diseases among the Jewish people.* Oxford: Oxford University Press; 1992.
70. Eberlein WR, Bongiovanni AM. Plasma and urinary corticosteroids in the hypertensive form of congenital adrenal hyperplasia. *J Biol Chem* 1956;223:85–94.
71. New MI, Levine LS. Congenital adrenal hyperplasia In: Harris H, Hirschhorn K, eds. *Advances in human genetics.* Vol 4. New York: Plenum Press; 1973:251–376.
72. Levine LS, Rauh W, Gottesdiener K, et al. New studies of the 11β-hydroxylase and 18-hydroxylase enzymes in the hypertensive form of congenital adrenal hyperplasia. *J Clin Endocrinol Metab* 1980; 50:258–263.
73. New MI, Seaman MP. Secretion rates of cortisol and aldosterone precursors in various forms of congenital adrenal hyperplasia. *J Clin Endocrinol Metab* 1970;30:361–371.
74. Rösler A, Leibermann E, Sack J, et al. Clinical variability of congenital adrenal hyperplasia due to 11β-hydroxylase deficiency. *Horm Res* 1982:16:133–141.
75. Zachmann M, Tassinari D, Prader A. Clinical and biochemical variability of congenital adrenal hyperplasia due to 11β-hydroxylase deficiency. *J Clin Endocrinol Metab* 1983;56:222–229.
76. Chua SC, Szabo P, Vitek A, Grzeschik K-H, John M, White PC. Cloning of cDNA encoding steroid 11β-hydroxylase (P450c11). *Proc Natl Acad Sci USA* 1987;84:7193–7197.
77. Mornet E, Dupont J, Vitek A, White PC. Characterization of two genes encoding human steroid 11β-hydroxylase deficiency (P45011β). *J Biol Chem* 1989;264:20,961–20,967.
78. Wada A, Okamoto M, Nonaka Y, Yamano T. Aldosterone biosynthesis by a reconstituted cytochrome P45011 beta system. *Biochem Biophys Res Commun* 1984;119:365–371.
79. Curnow KM, Tusie-Luna MT, Pascoe L, et al. The product of the CYP11B gene is required for aldosterone biosynthesis in the human adrenal cortex. *Mol Endocrinol* 1991;5:1513–1522.
80. Ogishima T, Shibata H, Shimada H, Mitani F, Suzuki H, Saruta T, Ishimura Y. Aldosterone synthase cytochrome P-450 expressed in the adrenals of patients with primary aldosteronism. *J Biol Chem* 1991;266:10,731–10,734.
81. White PC, Dupont J, New MI, Leiberman E, Hochberg Z, Rosler A. A mutation in CYP11B1 (Arg-448→His) associated with steroid 11β-hydroxylase deficiency in Jews of Moroccan origin. *J Clin Invest* 1991;87:1664–1667.
82. Helmberg A, Ausserer B, Kofler R. Frame shift by insertion of 2 basepairs in codon 394 of CYP11B1 causes congenital adrenal hyperplasia due to steroid 11β-hydroxylase deficiency. *J Clin Endocrinol Metab* 1992;75:1278–1281.
83. Curnow CM, Slutsker L, Vitek J, et al. Mutations in the CYP11B1 gene causing congenital adrenal hyperplasia and hypertension cluster in exons 6, 7, and 8. *Proc Natl Acad Sci USA* 1993;90:4552–4556.
84. Naiki Y, Kawamoto T, Mitsuuchi Y, et al. A nonsense mutation (TGG[Trp[116]]→TAG[Stop]) in CYP11B1 causes steroid 11β-hydroxylase deficiency. *J Clin Endocrinol Metab* 1993;77:1677–1682.
85. Bongiovanni AM. Congenital adrenal hyperplasia due to 3β-hydroxysteroid deficiency. In: New MI, Levine LS, eds. *Adrenal disease in childhood.* Basel: Karger; 1984;72–82.
86. Kenny FM, Reynolds JW, Green OC. Partial 3β-hydroxysteroid dehydrogenase (3β-HSD) deficiency in a family with congenital adrenal hyperplasia: evidence for increasing 3β-HSD activity with age. *Pediatrics* 1971;48:756–765.
87. Pang S, Levine LS, Stoner E, Opitz JM, New MI. Non salt-losing congenital adrenal hyperplasia due to 3β-hydroxysteroid dehydrogenase activity with normal glomerulosa function. *J Clin Endocrinol Metab* 1983;56:808–818.
88. Jänne O, Perheentupa J, Vihko R. Plasma and urinary steroids in an eight year old boy with 3β-hydroxysteroid dehydrogenase deficiency. *J Clin Endocrinol Metab* 1970;31:162–165.
89. Schneider G, Genel M, Bongiovanni AM, Goldman AS, Rosenfield RL. Persistent testicular Δ5-isomerase-3β-hydroxysteroid dehydrogenase (D5-3β-HSD) deficiency in the D5-3β-HSD form of congenital adrenal hyperplasia. *J Clin Invest* 1975;55:681–690.

90. Pang S, Lerner AJ, Stoner E, et al. Late-onset adrenal steroid 3β-hydroxysteroid dehydrogenase deficiency I: cause of hirsutism in pubertal and postpubertal women. *J Clin Endocrinol Metab* 1985;60:428–439.
91. Simard J, Rhéaume E, Sanchez R, et al. Molecular basis of congenital adrenal hyperplasia due to 3β-hydroxysteroid dehydrogenase deficiency. *Mol Endocrinol* 1993;7:716–728.
92. Chang YT, Kappy MS, Iwamoto K, Wang J, Yang X, Pang S. Mutations in the type II 3β-hydroxy-steroid dehydrogenase gene in a patient with classic salt-wasting 3β-hydroxysteroid dehydrogenase deficiency congenital adrenal hyperplasia. *Pediatr Res* 1993;34:698–700.
93. Chang YT, Wang J, Yang X, Pang S. Molecular basis of the type II 3-beta-hydroxysteroid dehydro-genase (3β-HSD) gene in patients with mild nonclassic (late-onset) 3β-HSD deficiency congenital adrenal hyperplasia (CAH). Program and Abstracts, 75th Annual Meeting of the Endocrine Society, Las Vegas, NV, June 1993; abstract N 1384.
94. New MI. Male pseudohermaphroditism due to 17α-hydroxylase deficiency. *J Clin Invest* 1970;49: 1930–1941.
95. Yanase T, Simpson ER, Waterman MR. 17α-hydroxylase/17,20-lyase deficiency: from clinical in-vestigation to molecular definition. *Endocr Rev* 1991;12:91–108.
96. Chung BC, Matteson KJ, Voutilainen R, Mohandas TK, Miller WM. Human cholesterol side-chain cleavage enzyme, P450scc: cDNA cloning, assignment of the gene to chromosome 15, and expres-sion in the placenta. *Proc Natl Acad Sci USA* 1986;83:8962–8966.
97. Lin D, Gikelman SE, Saenger P, Miller WL. Normal genes for the cholesterol side-chain cleavage enzyme, P450SCC, in congenital lipoid adrenal hyperplasia. *J Clin Invest* 1991,88:1955–1962.
98. New MI, Dupont B, Grumbach K, Levine LS. Congenital adrenal hyperplasia and related disorders. In: Stanbury JB, Wyngaarden JB, et al., eds. *The metabolic basis of inherited disease*, 5th ed. New York: McGraw-Hill; 1983:973–1000.
99. White PC, New MI. Genetic basis of endocrine disease. 2: Congenital adrenal hyperplasia due to 21-hydroxylase deficiency. *J Clin Endocrinol Metab* 1992;74:6–11.

Androgenic Disorders,
edited by G. P. Redmond.
Raven Press, Ltd., New York © 1995.

9

Adrenal Androgen Excess in Women with Cushing's Syndrome and Adrenal Tumors

Leslie R. Sheeler

Department of Endocrinology, Innova Medical Services, Brooklyn, Ohio 44144.

Since Harvey Cushing first described the clinical features of the disorder which now bears his name (1,2), androgen excess has been recognized as a major manifestation of Cushing's syndrome. Acne, hirsutism, and androgenic alopecia are often present in women with Cushing's syndrome. Frank virilization with decrease in breast and hip size, muscular hypertrophy, clitoromegaly, deepening of the voice, etc., even occurs in some women with androgen and cortisol excess.

The diagnosis and therapy of Cushing's syndrome are fraught with many problems (3–5). It is imperative that the patient be correctly classified with the right diagnosis since therapy must be directed at what is causing the problem. The pituitary gland, the adrenal gland, both adrenal glands, or tumors that cause Cushing's syndrome via the ectopic production of adrenocorticotropic hormone (ACTH) or corticotropin releasing factor (CRF) may need to be treated. There are a number of diagnostic difficulties that sometimes make accurate diagnosis difficult. Our attempts at therapy remain imperfect. Because Cushing's syndrome is a rare disorder and the clinical features have an insidious onset, it often goes undetected for months or years before the correct diagnosis is made (6,7). Yet as a health-threatening and even life-threatening disorder, Cushing's syndrome needs to be diagnosed when it is present.

CLINICAL FEATURES

Cushing's syndrome occurs mostly in women between ages 20 and 50, but it does occur in both sexes at all ages. Cushing's syndrome is rare in children—only 3% to 5% of all cases occur in childhood. The approximate occurrence of the most common signs and symptoms are summarized in Table 1.

Hypertension occurs about 80% of the time in Cushing's syndrome, while glucose intolerance or clinical diabetes occurs about half the time. Since both are so common in obese subjects with normal cortisol production, they are not very helpful as discriminatory clues to the diagnosis of Cushing's syndrome (6). More specific

TABLE 1. *Clinical features of Cushing's syndrome*

Sign or symptom	Approximate incidence (%)
Round face	85
Proximal weakness	80
Truncal weight gain	80
Thin skin	80
Hirsutism	80
Facial plethora	80
Amenorrhea/oligomenorrhea	75
Psychiatric symptoms (depression, psychosis, somatization disorder, etc.)	70
Acne	50
Purple striae	50
Osteopenia	50

indicators include proximal muscle weakness, round plethoric facies, presence of a hump and supraclavicular fat pads, thin skin, and truncal obesity. Hirsutism, acne, or androgenic alopecia occur in the majority of female patients. Increased lanugo hair on the face is also common and is attributed to cortisol excess rather than androgen excess.

Oligo- or amenorrhea occurs in three-fourths of premenopausal women. Most women with active Cushing's syndrome are also infertile, but 67 pregnancies in 58 women with Cushing's syndrome have been reported to date (9).

PATHOPHYSIOLOGY AND CLASSIFICATION OF CUSHING'S SYNDROME

An important pathophysiologic point is the distinction between ACTH-dependent and ACTH-independent Cushing's syndrome. Table 2 lists the various forms of Cushing's syndrome.

TABLE 2. *Types of Cushing's syndrome*

ACTH-dependent		ACTH-independent	
Entity	% of cases	Entity	% of cases
ACTH-secreting pituitary tumor	80	Adrenal adenoma	10
Eutopic CRF excess	?	Adrenal carcinoma	5
Ectopic CRF excess	<1	Micronodular adrenal hyperplasia	<1
Ectopic ACTH syndrome	3	Some cases of macronodular hyperplasia	<1
Some cases of macronodular hyperplasia	3–10 (part of 80% above)		

The most common type of cortisol excess is pituitary-dependent, ACTH over-production, i.e., Cushing's disease. Cushing's disease is usually due to a pituitary microadenoma (less than 10 mm in size) that secretes ACTH. Hyperplasia of cor-ticotrope cells is relatively rare (5,10), as is the finding of no definite abnormality despite very careful pathologic examination of the resected pituitary tissue (11). Very large adenomas that are locally invasive, and thus are nearly impossible to resect for a cure, occur in roughly 5% of patients with Cushing's disease.

The pathophysiology of the cortisol and androgen excess in Cushing's disease is fairly straightforward. The excess ACTH stimulates the adrenal cortex to make excess cortisol. There are more secretory bursts of ACTH in Cushing's disease, cortisol production rates increase as a result, and diurnal variation of ACTH and cortisol are usually lost. These tumors are often suppressible with glucocorticoids, which allowed Dr. Liddle (12) to devise his classic dexamethasone suppression test.

Adrenal androgens are hypersecreted in Cushing's disease. The secretion of de-hydroepihydrosterone (DHEA), DHEA-sulfate (DHEA-S) (13), androstenedione (which is converted to testosterone in the periphery), and adrenal testosterone itself are often increased due to the ACTH excess (14). Fig. 1 shows testosterone levels in a series of 23 women before and after therapy for Cushing's disease. These high androgen levels cause the androgen-excess manifestations frequently seen in women with Cushing's disease. Fig. 2 shows DHEA-S levels in patients with Cush-ing's disease and patients with adrenal adenomas and Cushing's syndrome. Note the suppressed DHEA-S levels in the patients with adrenal adenomas. Glucocorticoids suppress gonadotropin secretion (15), presumably resulting in the frequently ob-served menstrual abnormalities and relative infertility in affected women.

There has been a long-standing debate about all of the hormone-secreting pitu-itary adenomas: Are these primary tumors? (16) Or are these secondary to a hypo-thalamic abnormality (17) (e.g., CRF excess) that eventually results in the pituitary tumor that causes the adrenal hypersecretion? Although there is no absolutely de-finitive answer in Cushing's disease, the weight of evidence currently favors the primary tumor enthusiasts. Almost all patients with Cushing's disease have distinct corticotrope adenomas. If hypothalamic CRF overproduction causes the tumors, why do we not find more hyperplasia? And why does it take a year for the hypo-thalamic–pituitary–adrenal axis to recover? There are some recurrences; we re-cently reported the highest percentage to date: 20% (18). Even if our series has about the same percentage as others will eventually find, about 80% remain cured. In our series, two patients had repeat surgery. Both had tumors that appeared the same histologically as the original ones and both tumors were in the same location. This implies that in these two individuals, incomplete resection, rather than entirely new tumor formation, caused the recurrence of the Cushing's disease.

Additional forms of ACTH-dependent Cushing's syndrome include ectopic se-cretion of ACTH (4), or CRF (19), and some cases of macronodular adrenal hyper-plasia (20,21). Ectopic production of ACTH has been reported in many kinds of tumors (22). Classical ectopic ACTH syndrome is usually characterized by marked ACTH and cortisol excess, wasting with weight loss and weakness, and hypo-

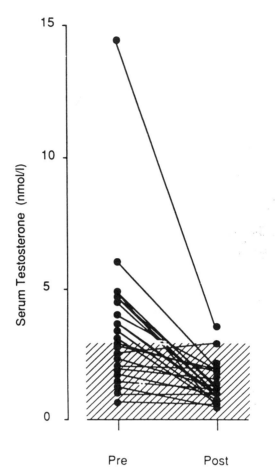

FIG. 1. Serum testosterone concentrations in 23 patients before and after treatment with ^{90}Y interstitial irradiation. The upper limit of normal is shown at 3nmol/L. (From ref. 91, with permission.)

kalemia. These patients often get ill so fast that they do not have many, if any, of the clinical features noted in Table 1. These patients usually have fairly malignant tumors, such as, oat cell cancer. However, some patients with benign or malignant tumors (e.g., thymoma, carcinoid, islet cell, pheochromocytoma, etc.) may have features of classic Cushing's syndrome and, in fact, may have clinical and laboratory features identical to those seen in patients with Cushing's disease. Correctly identifying these patients with occult ectopic ACTH syndrome is critical (23). This will be discussed in detail in the section on laboratory diagnosis.

Tumors have been described that make CRF in addition to ACTH (24). The case described by Asa et al. (25) of an intrasellar gangliocytoma was unique because the patient was curable with resection of the tumor which made CRF.

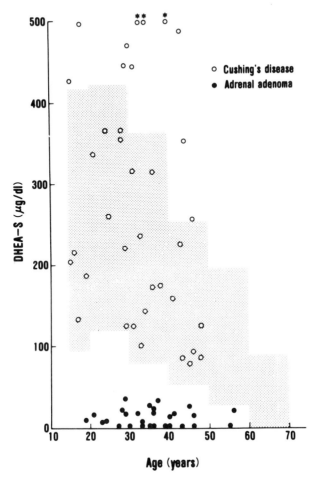

FIG. 2. Serum DHEA-S levels in patients with Cushing's disease (○) and in patients with hyper-adrenocorticism due to benign adrenocortical adenoma (●). The shaded area represents the 95% confidence limits of serum DHEA-S levels in normal individuals. *, over 500 μg/dL. (From ref. 13, with permission.)

Some patients with macronodular adrenal hyperplasia are clearly ACTH-dependent (20). Macronodular hyperplasia is characterized by bilateral, often massive, adrenal enlargement: often the total adrenal weight is 10 to 20 times the normal adrenal weight.

Since each of the disorders described above is ACTH dependent, adrenal androgen excess may accompany the cortisol excess.

Benign adrenal tumors which cause Cushing's syndrome usually make glucocorticoids only. Conversely, malignant adrenal tumors causing Cushing's syndrome may make androgens or mineralocorticoids (26). In patients who have tumors that make only cortisol, ACTH becomes quite suppressed. In turn, adrenal androgens are often quite low (13) (see Fig. 2). Adrenal cancers that make androgens and cortisol may have very high androgen levels and severe androgen excess manifestations clinically.

Micronodular adrenal hyperplasia refers to a unique subtype of Cushing's syndrome (27). The patients are usually young, and they usually have mild or atypical features of Cushing's syndrome and small or normal sized adrenals with hyperplastic/dysplastic nests of glucocorticoid-secreting cells (28). These cases often occur in association with Carney's complex (29), that is, they often have atrial myxomas, nerve tumors, micronodular adrenal hyperplasia, etc. This type of Cushing's syndrome is ACTH-independent, and thus low androgen levels might be found (30). Some have reported the presence of an adrenal-stimulating antibody (31). If this is correct, micronodular hyperplasia may be analogous to Grave's disease with hyperthyroidism.

Just as there are cases of macronodular hyperplasia with ACTH dependency, there are some cases that have ACTH independence (32,33). Androgen levels are variable in these patients.

LABORATORY DIAGNOSIS OF HYPERCORTISOLISM

Once Cushing's syndrome is suspected on clinical grounds, the diagnosis depends on documentation of endogenous cortisol excess. The best index of an excess cortisol production rate is the measurement of the amount of free cortisol in a 24-hour urine collection (34). This test is usually positive in patients with active Cushing's syndrome. Another commonly used screening test is the overnight dexamethasone test: 1 mg of dexamethasone at midnight followed by measurement of plasma cortisol at 8 or 9 AM (a normal result is less than 5 μg/dL). False negatives may occur in up to 10% of cases (35), making this an unacceptable screening test, especially for this serious disorder. False positives are also very common, occurring in up to 25% of cases (36).

About 10% of patients with actual Cushing's syndrome hypersecrete in episodes (37,38). Thus, if there are reasons to continue to suspect active Cushing's, one or more additional 24-hour urine samples for free cortisol levels should be collected if the first is negative (Fig. 3).

Once cortisol excess is documented by finding elevated free cortisol in the urine (usually greater than or equal to 150% of the upper limit of normal), two or more plasma ACTH (39) levels should be obtained. ACTH levels too low to measure indicate adrenal disease should be present. Levels from normal to twice normal suggest Cushing's disease, while levels greater than twice normal suggest ectopic ACTH syndrome. Invasive pituitary macroadenomas may have ACTH levels in the range found in ectopic ACTH syndrome (40).

The suppressibility of urine free cortisol with administration of dexamethasone (0.5 mg every 6 hours for 2 days, followed by 2.0 mg every 6 hours for 2 days) is the best single test (See Figs. 3, 4) to classify the type of Cushing's syndrome.

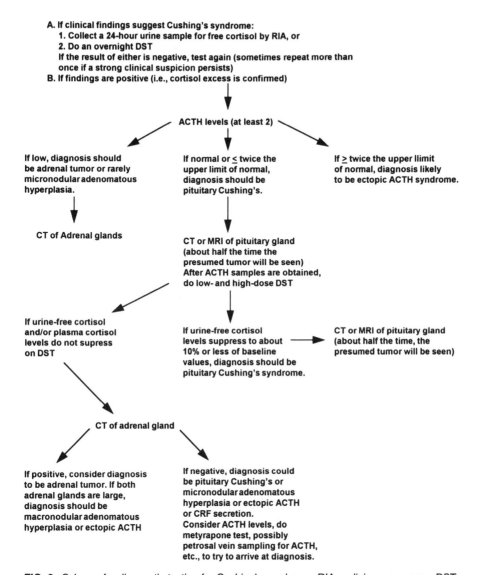

A. If clinical findings suggest Cushing's syndrome:
   1. Collect a 24-hour urine sample for free cortisol by RIA, or
   2. Do an overnight DST
   If the result of either is negative, test again (sometimes repeat more than
   once if a strong clinical suspicion persists)
B. If findings are positive (i.e., cortisol excess is confirmed)

ACTH levels (at least 2)

If low, diagnosis should
be adrenal tumor or rarely
micronodular adenomatous
hyperplasia.

If normal or ≤ twice the
upper limit of normal,
diagnosis should be
pituitary Cushing's.

If ≥ twice the upper llimit
of normal, diagnosis likely
to be ectopic ACTH syndrome.

CT of Adrenal glands

CT or MRI of pituitary gland
(about half the time the
presumed tumor will be seen)
After ACTH samples are obtained,
do low- and high-dose DST

If urine-free cortisol
and/or plasma cortisol
levels do not supress
on DST

If urine-free cortisol
levels suppress to about
10% or less of baseline
values, diagnosis should be
pituitary Cushing's syndrome.

CT or MRI of pituitary gland
(about half the time, the
presumed tumor will be seen)

CT of adrenal gland

If positive, consider diagnosis
to be adrenal tumor. If both
adrenal glands are large,
diagnosis should be
macronodular adenomatous
hyperplasia or ectopic ACTH

If negative, diagnosis could
be pituitary Cushing's or
micronodular adenomatous
hyperplasia or ectopic ACTH
or CRF secretion.
Consider ACTH levels, do
metyrapone test, possibly
petrosal vein sampling for ACTH,
etc., to try to arrive at diagnosis.

FIG. 3. Scheme for diagnostic testing for Cushing's syndrome. RIA, radioimmune assay; DST, dexamethasone test. (From ref. 8, with permission.)

Other tests include measurement of plasma cortisol values during the dexamethasone testing, measuring urine 17-hydroxysteroids at baseline and on the second and fourth days [the original test of Dr. Liddle (12)], giving 8 mg of dexamethasone at midnight and checking cortisol the next AM (42) (> 50% suppression compared to the baseline cortisol indicates Cushing's disease), and infusing dexamethasone i.v. (43). This last test involves continuous infusion of dexamethasone at a rate of 1 mg/

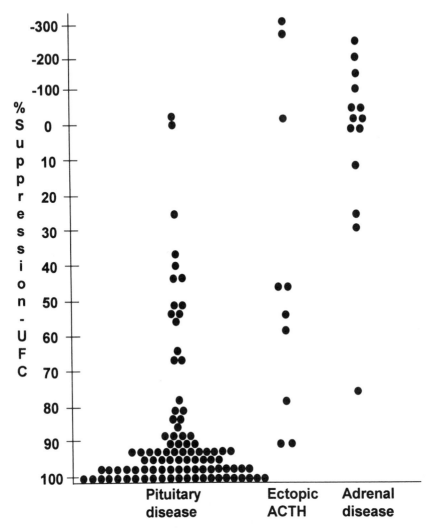

FIG. 4. Results of dexamethasone suppression of urine levels of free cortisol in pituitary disease, ectopic ACTH syndrome, and adrenal disease. (From ref. 41, with permission.)

hour for 7 hours. A positive test indicating Cushing's disease is a cortisol decrease of at least 190 nmol/L (44).

The best-studied test is the first of these choices. Fig. 4 shows that suppression of 24-hour urine free cortisol levels by 90% correctly separates the patients with Cushing's disease from the other forms of cortisol excess. Patients with some suppression, but not 90%, may have either Cushing's disease or occult ectopic ACTH syndrome. Further testing including inferior petrosal sinus sampling (45) may be needed to allow the physician to make a definite diagnosis.

Other tests or procedures are less reliable at making a diagnosis. Urinary 17-OH corticosteroids are often falsely normal in patients with Cushing's syndrome. Lack of diurnal variation in AM and PM cortisols is a notoriously inconclusive test because of the episodic secretory bursts of ACTH and cortisol in normal individuals and in patients with Cushing's disease. The ACTH response to CRF infusion (46), or responses to metyrapone administration (47), may fail to discriminate Cushing's disease from the other forms of Cushing's syndrome.

PROBLEMS IN DIAGNOSIS

Stress, depression (48), and alcoholism (49,50) are among the conditions that may mimic Cushing's syndrome biochemically: urine free cortisol levels may be high and suppression with dexamethasone may be abnormal. Some individuals have a reduced metabolic clearance of dexamethasone (51), which likely accounts for at least some of the false-negative overnight dexamethasone tests noted above. Fast clearance of dexamethasone, either spontaneous or secondary to drugs such as phenytoin or barbiturates, may account for false-positive dexamethasone suppression tests. If unsatisfactory dexamethasone testing is suspected, simultaneous measurement of dexamethasone and cortisol levels is possible (52).

High estrogen states, such as pregnancy (53) or estrogen therapy (54), raise cortisol-binding globulin levels and thus raise plasma cortisol levels. Urine free cortisol levels may even increase to high values (54). Decadron suppression of plasma cortisol may be abnormal in these patients.

Alcoholism, especially with liver disease, may mimic Cushing's disease clinically and chemically (55,56). Hidden alcohol abuse thus may be a major diagnostic problem.

Intermittent or cyclic Cushing's syndrome (57) is a common occurrence, seen in roughly 10% of those with the disorder. This can occur in a regular pattern of days to weeks or months (58), or it may be totally episodic with no pattern (59). In between the bursts of hypercortisolism, levels may be normal. Frequent sampling is the only way to make the diagnosis in these patients with periodic hormonogenesis.

The major difficulty is separating the patients with occult ectopic ACTH syndrome from those with Cushing's disease. Results from the NIH group suggest that if there is not 90% suppression of urine cortisol levels with the high dose of dexamethasone, petrosal sinus sampling (with CRF administration to maximize surges of ACTH) may be the wisest course of action (41,45).

RADIOLOGIC STUDIES

Another very important caveat is to select the radiologic procedures indicated by the results of biochemical tests. Misinterpretation of images of the pituitary and adrenal glands before one knows what to look for has needlessly caused many therapeutic problems for patients.

When primary adrenal disease is suggested by testing, adrenal computed tomography (CT) or magnetic resonance imaging (MRI) will reveal nearly all tumors associated with Cushing's syndrome (5). If normal adrenal glands are seen, the patient may have micronodular adrenal hyperplasia. Patients with Cushing's disease have unilateral or bilateral adrenal enlargement 10% to 30% of the time (8), yet nearly all respond totally to selective pituitary adenomectomy (45,60).

If the pituitary is the source of the problem, imaging with MRI (or sector CT) should be done. About 40% to 50% of the pituitary microadenomas are too small to definitely visualize. Enthusiasts of petrosal sinus sampling cite this problem as one additional reason to do the sampling, which can document the source as pituitary and can localize for the neurosurgeon the side that harbors the tiny adenoma (45).

Between 10% to 25% of pituitary glands examined at autopsy can contain microadenomas. Small cysts are common in the pituitary, as is unevenness in the thickness of the gland. For these reasons, false positive pituitary images can be a problem. Again, the physicians directing the diagnostic studies need to refrain from the impulse to image the pituitary before they know what they expect to find.

The tumors that cause occult ectopic ACTH syndrome can be fiendishly difficult to find (4). CT or MRI of the chest has correctly identified some of the carcinoids responsible for this syndrome (47). Sometimes, repeated searches over many years have been needed to finally find the tumor responsible (4,23,57).

THERAPY OF CUSHING'S SYNDROME

Therapy is directed at the source of the problem. Pituitary microsurgery via the transsphenoidal approach with selective adenomectomy is now used as the primary therapy for Cushing's disease at most major medical centers. The problems with this approach include failure to cure some of the patients [the lowest initial success rate is about 70% (62) and the highest success rate is about 95% (45)], recurrences later at 3 to 5 years after the first surgery (up to 20% of cases), and complications from the surgery itself such as CSF leaks, hypopituitarism, and perforated nasal septum. Complications other than ACTH deficiency are usually under 5% when the surgery is performed by an experienced team (60,61,63). Postoperative death is rare (under 1%). Cured patients need to be assessed yearly for at least 6 years since recurrence may occur up to 5 years after surgery (18). A necessary and desirable complication is selective ACTH deficiency, which lasts about a year in most patients. Failure to achieve this deficiency means that the patient almost certainly will have persistence of the Cushing's disease. Under 5% of patients have permanent ACTH deficiency. Failure to achieve an initial cure after pituitary surgery is due to many factors including incomplete removal of a tumor, inability to find the tumor, misdiagnosis, or the location of the adenoma in an aberrant area, for example, in an extra (or accessory) pituitary gland (64,65). An example of the last situation occurred in at least one of the patients in the NIH series (45), a woman whose two petrosal sinus samplings placed the ACTH source as the sella. Despite this, three pituitary surgeries failed to cure the Cushing's disease, despite leaving her with profound hypopituitarism. No ACTH-secreting tumor or corticotrope hyperplasia was ever identified in the surgical material.

One question that is inevitably raised when cure is not achieved is whether to reoperate or treat in some other way. Perhaps the best situation for a second operation is when an incidental adenoma or cyst that was not responsible for the Cushing's disease was found and removed at the first surgery. When this tissue is found not to stain for ACTH, there is some hope that the ACTH-secreting adenoma might still be found and removed at a second surgery. Otherwise, second operations have a low success rate (60,61). The majority of patients treated with radiation therapy after failed pituitary surgery have responded (66–68). Our experience with control of the disease with radiation therapy after unsuccessful initial surgery or after recurrence of disease has been surprisingly good: normal urine free cortisol levels within 2 years in 6 of 8 patients (69). Radiation therapy directed at the pituitary should be used only when there was proof of an ACTH-secreting adenoma or corticotrope hyperplasia.

Finding and successfully treating the tumors that cause occult ectopic ACTH syndrome is difficult. Several groups including Saint Bartholomew's in London (4,70), the University of California at San Francisco (23), and the NIH (71) have reported their experiences. About half the time, sometimes only after multiple studies over many years, the carcinoid tumor, thymoma, or islet cell tumor was discovered and removed. This also results in ACTH deficiency which lasts about a year. The only curable CRF-producing tumor known to the author was reported by Asa et al. (25). A detailed discussion about the endocrine recovery was not contained in this paper, but the patient's steroid replacement therapy was discontinued within a few months after the gangliocytoma was removed.

When the adrenal gland is the problem, either from a tumor or from bilateral ACTH-independent macronodular or micronodular hyperplasia, adrenal surgery is the preferred approach. Bilateral adrenalectomy obviously will cause permanent adrenal failure. Curative removal of a benign or malignant adrenal tumor will result in temporary adrenal failure lasting roughly 1 year, much like successful pituitary surgery for Cushing's disease. Treating with replacement steroids until the pituitary–adrenal axis recovers is necessary. Adrenal carcinoma often exhibits very aggressive behavior (26). When metastases are already present at the time of diagnosis, five-year survival is unusual (less than 5%) (72).

Although there are reports in the literature of excellent outcome with bilateral adrenalectomy for Cushing's syndrome, our group and others (73) have found a disturbingly high operative mortality. For example, from the 1960s through the 1990s, we have had at least a 10% operative mortality in each of the four decades (8).

A number of drugs have been developed that block the formation of cortisol and thus have been employed as medical therapy for Cushing's syndrome. Table 3 summarizes the drugs available in the USA. Drug therapy for Cushing's syndrome is especially useful in several clinical settings: while waiting for radiation therapy to be effective (74), while waiting to discover the tumor causing occult ectopic ACTH

TABLE 3. *Medical therapy for Cushing's syndrome*

Drug	Usual dose	Need to use glucocorticoid with the drug?	Effectiveness	Special comments
Cyproheptadine	24 mg/d	No	Quite variable	Few patients respond well.
Trilostane	200–360 mg/d	No	Generally effective	
Aminoglutethimide	1–2 g/d	Yes	Usually effective	A skin rash or drowsiness may limit use. Need to use more dexamethasone than one would expect.
Metyrapone	1–2 g/d	No	Usually effective	Least side effects of any of the effective agents.
o, p'-DDD (mitotane)	1.5–2 g	Yes	Usually effective	Used mostly for adrenal cancer. Can be used for hyperplasia; side effects frequent.
Ketoconazole	400 mg to 1 g/d	No	Usually effective	Newest agent used for medical therapy.
RU486	5–22 mg kg/d	No	Usually effective	1. May never be released due to abortion controversy. 2. Assays cannot be used to assess improvement—patient must be followed clinically.

From Sheeler, ref. 8.

syndrome, to palliate patients with incurable cancer-causing ectopic ACTH syndrome (75) or with incurable adrenal cancer (76), or to improve the status of quite ill patients prior to pituitary or adrenal surgery. Ketoconazole has some advantages over the other drugs: lower cost, ready availability, and low side effect and toxicity profiles (77).

In summary, physicians involved with the evaluation and therapy of women who are plagued by androgenic disorders need to be familiar with Cushing's syndrome. A small fraction of the women who present for evaluation of androgen excess will actually have cortisol excess as well as androgen excess. Old photographs may help the physician decide which women to investigate for Cushing's syndrome when suspicious features are present upon examination. If the patient did not appear cushingoid 2, 3, or 5 years ago but does now, investigation for possible Cushing's syndrome is warranted. A 24-hour urine collection for free cortisol is the best screening test. The diagnosis and therapy of Cushing's syndrome are often complex and difficult. Most patients are best managed by physicians with a special interest in dealing with Cushing's syndrome.

ANDROGEN-SECRETING ADRENAL TUMORS

Adrenal tumors that secrete only androgens are rare. The classic series from Vanderbilt University (26) contains only eight such patients among the 58 reported. This series spanned nearly three decades. In the last 25 years at the Cleveland Clinic, we have had three patients with pure androgen-producing tumors. In the same time interval we have had more than 170 patients with Cushing's syndrome, more than 200 with pheochromocytomas, and more than 100 with aldosterone-secreting tumors. Despite the rarity of androgen-secreting adrenal tumors, they are important because malignancy is common (26,78) and the benign adenomas are obviously curable with an adrenalectomy.

Most of the cases reported in the literature present with androgen excess that varies clinically from acne, hirsutism, or male-pattern baldness to frank virilization. Usually serum testosterone levels are quite elevated with values of greater than 400 ng/dL (79,80) (typical normal range 20 to 70 ng/dL). Most patients have high serum DHEA-S levels and/or high urine 17-keto steroid levels (78,80,81). However, there have been some cases reported of tumors that secrete testosterone but have normal serum DHEA-S or normal urine 17-keto steroid levels (78,80). In some patients this may be due to the presence of cells within the adrenal tumor which resemble Leydig cells (80). One patient with normal urine 17-keto steroids had an adrenal adenoma under gonadotropin control (82). A patient also has been described with human chorionic gonadotropin receptors in the androgen-secreting tumor (83).

The adrenal tumors that secrete androgens are usually large enough to easily identify with coned-down CT views of the adrenal gland. However, there still is some role for adrenal and ovarian vein sampling for testosterone and DHEA-S in selected patients (84,85). A case that illustrates the usefulness of venous sampling was seen at the Cleveland Clinic a few years ago. The patient was a 70-year-old woman referred for evaluation of virilization with a serum testosterone of 2,000 ng/dL and a 3 cm left adrenal adenoma. Because the serum DHEA-S levels and urine 17-keto steroids were normal, we thought it best to do the selective catheterization. An ovarian source of the testosterone was proven. At surgery, a small arrhenoblastoma was identified and removed. Her serum testosterone fell to less than 20 ng/dL and has remained the same value on follow-up visits over the past 5 years.

Adrenalectomy is the treatment of choice for androgen-secreting adrenal tumors. Noninvasive (stage 1) adrenal cancers have roughly a 50% 5-year survival rate (72). There may be a role for adjuvant mitotane therapy in some patients with adrenal carcinoma who have no known disease after adrenalectomy (86). This, unfortunately, is not often successful at preventing a recurrence (87), and in addition, ten more patients with no known metastases following adrenalectomy for adrenal carcinoma experienced a recurrence despite adjuvant mitotane and died from metastatic adrenal cortical carcinoma (*unpublished data*).

Mitotane can control hormonal secretion about 75% of the time, but tumor regression is rare (13.5%) (88). There appears to be little if any effect of mitotane on survival in metastatic adrenal cancer (89,72). At this time, there is no chemotherapeutic regimen that significantly prolongs survival in metastatic adrenocortical carcinoma, although there have been responders to 5-fluorouracil, cisplatin, and doxorubicin (90).

REFERENCES

1. Cushing H. Dyspituitarism. *Harvey Lect* 1910;11:31–45.
2. Cushing H. The basophile adenomas of the pituitary body and their clinical manifestations. *Bull Johns Hopkins Hosp* 1932;50:127–195.
3. Aron D, Tyrrell JB, Fitzgerald PA, Findling JW, Forsham PH. Cushing's syndrome: problems in diagnosis. *Medicine* 1981;60(1):25–33.
4. Howlett TA, Drury PL, Perry L, Doniach I, Rees LH, Besser GM. Diagnosis and management of ACTH-dependent Cushing's syndrome: comparison of the features in ectopic and pituitary ACTH production. *Clin Endocrinol* 1986;24:699–713.
5. Carpenter PC. Cushing's syndrome: update of diagnosis and management. *Mayo Clin Proc* 1986; 61:49–58.
6. Ross EJ, Linch DC. Cushing's syndrome—killing disease: discriminatory value of signs and symptoms aiding early diagnosis. *Lancet* 1982:646–649.
7. Plotz CM, Knowlton AI, Ragan C. The natural history of Cushing's syndrome. *Am J Med* 1952: 597–614.
8. Sheeler LR. Cushing's syndrome—1988. *Cleve Clin J Med* 1988;55:329–337.
9. Aron DC, Schnall AM, Sheeler LR. Cushing's syndrome and pregnancy. *Am J Obstet Gynecol* 1990;162(1):244–252.
10. Young WF, Scheithauer BW, Hossein G, Laws ER, Carpenter PC. Cushing's syndrome due to primary multinodular corticotrope hyperplasia. *Mayo Clin Proc* 1988;63:256–262.
11. Taylor HC, Velasco ME, Brodkey JS. Remission of pituitary-dependent Cushing's disease after removal of nonneoplastic pituitary gland. *Arch Intern Med* 1980;140:1366–1368.
12. Liddle G. Tests of pituitary–adrenal suppressibility in the diagnosis of Cushing's syndrome. *J Clin Endocrinol Metab* 1960;20(12):1539–1559.
13. Yamaji T, Ishibashi M, Sekihara H, Itabashi A, Yanaihara T. Serum dehydroepiandrosterone sulfate in Cushing's syndrome. *J Clin Endocrinol Metab* 1984;59:1164–1168.
14. Smals AGH, Kloppenborg PWC, Benraad THJ. Plasma testosterone profiles in Cushing's syndrome. *J Clin Endocrinol Metab* 1977;45:240–245.
15. Melis B, Mais V, Gambacciani M, Paoletti AM, Antinori D, Fioretti P. Dexamethasone reduces the postcastration gonadotropin rise in women. *J Clin Endocrinol Metab* 1987;65:237–241.
16. Fitzgerald PA, Aron DC, Findling JW, Brooks RM, Wilson CB, Forsham PH, Tyrell JB. Cushing's disease: transient secondary adrenal insufficiency after selective removal of pituitary microadenomas; evidence for a pituitary origin. *J Clin Endocrinol Metab* 1984;54(2):413–422.
17. Krieger DT, Glick SM. Growth hormone and cortisol responsiveness in Cushing's syndrome. *Am J Med* 1972;52:25–40.
18. Tahir AH, Sheeler LR. Recurrent Cushing's syndrome after transsphenoidal surgery. *Arch Intern Med* 1992;152:977–981.
19. Carey RM, Varma SK, Drake CR, Thorner MO, Kovacs K, Rivier J, Vale W. Ectopic secretions of corticotropin-releasing factor as a cause of Cushing's syndrome. *N Engl J Med* 1984;311:13–20.
20. Aron DC, Findling JW, Fitzgerald PA, Brooks RM, Fisher FE, Forsham PH, Tyrrell JB. Pituitary ACTH dependency of nodular adrenal hyperplasia in Cushing's syndrome. *Am J Med* 1981;71:302–306.

21. Smals AGH, Pieters FFM, Van Haelst UGJ, Kloppenborg PWC. Macronodular adrenocortical hyperplasia in long-standing Cushing's disease. *J Clin Endocrinol Metab* 1984;58(1):25–31.
22. Coates PJ, Doniach I, Howlett TA, Rees LH, Besser GM. Immunocytochemical study of 18 tumors causing ectopic Cushing's syndrome. *J Clin Pathol* 1986;39:955–960.
23. Findling JW, Tyrrell JB. Occult ectopic secretion of corticotropin. *Arch Intern Med* 1986;146:929–933.
24. Schteingart DE, Lloyd RV, Akil H, Chandler WF, Ibarra-Perez G, Rosen SG, Ogletree R. Cushing's syndrome secondary to ectopic corticotropin-releasing hormone–adrenocorticotropin secretion. *J Clin Endocrinol Metab* 1986;63(3):770–775.
25. Asa SL, Kovacs K, Tindall G, Barrow D, Horvath E, Vecsie P. Cushing's disease associated with an intrasellar gangliocytoma producing corticotrophin-releasing factor. *Ann Intern Med* 1984;101:789–793.
26. Bertagna C, Orth DN. Clinical and laboratory findings and results of therapy in 58 patients with adrenocortical tumors admitted to a single medical center. *Am J Med* 1981;71:855–875.
27. Young WF, Carney JA, Musa BU, Wulffraat NM, Lens JW, Drexhage HA. Familial Cushing's syndrome due to primary pigmented nodular adrenocortical disease. *N Engl J Med* 1989;321(24):1659–1664.
28. Travis WD, Tsokos M, Doppman JL, Nieman L, Chrousos GP, Cutler GB, Loriaux DL, Norton JA. Primary pigmented nodular adrenocortical disease: a light and electron microscopic study of eight cases. *Am J Surg Pathol* 1989;13(11):921–930.
29. Carney JA, Hruska LS, Beauchamp GD, Gordon G. Dominant inheritance of the complex of myxomas, spotty pigmentation, and endocrine overactivity. *Mayo Clin Proc* 1986;61:165–172.
30. Braithwaite SS, Collins S, Prinz RA, Walloch JL, Winters GL. Decreased dehydroepiandrosterone sulfate in pigmented nodular adrenal dysplasia. *Clin Chem* 1989;35(11):2216–2219.
31. Wullfraat NM, Drexhage HA, Wiersinga WM, Van Der Gaag RD, Jeucken P, Mol JA. Immunoglobulins of patients with Cushing's syndrome due to pigmented adrenocortical micronodular dysplasia stimulate in-vitro steroidogenesis. *J Clin Endocrinol Metab* 1988;66:301–307.
32. Findlay JC, Sheeler LR, England WC, Aron DC. Familial adrenocorticotropin-independent Cushing's syndrome with bilateral macronodular adrenal hyperplasia. *J Clin Endocrinol Metab* 1993; 76:189–191.
33. Malchoff CD, Roas J, DeBold CR. Adrenocorticotropic hormone-independent bilateral macronodular hyperplasia: an unusual case of Cushing's syndrome. *Endocrinol Jpn* 1989;68:855–860.
34. Eddy RL, Jones AL, Gilliland PF, Ibarra JD, Thompson JQ, McMurry JF. Cushing's syndrome: a prospective study of diagnostic methods. *Am J Med* 1973;55:621–630.
35. Sheeler LR, Bay JW. Normal overnight dexamethasone suppression tests (ODST) in patients with proven Cushing's syndrome. *Adv Pituitary Adenoma Res* 1987;69:373–374.
36. Crapo L. Cushing's syndrome: a review of diagnostic tests. *Metabolism* 1979;28(9):955–977.
37. Vagnucci AH, Evans E. Cushing's disease with intermittent hypercortisolism. *Am J Med* 1986;80:83–88.
38. Thorner MO, Martin WH, Ragan GE, MacLeod RM, Feldman PS, Bruni C, Williamson BRJ, Orth DN. A case of ectopic ACTH syndrome: diagnostic difficulties caused by intermittent hormone secretion. *Acta Endocrinol* 1982;99:362–370.
39. Kuhn JM, Proeschel MF, Seurin DJ, Bertagna XY, Luton JP, Girard FL. Comparative assessment of ACTH and lipoprotein plasma levels in the diagnosis and follow-up of patients with Cushing's syndrome: a study of 210 cases. *Am J Med* 1989;86:678–684.
40. Newton RW, Semple P, Browning MCK, Gunn A. Misleading corticotropin levels in Cushing's disease. *JAMA* 1978;240(8):770–772.
41. Flack MR, Oldfield EH, Culter GB, Zwieg MH, Malley JD, Chrousos GP, Loriaux DL, et al. Urine free cortisol in the high-dose dexamethasone suppression test for the differential diagnosis of the Cushing's syndrome. *Ann Intern Med* 1992;116(3):211–217.
42. Ashcraft MW, Van Herle AJ, Stuart SL, Geffner DL. Serum cortisol levels in Cushing's syndrome after low- and high-dose dexamethasone suppression. *Ann Intern Med* 1982;97:21–26.
43. Tyrrell JB, Findling JW, Aron DC, Fitzgerald PA, Forsham PH. An overnight high-dose dexamethasone suppression test for rapid differential diagnosis of Cushing's syndrome. *Ann Intern Med* 1986;104:180–186.
44. Biemond P, De Jong FH, Lamberts SWJ. Continuous dexamethasone infusion for seven hours in patients with Cushing's syndrome. *Ann Intern Med* 1990;112:738–742.
45. Oldfield EH, Doppman JL, Nieman LK, Chrousos GP, Miller DL, Katz DA, Cutler GB, Loriaux

DL. Petrosal sinus sampling with and without corticotropin-releasing hormone for the differential diagnosis of Cushing's syndrome. *N Engl J Med* 1991;325(13):897–906.

46. Orth DN. Corticotropin-releasing hormone in humans. *Endocr Rev* 1992;13(2):164–191.

47. Limper AH, Carpenter PC, Scheithauer B, Staats BA. The Cushing's syndrome induced by bronchial carcinoid tumors. *Ann Intern Med* 1992;117:209–214.

48. Gold PW, Loriaux DL, Roy A, Kling MA, Calabrese JR, Kellner CH, Nieman LK, et al. Response to corticotropin-releasing hormone in the hypercortisolism of depression and Cushing's disease. *N Engl J Med* 1986;314:1329–1335.

49. Rees LH, Besser GM, Jeffcoate WJ, Goldie DJ, Marks V. Alcohol-induced pseudo-Cushing's syndrome. *Lancet* 1977;1:726–728.

50. Lamberts SWJ, Klinj JGM, de Jong FH, Birkenhager JC. Hormone secretion in alcohol-induced pseudo-Cushing's syndrome. *JAMA* 1979;242(15):1640–1643.

51. King LW, Post KD, Yust I, Reichlin S. Suppression of cortisol secretion by low-dose dexamethasone testing in Cushing's disease. *J Neurosurg* 1983;58:129–132.

52. Meikle AW. Dexamethasone suppression tests: usefulness of simultaneous measurement of plasma cortisol and dexamethasone. *Clin Endocrinol* 1982;16:401–408.

53. Nolten WE, Lindheimer MD, Rueckert PA, Oparil S, Ehrlich EN. Diurnal patterns and regulation of cortisol secretion in pregnancy. *J Clin Endocrinol Metab* 1980;51:466–472.

54. Lindholm J, Schultz-Moller N. Plasma and urinary cortisol in pregnancy and during estrogen-gestation treatment. *Scand J Clin Lab Invest* 1973;31:119–122.

55. Smals AGH, Njo KT, Knoben JM, Ruland CM, Kloppenborg PWC. Alcohol-induced Cushingoid syndrome. *J R Coll Physicians* 1977;12(1):36–41.

56. Kapcala LP. Alcohol-induced pseudo-Cushing's syndrome mimicking Cushing's disease in a patient with an adrenal mass. *Am J Med* 1987;82:849–856.

57. Brown RD, Van Loon GR, Orth DN, Liddle GW. Cushing's disease with periodic hormonogenesis: one explanation for paradoxical response to dexamethasone. *J Clin Endocrinol Metab* 1973;36:445.

58. Sakiyama R, Ashcraft MW, Van Herle AJ. Cyclic Cushing's syndrome. *Am J Med* 1984;77:944–946.

59. Atkinson AB, Kennedy AL, Carson DJ, Hadden DR, Weaver JA, Sheridan B. Five cases of cyclical Cushing's syndrome. *Br Med J* 1985;291:1453–1457.

60. Mampalam TJ, Tyrrel JB, Wilson CB. Transsphenoidal microsurgery for Cushing's disease: a report of 216 cases. *Ann Intern Med* 1988;109:487–493.

61. Flint LD, Jacob EC. Belated recognition of adrenocorticotropic hormone–producing tumors in post-adrenalectomized Cushing's syndrome. *J Urol* 1974;112:688.

62. Bigos ST, Somma M, Rasio E, Eastman RC, Lantheir A, Johnston HH, Hardy J. Cushing's disease: management by transsphenoidal pituitary microsurgery. *J Clin Endocrinol Metab* 1980;50:348–354.

63. Bay JW, Sheeler LR. Results of transsphenoidal surgery for Cushing's disease. *Cleve Clin J Med* 1988;55:357–364.

64. Kammer J, George R. Cushing's disease in a patient with an ectopic pituitary adenoma. *JAMA* 1981;246(23):2722–2724.

65. Schteingart DE, Chandler WF, Lloyd RV, Ibarra-Perez G. Cushing's syndrome caused by an ectopic pituitary adenoma. *Neurosurgery* 1987;21(2):223–227.

66. Burch WM. Cushing's disease; a review. *Arch Intern Med* 1985;15:1106–1111.

67. Vicente A, Estrada J, de la Cuerda C, Stigarraga B, Marazueal M, Blanco C, Lucas T, Barcelo B. Results of external pituitary irradiation after unsuccessful transsphenoidal surgery in Cushing's disease. *Acta Endocrinol* 1991;125:470–474.

68. Howlett TA, Plowman PN, Wass JAH, Rees LH, Jones AE, Besser GM. Megavoltage pituitary irradiation in the management of Cushing's disease and Nelson's syndrome: long-term follow-up. *Clin Endocrinol* 1989;31:309–323.

69. King TM, Sheeler LR. Radiation therapy for recurrent or persistent Cushing's disease. *The Endocrine Society 75th Annual Meeting*, Las Vegas, 1993;786:242.

70. White FE, White MC, Drury PL, Kelsey Frey I, Besser GM. Value of computed tomography of the abdomen and chest in investigation of Cushing's syndrome. *Br Med J* 1982;284:771–774.

71. Leinung MC, Young WF, Whitaker MD, Trastek VF, Kvols LK. Diagnosis of corticotropin-producing bronchial carcinoid tumors causing Cushing's syndrome. *Mayo Clin Proc* 1990;65;1314–1321.

72. Bodie B, Novick AC, Pontes JE, Straffon RA, Montie JE, Babiak T, Sheeler LR, Schumacher OP. The Cleveland Clinic experience with adrenal cortical carcinoma. *J Urol* 1989;141:257–260.

73. Grabner P, Hauer-Jensen M, Jervell J, Flatmark A. Long term results of treatment of Cushing's disease by adrenalectomy. *Eur J Surg* 1991;157:461–464.

74. Luton JP, Mahoudeau JA, Bouchard PH, Thieblot PH, Hautecouverture M, Simon D, Laudat MH, et al. Treatment of Cushing's disease by *o,p'*DDD: survey of 62 cases. *N Engl J Med* 1979;300(9): 459–464.
75. Sheperd FA, Hoffert B, Evans WK, Emery G, Trachtenberg J. Ketokonazole: use in treatment of ectopic adrenocorticotropic hormone production and Cushing's syndrome in small-cell lung cancer. *Arch Intern Med* 1985;143:863–864.
76. Komanicky P, Spark RF, Melby JC. Treatment of Cushing's syndrome with trilostane (WIN24, 540), an inhibitor of adrenal steroid biosynthesis. *J Clin Endocrinol Metab* 1978;47(5):1042–1051.
77. Oates JA, Wood AJ. The use of ketoconazole as an inhibitor of steroid production. *N Engl J Med* 1987;317(13):812–818.
78. Del Gaudio A, Del Gaudio GA. Virilizing adrenocortical tumors in adult women. *Cancer* 1993; 72(6):1997–2003.
79. Gabrilove JL, Seman AT, Mitty HA, Nicolis GL. Virilizing adrenal adenoma with studies on the steroid content of the adrenal venous effluent and a review of the literature. *Endocr Rev* 1981;2(4): 462–469.
80. Vasiloff J, Chideckel EW, Boyd CB, Foshag LJ. Testosterone-secreting adrenal adenoma containing crystalloid characteristic of Leydig cells. *Am J Med* 1985;79:772–776.
81. Schteingart DE, Woodbury MC, Tsao HS, McKenzie AK. Virilizing syndrome associated with an adrenal cortical adenoma secreting predominantly testosterone. *Am J Med* 1979;67:140–146.
82. Werk EE, Sholiton EJ, Kalejs L. Testosterone-secreting adrenal adenoma under gonadotropin control. *N Engl J Med* 1973;289(15):767–770.
83. Leinonen P, Ranta T, Sieberg R, Pelkonen R, Heikkila P, Kahri A. Testosterone-secreting virilizing adrenal adenoma with human chorionic gonadotrophin receptors and 21-hydroxylase deficiency. *Clin Endocrinol* 1991;34(1):31–35.
84. Bricaire C, Raynaud A, Benotmane A, Clair F, Paniel B, Moskowicz I, Wright F, et al. Selective venous catheterization in the evaluation of hyperandrogenism. *J Clin Endocrinol Invest* 1991;14: 949–956.
85. Chen A, Bookstein JJ, Meldrum DR. Diagnosis of a testosterone-secreting adrenal adenoma by selective venous catheterization. *Fertil Steril* 1991;55(6):1202–1203.
86. Becker D, Schumacher OP. *o,p'*DDD therapy in invasive adrenocortical carcinoma. *Ann Intern Med* 1975;82:677–679.
87. Fishler DF, Nunez C, Levin HS, McMahon JT, Sheeler LR, Adelstein DJ. Adrenal carcinosarcoma presenting in a woman with clinical signs of virilization. *Am J Surg Path* 1992;16(6):626–631.
88. Luton JP, Cerdas S, Billaud L, Thomas G, Guilhaume B, Bertagna X, Laudat MH, et al. Clinical features of adrenocortical carcinoma, prognostic factors, and the effect of mitotane therapy. *N Engl J Med* 1990;322:1195–1201.
89. Kruimet JW, Smals AG, Beex LV, Swinkels LM, Pieters GF, Kloppenborg PW. Favorable response of a virilization adrenocortical carcinoma to preoperative treatment with ketokonazole and postoperative chemotherapy. *Acta Endocrinol* 1991;124(4):492–496.
90. Schlumberger M, Ostronoff M, Bellaiche M. 5-fluorouracil, doxorubicin and cisplatin regimen in adrenal cortical carcinoma. *Cancer* 1988;61:1492–1494.
91. Halpin DMG, Burrin JM, Joplin GF. Serum testosterone levels in women with Cushing's disease. *Acta Endocrinol* 1990;122:71–75.

Androgenic Disorders,
edited by G. P. Redmond.
Raven Press, Ltd., New York © 1995.

10

Acne Vulgaris

Karen F. Rothman

Departments of Medicine and Pediatrics, University of Massachusetts Medical School, Worcester, Massachusetts 01605.

Acne vulgaris is the most frequently occurring skin disorder in humans. Both primary care physicians and specialists in dermatology and endocrinology need a good understanding of the pathophysiology of and treatment options for afflicted patients. In this chapter these issues as well as the epidemiology and differential diagnosis of acne vulgaris will be discussed.

DEFINITIONS

Acne is more properly referred to as acne vulgaris, or common acne, to distinguish it from a variety of acneiform disorders with which it can sometimes be confused (Table 1). Acne vulgaris is characterized by lesions of various morphologies occurring at the same or different times in the same patient. Acne lesions may occur on the face, neck, chest, and back. The primary lesions which occur in acne patients are open and closed comedones, papules, pustules, and nodules. Comedones are noninflammatory acne lesions which persist for weeks to months. Closed comedones, commonly referred to as whiteheads, are firm, white 1 to 3 mm papules. Open comedones, also known as blackheads, contain a dilated sebaceous follicle filled with a keratin plug. The dark color at the surface of the open comedo is due to the oxidation of surface lipids rather than an accumulation of dirt, as is commonly supposed. Papules are inflamed lesions less than 5 mm in diameter. Pustules are pus-filled, elevated lesions. Individual papules and pustules usually persist for 1 to 4 days. Nodules are inflamed lesions larger that 5 mm in size. Nodules may protrude above the skin or may be largely subcutaneous. They may persist for weeks to months without ever draining. Cysts, which are epithelial-lined subcutaneous nodules, are occasionally seen in acne patients. However, since true cysts are rare in acne patients, the terms nodular acne and nodulocystic acne have replaced the term cystic acne in the dermatologic literature. Factors that lead to the development of comedones or papules in one patient but nodules in another patient are not known, although the tendency to have nodular acne may be hereditary. Why

TABLE 1. *Acne vulgaris: differential diagnosis*

Disease	History	Physical findings
Acne rosacea	Easy flushing; exacerbation with certain foods and beverages.	Erythema medial cheeks, nose, and/or chin + inflammatory lesions. No comedones.
Perioral/orbital/nasal dermatitis	Medium or potent topical and/or inhaled steroid use.	Groups of 1–2-mm inflammatory lesions. Underlying skin may be erythematous and/or scaly.
Steroid acne	p.o. steroid ingestion.	Monomorphic 1–3-mm papules or pustules on back, shoulders, and/or chest.
Gram-negative folliculitis	Long-term antibiotic therapy.	Inflammatory and/or nodular lesions.
Pityrosporum folliculitis	Lack of response to acne medications.	1–3-mm papules and pustules on back, shoulders, and/or chest.
Pyoderma faciale	Sudden onset pustules.	Multiple 2–5-mm pustules covering a large portion of the face.
Acne cosmetica	Long-term oil-based cosmetic use.	Usually numerous closed comedones; inflammatory papules less common.
Eosinophilic folliculitis	Usually H.I.V. or other underlying immune-compromising illness.	Pruritic 2–4-mm papules and pustules, usually most numerous on the trunk.

some patients are most afflicted on the face and others on the chest and/or back is also unknown.

Most acne lesions are neither tender nor pruritic. However, acne nodules may be exquisitely tender to touch. Although acne is not pruritic, many patients with acne pick and/or excoriate their skin in an attempt to make a lesion go away. This phenomenon, referred to as acnée excoriée, is particularly common in young women and teenage girls with acne.

While acne lesions are healing, erythema may persist for days to months. Post-inflammatory hypo- and/or hyperpigmentation may also occur, especially in patients who are darker skinned. True scarring may also occur. Scars from acne are most commonly 0.5 to 1 mm wide by 0.5 to 1 mm deep depressions resembling dilated pores. These are referred to as ice pick scars. Gently sloping contoured scars, referred to as crateriform, are also common. Numerous 2- to 3-mm white firm scars may develop in individuals with chest and/or back acne. Smooth, erythematous, elevated keloid scars that are larger than the patient's original acne lesions occasionally develop, particularly on the upper back. Nodular lesions commonly scar. However, even comedonal lesions resolve with scars in some patients. The tendency to have acne scarring is probably hereditary, although this has not been well studied.

PREVALENCE

Acne is commonly thought of as almost a rite of passage of teenagers. Although it is true that the incidence of acne is highest during the middle to late teenage years, acne is by no means confined to this age group. More than 2 million people in the United States between the ages of 15 and 44 are affected (1). The disease causes considerable shame and embarrassment (2). Patients with acne have higher unemployment rates than those who are unaffected (3).

Acne neonatorum is common. It is often attributed to the withdrawal of maternal estrogens that occurs at birth. However, androgen production by the fetal and newborn adrenal gland and, in the male, by the testes, contributes to neonatal acne. The newborn adrenal gland continues to produce androgenic hormones such as dehydroepiandrosterone sulfate (DHEA-S) at midpubertal level for the first 6 months or so after birth (4). The newborn male responds to the withdrawal of maternal estrogens at birth with a burst of luteinizing hormone, stimulating the testes to produce testosterone at early pubertal levels for 6 to 12 months after birth (5,6). These androgenic hormones account for the presence and persistence of neonatal acne and probably explain the greater incidence and severity of acne in newborn males than in newborn females. Comedones, papules, pustules, and rarely, nodules may occur. Lesions usually stop occurring by age 6 to 12 months, but may persist until age 3 (7). Between ages 2 and 6, acne lesions are distinctly unusual and may signal an underlying androgenic disorder. In young children with acne, careful genital examination should be performed to look for signs of adrenal hyperplasia or other androgen-excess disorders or precocious puberty.

Comedonal acne lesions begin in very early puberty in about 75% of girls (8) and boys (9). Inflammatory lesions begin somewhat later, peaking in prevalence at age 16 or so (10). Nodular lesions are much less commonly encountered and usually begin in the late teenage years or even later. Comedonal and/or inflammatory acne lesions persist or develop in about 60% of people in their early 20s, 30% of women and less than 5% of men in their 30s, about 20% of women and 6% of men in their 40s, and about 7% to 8% of women and men in their early 50s (11). Postmenopausal acne is distinctly uncommon in women, although patients with perimenopausal flares are not infrequently encountered (12). Acne persists in about 2% of men after age 55.

PATHOPHYSIOLOGY

Acne occurs in the pilosebaceous follicle, a specialized epidermally-derived unit which is composed of a large sebaceous gland, a small vellus hair, and a follicular canal. Factors known to contribute to the development and persistence of acne are listed in Table 2 and are detailed below.

Sebum

Sebum is the oil produced by sebaceous glands. Sebaceous glands develop in humans early in the second trimester in utero as outpouches of follicles. The growth

TABLE 2. *Factors that cause acne*

Sebum
Bacteria
Hormones
Genetic factors
Medications
External factors

of sebaceous glands in utero is stimulated by maternal hormones as well as by hormones produced by the fetal adrenal gland and, in males, the testes. At birth, sebaceous glands are about the same size that they are in adulthood. Sebaceous glands involute over the first year of life, presumably in response to decreasing serum androgen levels. By age 8, androgen output by the adrenals and gonads stimulates sebaceous glands to grow, and sebum production increases (13). Sebum production rates reach their maximum in 16- to 19-year-olds (14). After age 20, there is a slow, steady decrease in the rate of sebum excretion, with a faster rate of decline in women than in men (15). The rate of sebum excretion is identical in identical twins and different in fraternal twins, indicating that the rate of sebum production is genetically predetermined (16).

Patients with severe acne usually have high sebum excretion rates (17). Linoleic acid levels in sebum are lower in patients with acne than in people without acne (18). This may cause the abnormal keratinization within the follicular canal that is characteristic of acne lesions (19). When sebum is ingested by *Propionibacterium acnes*, free fatty acids are liberated that are irritants and increase the inflammatory response. When applied to rabbit ears, sebum induces comedone formation.

Bacteria

The anaerobic diptheroid *P. acnes* lives in the sebaceous follicle. Colonization of the sebaceous follicle begins in mid childhood, after sebum production begins to rise. Patients with acne have more *P. acnes* colonies residing in their sebaceous follicles than patients without acne.

P. acnes is responsible for the initiation of much of the inflammation that occurs in acne lesions. *P. acnes* attracts polymorphonuclear leukocytes (20), which migrate into the sebaceous follicle, ingest the bacteria, and cause the release of hydrolytic enzymes and free fatty acids (21). The follicular wall is broken down by the hydrolytic enzymes, and the follicular contents enter the dermis. Monocytes, macrophages, and giant cells surround the follicle. Both cell-mediated and humoral immunity are involved in the inflammatory response (22). C_{5a}, which attracts polymorphonuclear leukocytes, is produced. Interleukin-1α may also help to initiate the inflammatory response (23).

Hormones

Although there is no endocrine profile unique for patients with acne and the majority of patients with acne have no detectable hormone abnormality, many studies point to the importance of hormones in acne production. In some cases, identical tests performed on different groups of patients have yielded different results. Although this leads to some confusion, different results can sometimes be explained by understanding that acne is a clinical endpoint of a heterogeneous group of androgenic disorders. In addition, more sophisticated assays may detect subtle abnormalities missed in older assays.

Androgens are produced and metabolized in the adrenals, the gonads, and, to a smaller extent, in the liver, skin, and fatty tissue (24). Androgens increase sebum production by increasing cell division within the sebaceous gland (25). Androstenedione (A), dehydroepiandrosterone (DHEA), and DHEA-S are metabolized into testosterone (T). Ninety-seven percent of T circulates bound to sex hormone–binding globulin (SHBG), which is produced in the liver. When unbound T reaches androgen-sensitive end organs, including sebaceous glands, it is metabolized by 5α-reductase to form dihydrotestosterone (DHT), which is a much more potent androgen than T (26). DHT then diffuses into the sebaceous gland cell membranes, where it interacts with a nuclear receptor protein, stimulating the production of sebum through the production of 3α-androstanediol and 3α-androstanediol glucuronide (24).

Men with acne have normal androgen levels. In men, the testes are the primary source of T production. Castrated men produce less sebum than normal men (27) and do not have acne unless they are given exogenous T (28). Male pseudohermaphrodites, who are deficient in 5α-reductase, have the same sebum production rates as normal males and may also have acne (29). This apparent discrepancy can be explained by understanding that there are two isoenzymes of 5α-reductase, known as isoenzyme 1 and isoenzyme 2 (29). In male pseudohermaphrodites, 5α-reductase-1 is deficient and is responsible for the development and differentiation of the external male genitalia and prostate as well as for facial and body-hair growth; 5α-eductase-1 levels are normal. It is the type 1 isoenzyme that is responsible for sebum production and acne development in these patients.

In women, typically 50% of androgens are produced in the adrenal glands (30). The ovaries produce another 25%. Women with acne may have abnormalities in any of the androgen-producing organs. Thus, a large array of hormonal abnormalities may be seen. Women presenting for evaluation may have only acne or may also have a variety of menstrual abnormalities, and/or hirsutism. The patient's clinical picture does not differ with the hormone abnormality detected. In addition, even the most sophisticated testing will reveal no detectable hormone abnormalities in the majority of affected women.

A variety of adrenal problems may be seen in women with acne (Table 3). Patients with late-onset congenital adrenal hyperplasia have elevated levels of 17α-

TABLE 3. *Adrenal causes of acne in women*

congenital adrenal hyperplasia
adrenal tumors
hyperresponsiveness to ACTH
hypertrophic adrenals

hydroxyprogesterone, its precursors, and DHEA-S secondary to partial deficiency of the enzyme 21-hydroxylase. Markedly elevated levels of DHEA-S are seen in patients with adrenal tumors. Another group of women with acne appear to pour out greater than normal quantities of androgens in response to normal ACTH secretion (31). Other women without known enzymatic defects produce more androgens in response to ACTH because they have a larger amount of adrenal tissue to produce androgens (32). Levels of DHEA, DHEA-S, A, and T may all be elevated in patients with an adrenal cause for their acne, and an increased response to exogenous ACTH stimulation is characteristically seen. Dexamethasone will suppress adrenal androgen production.

Ovarian dysfunction, whether found alone or in association with adrenal dysfunction, may also cause a woman to produce greater amounts of androgens. Irregular menses, acne, and/or hirsutism may result. Although excess androgen production can very rarely be a result of an ovarian or adrenal tumor, the most common reason for the ovaries to produce higher levels of androgens is polycystic ovary syndrome (PCOS). In a recent study, 45% of women with acne had polycystic ovaries on ultrasound, as compared to 17% of women found to have PCOS who did not have acne (33). Laboratory evaluation will usually reveal elevated levels of free T, prolactin, and A, and an elevated luteinizing hormone (LH)/follicle-stimulating hormone (FSH) ratio, although normal hormone levels may also be seen (34). Dexamethasone will not suppress androgen production as it will in adrenal-derived androgen excess. Androgen production will, however, be reduced with long-term oral contraceptive pill use or with a gonadotropin-releasing hormone agonist such as nafarelin (35).

Most women with acne report a premenstrual flare. This has been attributed to the increase in progesterone levels which occurs during the luteal phase of the menstrual cycle. Progesterone has been claimed to have an androgenic effect within the sebaceous follicle (36), although sebum production rates do not rise in response to progesterone (37). The role, if any, of progesterone in acne requires further study.

A very small but clinically significant amount of androgens are produced in the skin. Androstenedione, which is quantitatively the major circulating androgen in women, is metabolized in the skin. Increased peripheral conversion to 3α-androsterone and 3α-androsterone glucuronide has been proposed as a specific marker for normoandrogenic women with acne (38).

Genetic Factors

Almost 100% of teenagers have acne. The tendency toward nodular acne with scarring may be genetic, but many factors may modify disease expression (39). Early and aggressive treatment of a child with acne may be particularly important for those with scarring or in whom there is a family history of severe acne scarring.

Medications

Any medication that has a direct or indirect androgenic effect may cause or exacerbate acne. Androgens are prescribed for many different medical conditions (40, 41) and may also be used illicitly by competitive athletes (42). Many medications that are not hormones may also cause acne in some individuals. Medications known to worsen acne are listed in Table 4.

External Factors

In the acne-prone individual, topical application of certain substances may exacerbate the problem. Certain cosmetics, sunscreens, and moisturizers cause papular and pustular acne lesions as well as comedones (43). These products have been referred to as comedogenic, or, more recently, as acnegenic (44). Substances which induce acne may be tested on rabbit ears, which develop follicular hyperkeratosis when acnegenic substances are applied (44). However, animal testing is frowned upon by certain animal rights groups and is not performed by certain cosmetic companies. Human testing can be done, but it is more costly and less reliable because of confounding external variables difficult to control in humans (44). Regardless of how testing is performed, many topically applied products are labeled by their manufacturer as noncomedogenic or nonacnegenic. Because of the extreme

TABLE 4. *Medications that exacerbate acne*

Androgens
    progestins (oral or implanted)
    testosterone
    anabolic steroids
    oral contraceptives (improve acne in some patients)
Nonhormonal medications
    azothioprine
    cyanocobalamin
    dactinomycin
    disulfuram
    gold
    halides
    halogenated hydrocarbons
    hydantoin
    isoniazid
    lithium
    maprotiline
    quinidine
    quinine
    rifampin
    tetracycline
    thiouracil
    thiourea
    vitamin D

From Rothman and Lucky, ref. 111.

awareness of the problem of acnegenicity in the cosmetics industry today, it is the author's opinion that the products of most reputable cosmetic and moisturizer manufacturers labeled as nonacnegenic are unlikely to cause acne in the majority of acne-prone patients. The fierce competition within the industry leads to so many new and refined products being introduced that it is unreasonable to expect us to be familiar with each one. General guidelines to the patient to avoid greasy emollients such as petroleum jelly, cocoa butter, cold creams, and oil-based makeup may be helpful. When patients ask about specific products, they should be told to look for labeling concerning acnegenicity. However, they should understand that even a product labeled as nonacnegenic may cause acne exacerbations in occasional patients.

Cutaneous exposure to halogenated hydrocarbons such as dioxin (45) will cause a severe form of nodulocystic acne termed chloracne in about 15% of people exposed. Young people and those with the largest exposure are most prone to developing the disease (46). Chlorophenol contaminants, coal tar, and petroleum products may also cause papular, pustular, comedonal, or nodular lesions (47,48).

Several physical factors may exacerbate acne. Devices which contact the skin for prolonged periods of time such as chin straps, shoulder pads, and telephones may cause comedonal and/or inflammatory acne (49). Such patients develop lesions primarily under the area of contact and only after they have used the offending device for a period of weeks to months. Acne patients who use harsh scrubs and compulsively pick, squeeze, and wash their skin increase the amount of inflammatory lesions they will get. Although most patients who have scarring acne do not excessively manipulate their lesions and most patients with acne who admit to picking their skin do not scar, occasional patients repeatedly gouge their skin, creating long, deep, linear or round scars.

PATIENT EVALUATION

Patients with acne should be asked about the course of their acne and about past and current therapies they have tried. Women should be questioned about their menstrual history, whether they experience premenstrual flares, and hirsutism. Sexually active females should also be questioned about the type of birth control they use, since this may influence the treatment chosen.

Physical examination should include the face, chest, and back. The type and number of acne lesions and presence of scarring should be noted. Excessive body and facial hair may be seen in some women with androgen excess.

Distinguishing which women with acne have an underlying treatable androgenic disorder is difficult. Serum-free T levels and DHEA-S levels are useful basic screens for distinguishing ovarian from adrenal causes of acne in women (50). However, testing is indicated only in women whose history or physical findings point to a hormonal abnormality or those women who fail to respond to usual acne treatment.

TREATMENT

Treatment of acne patients requires an understanding of the disease process as well as time and empathy. Acne patients may feel they have a problem too insignificant to bother a doctor about, and physicians may reinforce this by not taking the time necessary to evaluate and educate the patient. Even patients with mild acne may feel embarrassed to appear in public. Alternatively, some patients with severe acne or their parents may not appreciate the severity of scarring and may be reluctant to try appropriate treatments.

Patients should first understand that acne is a chronic but recurrent disease. With the exception of patients treated with isotretinoin, if an effective treatment is used and the patient stops it, acne will recur within a few months unless its natural course has ended. Patients should be told that acne is unrelated to eating or avoiding certain foods and is not caused by dirt. Astringents dry out the skin temporarily but do not improve acne. Acne patients should wash once or twice daily with a mild soap and avoid harsh scrubs. Facials have no beneficial effect on acne patients and may aggravate the disease in some patients.

Acne treatments may be conveniently divided into topical and systemic therapies. In general, using more than one topical therapy or combining topical and systemic therapies is more efficacious than using one form of therapy. However, oral medications may have undesirable side effects. Intensive topical therapies may be too drying to the skin for patients to use them comfortably. The major goal of therapy is to prevent the occurrence of new lesions. Patients must use the medications on a chronic basis, rather than waiting until lesions appear. Careful explanations, written instruction sheets, and scheduled follow-up visits all insure excellent patient compliance and maximally effective treatment.

Topical Treatments

Topical therapies are beneficial for acne patients with mild to moderate papular, pustular, or comedonal acne and as adjunctive therapy for patients with more severe disease. Topical therapies have very little efficacy for back and chest lesions, since the thicker trunkal skin absorbs so little of these medications. All topical treatments should be used all over the affected area, rather than applied to individual active lesions. Payment for topical acne medications is not covered by Medicaid and certain health maintenance organizations.

Benzoyl Peroxide

Benzoyl peroxide products are antibacterial and comedolytic (51). Preparations are available in concentrations of 2.5%, 4%, 5%, and 10% and may be purchased in lotion, gel, cream, and soap form. The 4% concentration is available only by prescription, but the others are available without prescription. All forms are equally efficacious for treating acne (51), but higher concentrations are more drying to the skin. Benzoyl peroxide preparations may decrease acne lesion counts as much as low dosages of oral tetracycline (52). Dry skin, irritant contact dermatitis, and staining of clothing are common side effects. True allergic contact dermatitis may also be seen. Benzoyl peroxide is not carcinogenic (53), teratogenic (54), or mutagenic.

Topical Antibiotics

Topical antibiotic preparations act both through decreasing the population of *P. acnes* and through lowering surface lipid concentration (55). All may be obtained only by prescription. Topical erythromycin is available in liquid and gel forms. It is available as a single agent, combined with zinc in a liquid preparation (56), or combined with 5% benzoyl peroxide in a gel (57). The combination preparations are more efficacious but are also more expensive. Topical erythromycin preparations may be safely used during pregnancy.

Topical tetracycline is as effective as topical erythromycin preparations. However, patients using them may notice their skin and nails will fluoresce green if they are exposed to black light such as is used in many dance clubs. Therefore, the author does not prescribe this preparation. Although it has not been tested, use during pregnancy should probably be avoided because of the theoretical risk of primary dentition staining from absorption of small amounts of tetracycline.

Topical clindamycin is available in liquid, gel, or lotion form. These are generally more expensive than other topical antibiotic preparations. Efficacy is equal to other topical antibiotic preparations. The lotion form of clindamycin is less drying to the skin than the other available preparations and is generally tolerated well even in acne patients with dry, sensitive skin. Topical clindamycin preparations have been reported to cause pseudomembranous enterocolitis in two patients (58,59), although very little of the preparation is absorbed into the skin (56). It may be safely used during pregnancy (54).

Sulfur-Containing Preparations

Various preparations containing sulfur, either as the sole active agent or combined with resorsinol, sulfacetamide, and/or salicylic acid, are available. Some may be obtained by prescription only. Although these preparations are quite drying to the skin, foul-smelling, and are generally considered by dermatologists to be less effective than some of the other topical preparations, a new preparation has recently been formulated which is both less irritating and less noisome (60). The author has found this new preparation quite useful in adult women with acne and dry skin. Topical sulfur preparations may be safely used except during the last couple of weeks of pregnancy, when there is a theoretical risk of kernicterus in the newborn from drug absorption through maternal skin (54). Allergic reactions, including toxic epidermal necrolysis, can occur in sulfa-sensitive patients (61).

Salicylic Acid

A number of preparations containing salicylic acid are available without a prescription. Salicylic acid washes may improve both comedonal and inflammatory acne lesions (62). Although these preparations are much less efficacious than topical tretinoin, they are considerably less irritating to the skin and are much more easily affordable.

Tretinoin

Tretinoin, a Vitamin A derivative, is available as a 0.01% gel, a 0.025% gel or cream, a 0.05% cream or liquid, and a 0.1% cream. Tretinoin acts by reducing adhesion of keratinocytes in the follicular canal, lysing the microcomedones from which acne lesions form (63). It is the most potent topical agent available, but its usefulness is limited in many patients because it may be irritating to the skin. Topical isotretinoin, an isomer of tretinoin, may be less irritating than tretinoin but is not available in the United States. Phototoxicity may also occur. Patients should be instructed to apply only a thin layer of medication. It should be worked away from the skin creases and eyes. Applying it every other night and using a moisturizer mixed with or following application may lessen irritant reactions. In most cases, the patient's skin becomes more tolerant to the medication after a week or 2 of use. Worsening of acne may occur in some patients for the first 1 to 2 months of use, and acne characteristically does not improve until the medication has been used for 2 to 3 months. Although less than 7% of the medication is absorbed (64), tretinoin is isomerized in the skin to isotretinoin (65). Since both isotretinoin and tretinoin are extremely potent teratogens at even low doses (66,67), use of tretinoin during pregnancy should be avoided. Nearly all instances where tretinoin was applied during pregnancy have resulted in healthy newborns, but there are occasional case reports of multiple congenital anomalies fitting the same pattern of abnormality seen after oral isotretinoin use (68). If a woman using tretinoin becomes pregnant, she should be reassured that there is very little risk to the fetus. However, intentional use of topical tretinoin preparations during pregnancy should be avoided.

Oral Medications

Oral antibiotics may be used in patients who have failed to respond to topical therapy, those with extensive back and chest acne, and those with scarring acne. The three major classes of oral acne therapy are antibiotics, hormones, and isotretinoin.

Antibiotics

Many oral antibiotics are effective for acne (Table 5). Oral antibiotics effective for acne decrease *P. acnes* colony counts and free fatty acid concentration in sebum

TABLE 5. *Oral antiobiotics efficacious for acne*

tetracycline
minocycline
doxycycline
erythromycin
clindamycin
trimethoprim
cephalexin

(69). They also inhibit neutrophil chemotaxis (70), thus lessening the inflammatory response. Patients may see some early improvement, but the maximum effect of a particular treatment is seen about 2 to 3 months after treatment is initiated. If treatment is discontinued, acne will usually recur within a few months. Thus, in deciding which medication to prescribe, the physician must consider the effectiveness of the treatment as well as potential short- and long-term side effects. The major side effects of the commonly prescribed medications will be discussed below, but all oral antibiotics share the common side effect of development of yeast infections in women and the uncommon risks of development of a secondary infection and pseudomembranous enterocolitis. Development of resistant strains of *P. acnes* may also occur (71,72). Patients may choose or be advised to discontinue treatment after a time on medication, but it is common practice among dermatologists to continue certain antibiotics for months to years. Routine laboratory testing is not necessary, since side effects are rare and can usually be detected clinically (73). However, periodic follow-up visits are essential to monitor for any potential ill effects.

Tetracycline, minocycline, and doxycycline are the antibiotics most commonly prescribed for acne treatment. The major side effects of treatment are gastrointestinal disturbance, photosensitivity, and, in women, yeast infections. An uncommon but more serious side effect of tetracyclines is pseudotumor cerebri (74). Permanent staining of teeth may occasionally occur in adults who use minocycline (75) or tetracycline (76) chronically. Grey skin pigmentation may also occur with chronic minocycline use (77,78). Factors which may help the prescribing physician decide which preparation to choose are listed in Table 6. If one medication is unsuccessful in a patient, another tetracycline preparation may be useful. Several studies attest to the long-term safety of oral tetracyclines as acne treatment in otherwise healthy patients. Tetracyclines must be avoided during pregnancy because of the risk of staining of the deciduous teeth if tetracycline is used during the second or third trimester of pregnancy (54). A variety of bony and other more serious side effects

TABLE 6. *Guide to prescribing a tetracycline for acne*

Medicine	Relative cost	GI distress*	Sunburn*	Efficacy	Pigmentation
Tetracycline	$	+ + +	+ +	+	−
Doxycycline	$$	+ +	+ +/+ + +	+ +	−
Minocycline	$$$**	+	+	+ +	occasional

*Author's experience.
**Generic formulation approximately equal to doxycycline.

have also rarely been reported with tetracycline use during pregnancy (79–81), but because there is no consistent pattern of malformation seen, it is unclear whether there is a causal relationship between tetracycline use and these more severe birth defects. Thus, women should be counseled to avoid pregnancy while on a tetracycline preparation. However, if pregnancy exposure occurs and the tetracycline is stopped very early in the pregnancy, there is probably very little risk to the fetus.

Tetracyclines may slightly decrease the efficacy of oral contraceptive agents by decreasing the concentration of gut flora (82). Less bacteria are available to absorb estrogens, reducing serum estrogen concentration. Physicians who have studied this interaction feel that there is very little increased risk of pregnancy when antibiotics are administered to women on birth control pills (83–85).

It is the author's belief that, although there is a slight decrease in pill efficacy with concomitant administration of antibiotics, the combination of birth control pill plus antibiotics is still a more effective method of birth control than any other single method available except levonorgestrel implants (norplant). Since levonorgestrel commonly causes acne (86), it is not a method suitable for many women with acne. The oral antibiotic–oral contraceptive interaction is discussed in the package inserts of these medications and is well known by pharmacists. The author has even had pharmacists refuse to fill an antibiotic prescription for a woman on an oral contraceptive agent. The issue of potential interaction must be discussed with each patient. Signs of decreased birth control efficacy, such as spotting, must be understood by the patient. It is the author's practice to have the woman sign a statement that she understands that there is a potential interaction between the medications. She then checks off her decision to use an alternative or additional method of contraception, to not use oral antibiotics, or to assume the risk of potential pregnancy.

Oral erythromycin preparations are somewhat effective in treating acne (87). Their long-term administration is often hampered by gastrointestinal distress, a common side effect. Several enteric-coated preparations are available and these are tolerated somewhat better. Although prolonged use for more than 6 weeks during pregnancy has never been studied, they are generally considered to be safe (54). However, most patients and obstetricians are infinitely more concerned about the potential well-being of the fetus than about acne. Therefore, except in cases of new-onset, severe-scarring acne during pregnancy, the author limits treatment to topical preparations. Any medication prescribed should be approved by the patient's obstetrician. The author uses erythromycin as the antibiotic of choice in women who use birth control inconsistently or use an unreliable method of birth control. Although there is a theoretical risk of interaction between any antibiotic and oral contraceptive agents, cases of pregnancy have not been reported with erythromycin use. Thus, this class of antibiotics is a useful alternative to the tetracyclines for patients on birth control pills.

Other oral antibiotics, such as trimethoprim/sulfa (88), cephalexin, and clindamycin, are also effective in treating acne. However, such broad-spectrum antibiotics have much greater potential for complications than the tetracyclines and erythromycins. In the author's opinion, they should be used for a 2- to 3-month time period only, to alleviate an extreme situation where other methods of treatment are not suitable or are failed.

Hormonal Treatment

Hormonal treatment may be successful in patients who have a demonstrable increase in androgens and in those in whom no abnormality can be detected. These agents are suitable only for women, because feminizing side effects are generally undesirable in men. These agents should not be used during pregnancy because they may inhibit genital masculinization in male fetuses.

As originally developed, oral contraceptive agents contained a large amount of estrogen and progestin. Birth control pills suppress ovarian production of androgen and increase the serum level of SHBG, lowering the amount of T that circulates unbound. These agents were excellent at controlling acne. However, because of the increased risk of heart disease and strokes, the medications were gradually modified to contain lower amounts of estrogen. As a result, current oral contraceptives are progestin dominant. These pills, especially those containing a relatively androgenic progestin, sometimes exacerbated acne. Levonorgestrel, which is inserted under the skin, contains unopposed progestin. From 5% to 25% of patients on levonorgestrel develop acne (86). In the last few years, estrogens have been combined with lower doses of less androgenic progestins (89). These preparations are efficacious for both acne control and birth control (90,91). Side effects, such as nausea and weight gain, are less common than with older preparations. Breakthrough bleeding or daily spotting is common but usually stops after one or two cycles. This newest generation of birth control pills does not seem to pose risk of heart disease or strokes, and they are not contraindicated in women with migraine. Probably the most potent of this new class of birth control pills is cyproterone acetate, which combines estrogen with an antiandrogen (92,93), but this medication is not available in the United States although it is in Canada. Preparations containing desogestrel (94) and norgestimate (95) are available in the United States as of this writing. Whether preparations containing gestodene (95) will become available in the United States is uncertain because of safety concerns. The author uses these newer oral contraceptive agents as first line oral treatment for women who desire effective acne and birth control. The author uses these agents after oral antibiotics have failed in some younger women who are not sexually active, although sometimes parents will not allow their children to use them.

Spironolactone, originally introduced as a potassium-sparing diuretic, competitively competes with androgens for their receptors to decrease production of 5α-reductase (96). When used alone in doses of 50 to 100 mg/day or when combined with oral contraceptive agents, spironolactone improves acne in women after 3 to 6 months of use (89). Common side effects include breast tenderness and menstrual irregularities. Less common side effects include hyperkalemia, headache, dizziness, confusion, and agranulocytosis. Tumors developed in rats given large doses of spironolactone, but this has not been reported in humans. Although some concerns have been raised about breast cancer after long-term use, there is no scientific basis for this fear.

Flutamide is a newer antiandrogen which also may control acne well. The usual dose is 250 mg 1 to 3 times daily (97–100). Although it is usually well tolerated, menstrual irregularities and xerosis may occur. Hepatic necrosis occurs rarely.

Ketoconazole is commonly used in dermatology for fungal infections. It blocks androgen synthesis, and may be useful in selected women with acne (101). Side effects include alopecia, nausea, headache, xerosis, and pruritus. Because of the risk of hepatitis and the extremely low risk of fulminent hepatic failure associated with the use of ketoconazole, extreme caution should be used when prescribing this medication for acne.

Finasteride (Proscar®) is a peripheral antiandrogen developed for the treatment of benign prostatic hypertrophy. It blocks the 5α-reductase conversion of T to DHT. Finasteride has much more activity against the type 2 isoenzyme of 5α-reductase, which is active in acne-prone areas of skin, than the type 1 isoenzyme, which is active in the scalp and prostate (29,102). It may be used alone or in combination with oral contraceptive agents. Gonadotropin-releasing hormone agonists may benefit acne patients with polycystic ovaries by lowering androgen production (103,104).

Patients with an adrenal cause for their acne may be treated with 2.5 to 5 mg of prednisone nightly, 4 mg of methylprednisolone nightly, or 0.25 mg of dexamethasone nightly. Patients must be followed for adrenal suppression with ACTH stimulation testing. Careful monitoring for glucocorticoid side effects is essential.

Isotretinoin

Isotretinoin, also known as 13-cis-retinoic acid, is a vitamin A derivative that has been available in the United States for acne treatment since the mid 1980s. Isotretinoin virtually stops sebum production by sebaceous glands. It interferes with the differentiation of follicular cells into sebocytes (105), destroying the architecture of sebaceous gland ducts (106). Sebum production ceases almost completely. Since the sebaceous glands are smaller in patients on isotretinoin, there is a decrease in 5α-reduction of androgens (107). These processes revert to normal when isotretinoin is discontinued. This drug has revolutionized the treatment of patients with severe, scarring, nodulocystic acne. After a 16- to 20-week course at a dose of 1 mg/kg/day, it is effective in 90% of patients, and for approximately 90% of patients in whom it is effective, the acne does not recur after treatment is stopped. Patients whose acne recurs after a single course may clear after a second course at a higher dose. A cumulative amount of 150 mg/kg may be required for permanent remission (108). Because of its remarkable success in patients with severe acne, the medication has also been used in patients with less severe forms of acne. Although isotretinoin usually does cause temporary clearing, acne commonly recurs in patients with milder forms of the disease and in those with endocrinopathies (109). Because of the severity of side effects that occur in patients on isotretinoin, the medication should be used only as a last resort in patients with less severe disease (110).

Nearly all patients on isotretinoin experience reversible side effects. Higher dosages are associated with more side effects. Patients should be monitored monthly.

Severe drying of mucous membranes is the most common side effect. Dry skin occurs in 90% of patients. Joint pains occur in 16% of patients. Hair loss, loss of night vision, headaches, pseudotumor cerebri, pyogenic granulomas, secondary staphylococcus infection, mood changes, and elevation of blood triglycerides are all uncommon reversible side effects which must be discussed with each patient at each visit. Persistence of dry eyes well after isotretinoin has been discontinued has recently been reported (112). By far the greatest problem with using isotretinoin is its extreme teratogenicity. As little as one dose of isotretinoin may cause severe birth defects. A distinctive pattern of malformations including the central nervous system, craniofacial structures, and midthoracic organs occurs in approximately 25% of babies exposed in utero to isotretinoin. About 25% of pregnancy exposures result in a spontaneous abortion. Even babies who seem normal at birth may have central nervous system anomalies which may severely impair brain function. Patients may safely get pregnant as little as 1 month after a course of isotretinoin is completed, since the drug is rapidly eliminated and is not stored in the tissues. A woman considering isotretinoin must understand the extreme risk to her fetus if she becomes pregnant while on the drug. Sexually active women must be on two extremely reliable methods of birth control and must understand that every method of birth control can occasionally fail. Women should have a serum pregnancy test performed at monthly visits. Because of the seriousness of side effects, many dermatologists, including the author, believe that only dermatologists should prescribe this medication, since we are most familiar with its use. The medication should be used only in the most reliable patients and only after other measures have failed.

REFERENCES

1. Stern RS. The prevalence of acne on the basis of physical examination. *J Am Acad Dermatol* 1992; 26:931–935.
2. Krowchuk DP, Stancin T, Keskinen R, Bass J, Anglin TM. The psychological effects of acne on adolescents. *Pediatr Dermatol* 1991;8:332–338.
3. Lowe JG. The stigma of acne. *Br J Hosp Med* 1993;49:809–812.
4. Deperetti E, Forest MG. Pattern of plasma dehydroepiandosterone sulfate levels in humans from birth to adulthood: evidence for testicular production. *J Clin Endocrinol Metab* 1978;47:572–577.
5. Winter JSD, Hughes IA, Reyes FI, Faiman C. Pituitary–gonadal relations in infancy: 2. Patterns of sebum gonadal steroid concentrations in man from birth to two years of age. *J Clin Endocrinol Metab* 1976;42:679–686.
6. Burger HG, Yamada Y, Banagah ML, McCloud PI, Warne GL. Serum gonadotropin, sex steroid, and immunoreactive inhibin levels in the first two years of life. *J Clin Endocrinol Metab* 1978;47: 572–577.
7. Chew EW, Bingham A, Burrows D. Incidence of acne vulgaris in patients with infantile acne. *Clin Exp Dermatol* 1990;15:376–377.
8. Lucky AW, Biro FM, Huster G, Leach AD, Morrison JA, Ratterman J. Acne vulgaris in premenarchal girls: an early sign of puberty associated with rising levels of dehydroepiandrosterone. *Arch Dermatol* 1994;130:308–314.
9. Lucky AW, Biro FM, Huster GA, Morrison JA, Elder N. Acne vulgaris in early adolescent boys. *Arch Dermatol* 1991;127:210–216.
10. Cunliffe WJ, ed. *Acne.* Chicago, IL: Year Book Medical Publishers; 1989:2–10.
11. Epstein E. Incidence of facial acne in adults. *Dermatol Digest* 1968;7:49–58.
12. Kligman AM. Postmenopausal acne. *Cutis* 1991;47:425–426.

13. Pochi PE, Strauss JS. Sebaceous gland response in man to the administration of testosterone, Δ^4-androstenedione, and dehydroepiandosterone. *J Invest Dermatol* 1969;52:32–36.
14. Pochi PE, Strauss JS. Endocrinologic control of the development and activity of the human sebaceous gland. *J Invest Dermatol* 1974;62:191–201.
15. Jacobsen E, Billings JK, Franz RA, et al. Age-related changes in sebaceous wax-ester secretion rates in men and women. *J Invest Dermatol* 1985;85:483–485.
16. Walton S, Wyatt EH, Cunliffe WJ. Genetic control of sebum excretion and acne: a twin study. *Br J Dermatol* 1988;118:393–396.
17. Rothman KF, Pochi PE. Acne in the mature woman. Upjohn monograph, 1986.
18. Morello AM, Downing DT, Strauss JS. Octadecadienoic acids in the skin surface lipids of acne patients and normal subjects. *J Invest Dermatol* 1976;66:319–323.
19. Lucky AW. Update on acne vulgaris. *Pediatr Ann* 1987;16:29–38.
20. Tucker SB, Rogers RS, Winkelmann RR, Privett OS, Jordan RE. Inflammation in acne vulgaris. Leukocyte attraction and cytotoxicity by comedonal material. *J Invest Dermatol* 1980;74:21–25.
21. Dalziel K, Dykes PJ, Marks R. Inflammation due to intracutaneous implantation of stratum corneum. *Br J Exp Pathol* 1984;65:107–115.
22. Webster GF, Leyden JJ, Norman ME, et al. Complement activation in acne vulgaris: in vitro studies with *Proprionibacterium acnes* and *Proprionibacterium granulosum*. *Infect Immunol* 1978; 22:523–529.
23. Ingham E, Eady A, Goodwin CE, Cove JH, Cunliffe WJ. Pro-inflammatory levels of interleukin-1 α-like bioactivity are present in the majority of open comedones in acne vulgaris. *J Invest Dermatol* 1992;98:895–901.
24. Lookingbill DP, Horton R, Dermer LM, et al. Tissue production of androgens in women with acne. *J Am Acad Dermatol* 1985;12:481–486.
25. Strauss JS, Pochi PE, Downing DT. The sebaceous glands: twenty-five years of progress. *J Invest Dermatol* 1976;67:90–97.
26. Hodgins MB, Hay JB. Steroid metabolism in the human skin: its relation to sebaceous gland growth and acne vulgaris. *Biochem Soc Trans* 1976;4:605–609.
27. Pochi PE, Strauss JS, Mescon H. Sebum secretion and urinary fractional 17-ketosteroid and total 17-hydroxycorticoid excretion in male castrates. *J Invest Dermatol* 1962;39:485–489.
28. Hamilton JB. Male hormone substance: a prime factor in acne. *J Clin Endocrinol* 1941;1:570–592.
29. Imperato-McGinley J, Gauthier T, Cai LQ, Yee B, Epstein J, Pochi P. The androgen control of sebum production: studies of subjects with dihydrotestosterone deficiency and complete androgen insensitivity. *J Clin Endocrinol Metab* 1993;76:524–528.
30. Cunliffe WJ, Bottomley WW. Antiandrogens and acne: a topical approach? *Arch Dermatol* 1992; 128:1261–1264.
31. Lucky AW, Rosenfield RL, McGuire J. Adrenal androgen hyperresponsiveness to adrenocorticotropin in women with acne and/or hirsutism: adrenal enzyme defects and exaggerated adrenarche. *J Clin Endocrinol Metab* 1986;62:840–848.
32. Laue L, Peck GL, Loriaux DL, Gallucci W, Chrousos GP. Adrenal androgen secretion in post-adolescent acne: increased adrenocortical function without hypersensitivity to adrenocorticotropin. *J Clin Endocrinol Metab* 1991;73:380–384.
33. Peserico A, Angeloni G, Bertoli P, Marini A, Piva G, Panciera A, Suma V. Prevalence of polycystic ovaries in women with acne. *Arch Dermatol Res* 1989;281:502–503.
34. Bunker CB, Newton JA, Conway GS, Jacobs HS, Greaves MW, Dowd PM. The hormonal profile of women with acne and polycystic ovaries. *Clin Exp Dermatol* 1991;16:420–423.
35. Ehrmann DA, Rosenfield RL, Barnes RB, Bringell DF, Sheikh Z. Detection of functional ovarian hyperandrogenism in women with androgen excess. *N Engl J Med* 1992;327:157–162.
36. Zeligman I, Hubener LF. Experimental production of acne by progesterone. *Arch Dermatol* 1957; 76:653–658.
37. Strauss JS, Pochi PE. The human sebaceous gland: its regulation by steroid hormones and its use as an end organ for assaying androgenicity *in vivo*. *Recent Prog Horm Res* 1963;19:385–444.
38. Carmina E, Lobo RA. Evidence for increased androsterone metabolism in some normoandrogenic women with acne. *J Clin Endocrinol Metab* 1993;76:1111–1114.
39. Pochi PE. The pathogenesis and treatment of acne. *Ann Rev Med* 1990;41:187–198.
40. Precious DS, Hoffman CD, Miller R. Steroid acne after orthognathic surgery. *Oral Surg Oral Med Oral Pathol* 1992;74:279–281.

41. Monk B, Cunliffe WJ, Layton AM, Rhodes DJ. Acne induced by inhaled corticosteroids. *Clin Exp Dermatol* 1993;18:148–150.
42. Scott MJ, Scott AM. Effects of anabolic-androgenic steroids on the pilosebaceous unit. *Cutis* 1992; 50:113–116.
43. Mills OH, Kligman AM. External factors aggravating acne. *Dermatol Clin* 1988;1:365–370.
44. Strauss JS, Jackson EM, Engasser PG, et al. American Academy of Dermatology Invitational Symposium on Comedogenicity. *J Am Acad Dermatol* 1989;20:272–277.
45. Crow KD. Significance of cutaneous lesions in the symptomatology of exposure to dioxins and other chloracnegens. In: Tucker RE, ed. *Human and environmental risks of chlorinated dioxins and related compounds.* New York: Plenum Press; 1983:605–612.
46. Bond GG, McLaren EA, Brenner FE, Cook RR. Incidence of chloracne among chemical workers potentially exposed to chlorinated dioxins. *J Occup Med* 1989;31:771–774.
47. Das M, Misra MP. Acne and folliculitis due to diesel oil. *Contact Dermatitis* 1988;18:120–121.
48. Mills OH, Kligman AM. External factors aggravating acne. *Dermatol Clin* 1988;1:365–370.
49. Shalita AR. Acne vulgaris: pathogenesis and treatment. *Cosmet Toiletries* 1983;98:57–60.
50. Jung-Hoffman C, Taubert HD, Kuhl H. Direct radioimmunoassay of free testosterone in the evaluation of androgenic manifestations in women. *Gynecol Endocrinol* 1987;1:83–92.
51. Mills OH, Kligman AM, Pochi PE, Comite H. Comparing 2.5%, 5%, and 10% benzoyl peroxide on inflammatory acne vulgaris. *Int J Dermatol* 1986;25:664–667.
52. Norris JFB, Basey AJ, Cunliffe WJ. A comparison of the effectiveness of topical tetracycline, benzoyl-peroxide gel and oral oxytetracycline in the treatment of acne. *Clin Exp Dermatol* 1991; 16:31–33.
53. Zbinden G. Scientific opinion on the carcinogenic risk due to topical administration of benzoyl peroxide for the treatment of acne vulgaris. *Pharmacol Toxicol* 1988;63:307–309.
54. Rothman KF, Pochi PE. Use of oral and topical agents for acne in pregnancy. *J Am Acad Dermatol* 1988;19:431–442.
55. Algra RJ, Rosen T, Waisman M. Topical clindamycin in acne vulgaris. *Arch Dermatol* 1977;113:1390–1391.
56. Schachner L, Pestana A, Kittles C. A clinical trial comparing the safety and efficacy of a topical erythromycin-zinc formulation with a topical clindamycin formulation. *J Am Acad Dermatol* 1990; 22:489–495.
57. Pochi PE. The pathogenesis and treatment of acne. *Annu Rev Med* 1990;41:187–198.
58. Milstone EB, McDonald AJ, Scholhamer CF. Pseudomembranous colitis after topical application of clincamycin. *Arch Dermatol* 1981;117:154–155.
59. Parry MF, Rha C-K Pseudomembranous colitis caused by topical clindamycin phosphate. *Arch Dermatol* 1986;122:583–584.
60. Breneman DL, Ariano MC. Successful treatment of acne vulgaris in women with a new topical sodium sulfacetamide/sulfur lotion. *Int J Dermatol* 1993;32:365–367.
61. Margolis DJ, Bondi EE. Toxic epidermal necrolysis associated with sulfonamides. *Int J Dermatol* 1990;29:153.
62. Shalita AR. Comparison of salicylic acid cleanser and a benzoyl peroxide wash in the treatment of acne vulgaris. *Clin Ther* 1989;11:264–267.
63. Leyden JJ, Shalita RN. Rational therapy for acne vulgaris: an update on topical treatment. *J Am Acad Dermatol* 1986;15:907–914.
64. Franz TJ. Percutaneous absorption of retinoic acid in monkey and man. *Am Acad Dermatol Symposium on Cutaneous Toxicol* (abst). 1988.
65. Lehman PA, Malany AM. Evidence for percutaneous absorption of isotretinoin from the photoisomerization of topical tretinoin. *J Invest Dermatol* 1989;93:595–599.
66. Kraft JC, Kochhar DM, Scott WJ, Nau H. Low teratogenicity of 13-cis retinoic acid (isotretinoin) in the mouse corresponds to low embryo concentrations during organogenesis: comparison to the all-trans isomer. *Toxicol Appl Pharmacol* 1987;87:474–482.
67. Kochhar DM, Penner JD, Tellone CI. Comparative teratogenic activities of two retinoids: effects on palate and limb development. *Teratogenesis Carcino Mutagen* 1984;4:377–387.
68. Lipson AH, Collins F, Webster WS. Multiple congenital defects associated with maternal use of topical tretinoin. *Lancet* 1993;341:1352–1353.
69. Freinkel RK, Strauss JS, Yip SY, et al. Effect of tetracycline on the composition of sebum in acne vulgaris. *N Engl J Med* 1965;273:850–854.

70. Esterly NB, Furey NL, Flanagan LE. The effect of antimicrobial agents on leukocyte chemotaxis. *J Invest Dermatol* 1978;70:51–55.
71. Eady EA, Jones CE, Gardner KJ, et al. Tetracycline-resistant Propionibacteria from acne patients are cross-resistant to doxycycline, but sensitive to minocycline. *Br J Dermatol* 1993;128:556–560.
72. Eady EA, Jones CE, Tipper JL, et al. Antibiotic resistant propionibacteria in acne: need for policies to modify antibiotic usage. *Br Med J* 1993;306:555–556.
73. Driscoll M, Rothe M, Abrahamia L, et al. Long-term oral antibiotics for acne: is laboratory monitoring necessary? *J Am Acad Dermatol* 1993;28:595–602.
74. Moskowitz Y, Leibowitz E, Ronen M, Aviel E. Pseudotumor cerebri induced by vitamin A combined with minocycline. *Ann Opthalmol* 1993;25:306–308.
75. Parkins FM, Furnish G, Bernstein M. Minocycline use discolors teeth. *J Am Dent Assoc* 1992;123:87–89.
76. Chiappinelli JA, Walton RE. Tooth discoloration resulting from long-term tetracycline therapy: a case report. *Quintessence Int* 1992;23:539–541.
77. Schofield JK, Tatnall FM. Minocycline induced skin pigmentation. *Br J Gen Pract* 1993;43:173–174.
78. Eady DJ, Burrows D. Minocycline-induced pigmentation occurring in two sisters. *Clin Exp Dermatol* 1991;16:55–57.
79. Carter MP, Wilson F. Tetracycline and congenital limb abnormalities. *Br J Med* 1962;2:407–408.
80. Corcoran R, Castles JM. Tetracycline for acne vulgaris and possible teratogenesis. *Br Med J* 1977;2:807–808.
81. Ruiz GM, Perez BF, Lopez SC, et al. Syndrome of hypomelia, hypotrichosis and facial hemangioma (pseudothalidomide syndrome) [abst]. *An Esp Pediatr* 1982;17:229–233.
82. Barnett ML. Inhibition of oral contraceptive effectiveness by concurrent antibiotic administration. *J Peridontol* 1985;56:18–20.
83. Fleisher AB, Resnick SD. The effect of antibiotics on the efficacy of oral contraceptives. *Arch Dermatol* 1989;125:1562–1564.
84. DeGroot AC, Eshuis H, Stricker BHC. Oral contraceptives and antibiotics in acne. *Br J Dermatol* 1991;124:212.
85. Rasmussen JE. The effect of antibiotics on the efficacy of oral contraceptives. *Arch Dermatol* 1989;125:1562–1564.
86. Shoupe D, Mishell DR. Norplant: subdermal implant system for long-term contraception. *Am J Obstet Gynecol* 1989;160:1286–1292.
87. Al-Mishari MA. Clinical and bacteriological evaluation of tetracycline and erythromycin in acne vulgaris. *Clin Ther* 1987;9:273–280.
88. Bottomly WW, Cunliffe WJ. Oral trimethoprim as a third-line antibiotic in the management of acne vulgaris. *Dermatol* 1993;187:193–196.
89. Lemay A, Dewailly SD, Grenier R, Huard J. Attenuation of mild hyperandrogenic activity in postpubertal acne by a triphasic oral contraceptive containing low doses of ethynyl estradiol and d,1,-norgestrel. *J Clin Endocrinol Metab* 1990;71:8–14.
90. Palatsi R, Hirvensalo E, Luikko P, et al. Serum total and unbound testosterone and sex hormone binding globulin (SHBG) in female acne patients treated with two different oral contraceptives. *Acta Derm Venereol (Stockh)* 1984;64:517–523.
91. Anderson KD. Selectivity and minimal androgenicity of norgestimate in monophasic and triphasic oral contraceptives. *Acta Obset Gynecol Scand Suppl* 1992;156:15–21.
92. Monk BE, Almeyda JA, Caldwell IW, et al. Efficacy of low-dose cyproterone acetate compared with minocycline in the treatment of acne vulgaris. *Clin Exp Dermatol* 1987;12:319–322.
93. Eden JA. The polycystic ovary syndrome presenting as resistant acne successfully treated with cyproterone acetate. *Med J Aust* 1991;155:677–680.
94. Kaunitz AM. Combined oral contraception with desogestrel/ethinyl estradiol: tolerability profile. *Am J Obstet Gynecol* 1993;168:1028–1033.
95. Weber-Diehl F, Lehnert J, Lachnit U. Comparison of two triphasic oral contraceptives containing either gestodene or norethindrone: a randomized, clinical trial. *Contraception* 1993;48:291–301.
96. Shaw JC. Spironolactone in dermatologic therapy. *J Am Acad Dermatol* 1991;24:236–243.
97. Lookingbill DP, Abrams BB, Ellis CN. Inocoterone and acne. *Arch Dermatol* 1992;128:1197–1200.
98. Cusan L, Dupont A, Belanger A, Tremblay R, Manhes G, Labrie F. Treatment of hirsutism with the pure antiandrogen flutamide. *Amer Acad Dermatol* 1990;23:462–469.

99. Motta T, Maggi G, Perra M, Azzolari E, Casazza S, D'Alberton A. Flutamide in the treatment of hirsutism. *Int J Gynecol Obstet* 1991;36:155–157.
100. Marcondes JA, Minnani SL, Luthold WW, Wajchenberg BL, Samojlik E, Kirschner MA. Treatment of hirsutism in women with flutamide. *Fertil Steril* 1992;57:543–547.
101. Venyuroli R, Fabbri L, Dal Prato B, et al. Ketoconazole therapy for women with acne and/or hirsutism. *J Clin Endocr Metab* 1990;71:335–339.
102. Thigpen AE, Silver RI, Guileyardo JM, Casey ML, McConnell JD, Russell DW. Tissue distribution and ontogeny of steroid 5 ALPHA-reductase isozyme expression. *J Clin Invest* 1993;92:903–910.
103. Adashi EY. Potential utility of gonadotropin-releasing hormone agonists in the management of ovarian hyperandrogenism. *Fertil Steril* 1990;53:765–769.
104. Chang RJ, Laufer LR, Meldrum DR, et al. Steroid secretion in polycystic ovarian disease after suppression by a long-acting gonadotropin-releasing hormone agonist. *J Clin Endocr Metab* 1983;56:897–903.
105. Landthaler M, Kummermehr J, Wagner A, Plewig G. Inhibitory effects of 13-cis-retinoic acid in human sebaceous glands. *Arch Dermatol Res* 1980;269:297–309.
106. Guy R, Ridden C, Barth J, et al. Isolation and maintenance of the human pilosebaceous duct: 13-cis retinoic acid acts directly on the duct in vitro. *Br J Dermatol* 1993;128:242–248.
107. Rademaker M, Wallace M, Cunliffe W, Simpson NB. Isotretinoin treatment alters steroid metabolism in women with acne. *Br J Dermatol* 1991;124:361–364.
108. Lehucher-Ceyrac D, Weber-Buisset WJ. Isotretinoin and acne in practice: a prospective analysis of 188 cases over 9 years. *Dermatol* 1993;186:123–128.
109. Macdonald Hull S, Cunliffe WJ, Hughes BR. Treatment of the depressed and dysmorphic acne patient. *Clin Exper Dermatol* 1991;16:210–211.
110. Rothman KF, Lucky AW. Acne vulgaris. In: Callen JP, Dahl MV, Golitz LE, Greenway HT, Schachner LA, eds. *Advances in dermatology*, vol 8. St. Louis, MO: Mosby Year Book; 1993; 347–375.
111. Goulden V, Layton AM, Cunliffe WJ. Long-term safety of isotretinoin as a treatment for acne vulgaris. *Br J Dermatol;* 1994;131:360–363.
112. Lerman S. Ocular side-effects of accutane therapy. *Lens Eye Toxic Res* 1992;9:429–438.

Androgenic Disorders,
edited by G. P. Redmond.
Raven Press, Ltd., New York © 1995.

11

Androgenetic Alopecia— An Autosomal-Dominant Disorder

Wilma F. Bergfeld

Department of Dermatology, Cleveland Clinic Foundation, Cleveland, Ohio 44195.

Androgenetic alopecia (AGA), an autosomal-dominant disorder, is the most common alopecia in man with a prevalence of 23 to 87% (1,2). In both men and women, it presents with a central scalp alopecia at puberty and is associated with clinical signs of sexual development and androgen excess such as acne, seborrhea, and hirsutism.

The central alopecia is more severe in men than in women; in men it presents with several distinct areas of partial or complete alopecia, while in women there is a more diffuse thinning (Fig. 1) (2–7).

MORPHOLOGY AND HISTOLOGY

In AGA, the follicular growth cycle is altered, with shortened anagen growth and a reduced diameter of the follicle, or miniaturization. This results in reduced terminal follicles and increased indeterminant and vellus follicles (Fig. 2) (8).

Other changes include patchy, chronic, perifollicular, and perivascular inflammation in late AGA. In chronic AGA, scarring may be seen (9).

CONTROL OF HAIR GROWTH

Regeneration of hair is dependent on recycling of the anagen terminal follicle (10). The primary follicle stem cells are within the bulge area (11), the site of contact of the external root sheath and the arrector pili muscle, inferior to the sebaceous canalway. The secondary site of regeneration is the anagen bulb composed of follicular epithelium and the dermal papillae. This interface of ectoderm and mesoderm regulates follicular size (12), hair diameter, hair color (13), and growth cycles. The larger follicles produce larger hairs (Fig. 3).

The dermal papillae contain androgen receptors whose numbers vary in different sites and are able to interact with several androgen precursors (14,15).

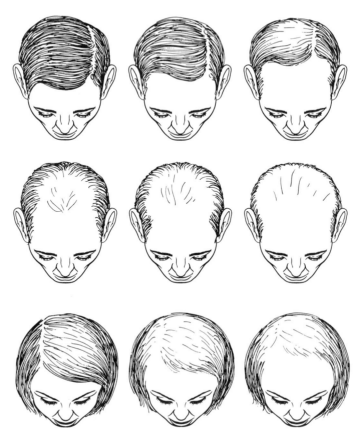

FIG. 1. Clinical presentation of androgenetic alopecia. The clinical patterns of AGA in men and women are similar in some respects. Both sexes usually demonstrate progressive hair loss, centered over the crown, and M-shaped frontotemporal recession. Hamilton divided the male pattern (*top two rows*) into eight stages. (The first stage, which precedes any loss, and the third, which is only marginally different from the second and fourth, are not shown here.) In contrast, Ludwig classified the typically more diffuse hair loss in women (*bottom row*) as mild, moderate, or severe. The frontal hairline recedes less markedly than in men and remains intact. Unlike men, women rarely develop total or near-total baldness.

Androgens

Androgens are the modulators of hair growth (16–19). In man, the follicular response to androgens is dependent upon the specific androgen, the amount present for peripheral metabolism, peripheral metabolism activity, and the presence and numbers of androgen receptors and androgen receptors sensitivity (Fig. 4).

In men, testosterone is the major precursor of dehydrotestosterone (DHT) while dehydroepiandrostenedione (DHEA) is more likely to be the major precursor in women (20,21). The conversion of these precursors to DHT is the important step in the production of the peripheral androgens that result in the clinical signs of andro-

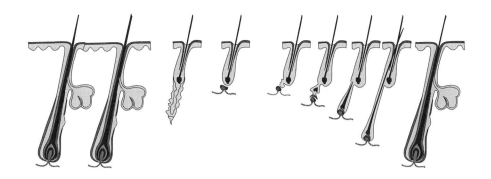

| Previous growing phase (anagen) | Involution phase (catagen) | Resting phase (telogen) | Regrowing phase (mid-anagen) | New growing phase (anagen) |

FIG. 2. Hair follicle growth cycles of the scalp.

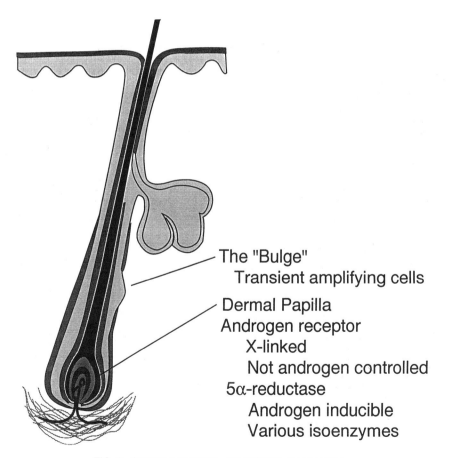

The "Bulge"
 Transient amplifying cells
Dermal Papilla
Androgen receptor
 X-linked
 Not androgen controlled
5α-reductase
 Androgen inducible
 Various isoenzymes

FIG. 3. Anagen hair follicle: site of follicle regeneration.

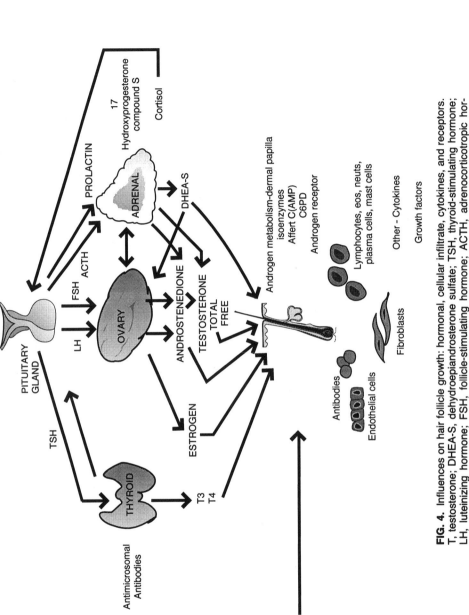

FIG. 4. Influences on hair follicle growth: hormonal, cellular infiltrate, cytokines, and receptors. T, testosterone; DHEA-S, dehydroepiandrosterone sulfate; TSH, thyroid-stimulating hormone; LH, luteinizing hormone; FSH, follicle-stimulating hormone; ACTH, adrenocorticotropic hormone.

gen excess such as seborrhea, alopecia, hirsutism, and acne (SAHA). The production of these androgens is facilitated by increased activity of three enzymes: 5α-reductase, aromatase, and 3β-hydroxysteroid dehydrogenase isomerase (3βHSD).

Specifically, testosterone is converted to DHT by 5α-reductase (22). In women, the major precursor, DHEA, is converted to androstenedione by 3βHSD and to testosterone by 17β-ol-dehydrogenase (17DH). Testosterone is then converted to DHT by 5α-reductase.

The present increased activity of aromatase in the female scalp facilitates conversion of androstenedione and estrone and is greater than its conversion to testosterone and DHT. This appears to protect women from severe AGA since aromatase is markedly decreased in the bald or balding areas of both men and women (Fig. 5) (23).

Increased activity of 3βHSD isomerase has been identified in balding scalp and sebaceous glands (24). This enzyme is responsible for conversion of 5-androstene-3β,17β-diol to testosterone, and DHEA to androstenedione and then to testosterone and DHT.

Increased circulation of androgens and precursors can affect the peripheral metabolism and results in signs of androgen excess. This mechanism results primarily in increased androgen diffusing into the cell nuclei and binding to the cytosolic or nuclear receptor proteins (17,23).

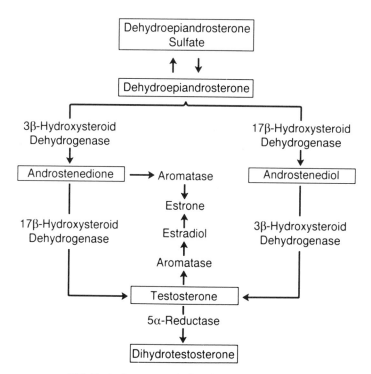

FIG. 5. Androgen metabolism in scalp hair follicle.

Androgen Receptors

Androgen receptors vary in number and are dependent on site, for example, the beard has more than the scalp in men. These cytosolic or nuclear receptor proteins are of two types: monomer and tetramer. In the balding areas of men, the monomer/tetramer ratio is increased (23).

Anagen receptors in follicles are mainly identified in the dermal papillae and within pilosebaceous keratocytes, but they are absent from the bulge area and the matrix. Extrafollicular androgen receptors are seen in many tissues and cells.

Androgens That Shorten Growth Cycles

DHT inhibits adenyl cyclase activity, interfering with the formation of cyclic adenosine monophosphate (cAMP), while estrone stimulates it. Glucose 6-phosphate dehydrogenase (G6PD) activity is then stimulated by cAMP, which increases during the anagen cycle (25).

DHEA inhibits G6PD, which shortens the anagen cycle. Both androgens, DHT and DHEA, therefore, are able to shorten the anagen cycle and are partially responsible for the miniaturization of the follicle in AGA.

Androgen Production

Central and peripheral production and metabolism are similar in men and women, but differ in type, amount, and enzyme activity.

In women, 40% to 50% of testosterone is produced by the ovaries and adrenals, while 50% to 60% is produced by peripheral conversion of androgen precursors. The result is lower plasma levels of testosterone and higher levels of DHEA and estradiol. Any elevated androgen levels in plasma produce greater peripheral metabolism.

Sex hormone binding globulin (SHBG) binds androstenediol, testosterone, and estradiol in plasma with different binding affinities. Its affinity for DHT is three times greater than that for testosterone, which is nine times greater than that for estradiol. Unbound testosterone or free testosterone produces greater peripheral metabolism and increased production of DHT.

Other Factors

The acute onset of alopecia in individuals with inflammatory disease of the scalp has a variety of etiologies which include the influence of the inflammatory cells, release of cytokines, presence of growth factors, and increased interaction of the stromal cells, i.e., fibroblasts, endothelial cells, and adnexal keratinocytes.

Alopecia has been noted in seborrheic dermatitis which frequently accompanies alopecia. Other conditions include psoriasis, pityriasis rubra pilaris, infections, and physical and chemical alopecia (26).

Animal Models

Animal models of AGA have included the chimpanzee, stump-tailed macaques, and South American red uacari. The stump-tailed macaque is the most frequently studied AGA model because of its similarities morphologically, histologically, and hormonally to man. In the macaque, puberty is noted at age 3 to 4 with the onset of secondary sex development and AGA in both males and females. Studies have demonstrated miniaturization of the follicle and increased follicular testosterone and DHT. The miniaturized follicular bulb area has shown decreased uptake and conversion of testosterone and DHT. In addition, the use of hair promoters, antiandrogens, and androgen blockade agents appear to have reversed AGA in this animal model (27,28).

Laboratory Screening Tests

Laboratory screening tests for elevated circulating androgens should include DHEA-S and free and total testosterone. If menstrual irregularities are noted, prolactin, luteinizing hormone, and follicle-stimulating hormone should be included. More elaborate androgen testing should be done if clinically indicated (1,20,29).

At the present time, measurements of peripheral androgen metabolism is not standardized. Urinary androstanediol is the best measurement available to assess increased peripheral DHT metabolism.

Therapies

Therapies for AGA are still unsatisfactory. Because of the knowledge of follicular growth cycles, androgen influence, and androgen receptors, therapies have included hair growth promoters, antiandrogens, and androgen blockade agents (30–33). These therapeutic modalities, which can be grouped as shown in Table 1, are best used in combination for enhanced therapeutic response.

TABLE 1. *Therapeutic modalities for AGA*

Antiandrogens	Topical	SHBG binding	5α-reductase	Unavailable
Estrogen	Minoxidil	Estrogen	Finasteride	Cyctol
Spironolactone	Tretinoin		Progestins	Cyproterone acetate
Progesterone	Diazoxide			
Cimetidine				
Flutamide				

SUMMARY

Androgenetic alopecia is a hereditary, androgen-driven disorder, which presents with mild-to-severe central alopecia in men and women.

In 40% to 50% of women, increased circulating androgens may be identified, while in 50% to 60% peripheral plasma metabolism of androgen precursors appears responsible for AGA. Certainly, greater understanding of androgen excess syndromes and mechanisms may lead to a better understanding of and improved therapies for androgenetic alopecia and other disorders of androgen excess.

REFERENCES

1. Kuster W, Hopple L. The inheritance of common baldness: two B or not to B. *J Am Acad Dermatol* 1984;11:921.
2. Olsen EA. Androgenetic alopecia. In: Olsen EA, ed. *Disorders of hair growth.* New York: McGraw-Hill; 1993:257–283.
3. Bergfeld WF. Androgenetic alopecia: an overview. Badin HP, ed. *Symposium on alopecia (7th): dermatologic capsule and comment.* New York: HP; 1988:1–10.
4. Bergfeld WF. Diffuse hair loss in women. *Cutis* 1978;22:190.
5. Hamilton JB. Patterned loss of hair in man: types and incidence. *Ann NY Acad Sci* 1951;53:708–728.
6. Ludwig E. Classification of the types of androgenetic alopecia (common baldness) occurring in the female sex. *Br J Dermatol* 1977;97:247–254.
7. Simpson NB. Diffuse alopecia: Endocrine, metabolic and chemical influences on the follicular cycle. In: Rook A, Dawber K, eds. Disease of the hair and scalp. Boston: Blackwell Scientific, 1991:136–166.
8. Uno H. The histopathology of hair loss. In: *Current concepts*, Upjohn Company, Kalamazoo, Michigan; 1988:1–47.
9. Abell E. Embryology and anatomy of the hair follicle. In: Olsen EA, ed. *Disorders of hair growth.* New York: McGraw-Hill; 1993:1–19.
10. Kligman AM. The human hair cycle. *J Invest Dermatol* 1959;33:307–316.
11. Cotsarelis G, Sun TT, Lavker RM. Label-retaining cells reside in the bulge area of pilosebaceous unit: implication for follicular stem cells, hair cycle and skin. *Cell* 1990;61:1329–1337.
12. Van Scott E, Kel TM. Geometric relationship between the matrix of the hair bulb and its dermal papilla in normal and alopecia scalp. *J Invest Dermatol* 1958;31:281–287.
13. Messenger AG. The control of hair growth and pigmentation. In: Olsen EA, ed. *Disorders of hair growth.* New York: McGraw-Hill; 1993:39–58.
14. Itami S, Kurata S, Sonada T, Takayasu S. Mechanism of action in dermal papilla cells. *Ann NY Acad Sci* 1991;642:385–395.
15. Killinger DW. The role of peripheral metabolism in androgenic action. *Semin Reprod Endocrinol Metab* 1986;4:101–108.
16. Randall VA, et al. Androgens and the hair follicle: cultured human dermal papilla cells as a model system. *Ann NY Acad Sci* 1991;641:355.
17. Sawaya ME. Steroid chemistry and hormone controls during hair follicle cycle. *Ann NY Acad Sci* 1991;642:376–384.
18. Schmeikirt HU, Wilson JD. Androgen metabolism in isolated human hair roots. In: Orfanos CE, Montagna W, Stuttgen G eds. *Hair res.* Berlin: Springer-Verlag; 1981:210–214.
19. Sperling LC, Heimer WL. Androgen biology as a basis for the diagnosis and treatment of androgenic disorders in women, II. *J Am Acad Dermatol* 1993;28:901–916.
20. Kasick JM, Bergfeld WF, Steck WD, Gupta MK. Adrenal androgenic female-pattern alopecia: sex hormones and the balding woman. *Cleve Clin J Med* 1983;50:111–122.
21. Fazekas AG, Sandor T. The metabolism of dihydroepiandrosterone by human scalp hair follicles. *J Clin Endocrinol Metab* 1973;36:582–586.
22. Thigpen AE, Silver RI, Guileyardo JM, Casey ML, McConnell JD, Russell DW. Tissue distribu-

tions and autogeny of steroid 5 alpha reductase isozyme expression. *J Clin Invest* 1993;92(2):903–910.

23. Sawaya ME, Penneys NS. Immunohistochemical distribution of aromatase and 3 beta-hydroxysteroid in human hair follicles and sebaceous gland. *J Cutan Pathol* 1991;19:309–314.

24. Sawaya ME, Homs LS, Garland LD, Hsia SL. Δ^5-3β Hydroxysteroid dehydrogenase activity in sebaceous glands of scalp in male-pattern baldness. *J Invest Dermatol* 1988;91:101–105.

25. Adachi K, Kano M. Adenyl cyclase in human hair follicles: its inhibition by dihydrotestosterone. *Biochem Biophys Res Commun* 1970;1:884–890.

26. DeVillez RL. Infections: physical and inflammatory causes of hair and scalp abnormalities. In: Olsen EA, ed. *Disorders of hair growth*. New York: McGraw-Hill; 1993:71–90.

27. Uno H, Adachi K, Montagna W. Morphological and biochemical studies of hair follicles in common baldness of stumptailed macaque (Macaca speciosa). In: Montagna W, Dobson RL, eds. *Advances in biology of skin, Vol 9, Hair growth*. Oxford: Pergamon Press; 1969:221–224.

28. Uno H. Stumptailed macaques as a model of male-pattern baldness. In: Maibach HI, Lowe NJ, eds. *Models in dermatology*. Basel: Karger; 1987:159–169.

29. Redmond GP, Bergfeld WF. Diagnostic approach to androgen disorders in women: Acne, hirsutism, and alapecia. *Cleve Clin J Med* 1990;57:423–427.

30. Redmond GP, Bergfeld WF. Treatment of androgenic diseases in women: acne, hirsutism and alopecia. *Cleve Clin J Med* 1990;57:423–427.

31. Sawaya ME, Hordinsky MK. The antiandrogens, when and how they should be used. *Dermatol Clin* 1993;11(1):65–72.

32. Sperling LC, Heines WL. Androgen biology as a basis for the diagnosis and treatment of androgenic disease in women, I. *J Am Acad Dermatol* 1993;28:669–683.

Androgenic Disorders,
edited by G. P. Redmond.
Raven Press, Ltd., New York © 1995.

12

Hyperandrogenism: Implications for Cardiovascular Disease

Robert A. Wild

Section of Research and Education in Women's Health, Department of Obstetrics and Gynecology, University of Oklahoma Health Science Center, Oklahoma City, Oklahoma 73190.

While our understanding of androgen disorders at the molecular, ovarian, physiologic, and genetic levels has improved remarkably in the past decade, it has become increasingly recognized that the metabolic alterations found in patients with disorders of androgen excess are important to recognize and are prevalent. These metabolic changes hold clues to pathophysiology, they have implications for individual patient management decisions, and they are relevant to development of public health strategies to prevent long-term sequelae of cardiovascular disease. Women with hirsutism, including those with polycystic ovary syndrome (PCOS), can be viewed as experiments of nature that provide opportunities to better understand complex interactions between genetic, gonadal, adrenal, and endocrine mechanisms and environmental interactions resulting in metabolic aberrations that determine cardiovascular risk. This has enormous public health implications because of the prevalent morbidity and mortality due to heart disease in women.

ANATOMY, PHYSIOLOGY, AND ETIOLOGY

Polycystic ovaries (Fig. 1) are found in many patients with many forms of androgen excess. Polycystic ovaries can result from androgen excess. Androgen therapy for disorders such as fibrocystic breast disease or endometriosis, or anabolic steroid use for improved athletic performance, or excess androgen of adrenal origin such as occurs in congenital adrenal hyperplasia, or excess androgen of ovarian origin, all can lead to PCOS. Because the etiologies of androgen excess are heterogeneous, the cardiovascular implications are heterogeneous (1). The pathophysiology of cardiovascular changes with exogenous anabolic hormone use is characteristic and includes an increased risk of coronary artery disease (CAD) and hence infarction secondary to changes in lipid metabolism, as well as concentric myocardial hypertrophy with decreased ventricular volume leading to alterations in pres-

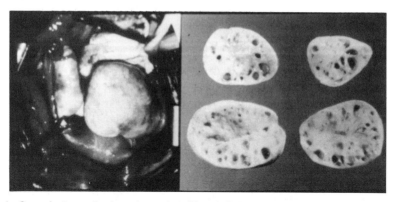

FIG. 1. Gross features of polycystic ovaries. (From ref. 40, with permission.)

sure–volume relationships within the heart. Exogenous androgens carry risks of hypertension. The pathophysiologies of cardiovascular effects of endogenous androgen excess may be entirely different from those due to exogenous androgens and may indeed be multiple and quite complex. The metabolic aberrations associated with congenital adrenal hyperplasia may or may not be different from those associated with the more common disorders that most endocrinologists refer to as garden variety PCOS. Because there is no uniform definition of PCOS, the reader is encouraged to pay particular attention to the exact characteristics of the patient population reported in the literature before making conclusions.

Patients with PCOS cluster cardiovascular risk factors. These clustered factors are thought to be additive and possibly multiplicative. Patients with these disorders were historically ignored. Because prospective incident data will take a lifetime of observation (a task for the population at large which is only partially addressed by the Framingham data in the cardiovascular literature) and because these studies are only beginning for androgenic disorders, the discussion regarding cardiovascular disease will be centered around risk factors commonly found in patients with PCOS.

IMPLICATIONS FOR CARDIOVASCULAR DISEASE

Hyperinsulinemia and Insulin Resistance, Hypertension, Hypercoagulation

Hyperinsulinemia is found frequently with disorders of androgen excess. Hyperinsulinemia is associated with underlying insulin resistance. Patients with PCOS frequently have insulin resistance whether or not they are obese (2). Obese patients with PCOS have higher insulin levels and/or insulin resistance than obese controls (3,4). A number of prospective epidemiological studies have established that hyperinsulinemia, both fasting and postprandial, is a risk factor for the development of CAD in nondiabetics (5). This association is independent of obesity, hypertriglyceridemia, hypercholesterolemia, physical inactivity, hypertension, and smoking. In prospective studies carried out in non–insulin dependent diabetic patients, a similar association between hyperinsulinemia and CAD has been observed. An association between elevated plasma insulin levels and CAD in both nondiabetic and diabetic subjects has been observed in cross-sectional studies. Asians who have migrated from India to England have been found to have an increased susceptibility to CAD not explained by known cardiovascular risk factors. Hyperinsulinemia and insulin resistance are common metabolic abnormalities in this population (6). Black patients with the insulin-sensitive variant of non–insulin dependent diabetes mellitus (NIDDM) have low risk for cardiovascular disease compared with those with insulin resistance (7).

Insulin is antherogenic. Its major effects on the arterial tree include: (a) increased formation and decreased regression of lipid plaques, (b) proliferation of smooth muscle cells, (c) stimulation of growth factors, and (d) enhanced cholesterol synthesis and increased low-density lipoprotein (LDL) receptor activity. All of these are important elements in the formation of atherosclerotic plaques. Hyperinsulinemia does not occur in isolation and almost always reflects underlying insulin resistance. Patients with PCOS are more likely to develop overt diabetes mellitus and hypertension earlier in life (8). NIDDM occurs in PCOS women at an earlier age (third and fourth decade) than in the general population (9,10). The development of overt diabetes mellitus carries very significant cardiovascular risk because it removes the selective female advantage against the development of cardiovascular disease (Table 1). Insulin resistance to carbohydrate metabolism is associated with resistance to insulin's effect to decrease skeletal muscular vascular resistance and therefore could act as a risk for hypertension. In a group of primary hypertensive and normotensive patients without drug treatment, clamped glucose disposal was correlated with blood pressure, fasting glucose, triglycerides, and very low-density lipoproteins (VLDL) and high-density lipoproteins (HDL) in both sexes, but it was strongest in women (11).

Increased concentrations of hemostatic variables, principally plasmogen-activator–inhibitor 1, accompany hyperinsulinemia, hypertriglyceridemia, hypertension, and obesity. All of these are associated with insulin resistance. This syndrome is associated with the development of CAD (as assessed by angiography) (12). Left ventricular mass has been found to be a powerful independent predictor of cardiovascular morbidity and mortality. Left ventricular mass in normotensive; nondia-

TABLE 1. *Cardiovascular disease in diabetic and nondiabetic subjects*

| | Annual mean incidence per 1,000 subjects | | | |
| | Women | | Men | |
Age (yr)	Diabetic	Nondiabetic	Diabetic	Nondiabetic
45–54	24.8	4.3	31.7	12.3
55–64	37.9	12.6	48.1	25.1
65–74	40.4	22.4	57.5	28.4

Adapted from Kannel et al., ref. 38.

betic obesity has been found to be associated with insulin resistance independent of body mass index and blood pressure (13).

Alteration in Apolipoprotein Lipid Metabolism

Women with PCOS commonly have higher triglyceride concentrations and lower HDL cholesterol concentrations than regularly menstruating, nonhirsute women matched for body weight (14). These qualitatively characteristic lipoprotein profiles are found in diabetic and nondiabetic patients with insulin resistance and hyperinsulinemia (Table 2). Insulin resistance measured by the euglycemic clamp technique is associated with similar adverse lipid and apolipoprotein changes favoring arteriosclerosis not only in nondiabetic subjects, but also in those patients with impaired glucose tolerance (15). A relationship between hyperinsulinemia and higher LDL cholesterol also has been described. Obese patients with PCOS have higher LDL cholesterol and total cholesterol than regular menstruating nonhirsute non-obese women (16). This relationship appears to be less impressive for cholesterol than for lower HDL cholesterol and hypertriglyceridemia. Utilizing a gonadotropin releasing hormone analog to remove gonadal hormonal androgen and estrogen, insulin resistance has been found to be more important than the apparently deleterious

TABLE 2. *Lipids, lipoprotein cholesterol, apolipoproteins, and ratios*

	Hirsute women (n = 47)		Normal women (n = 15)	
Triglycerides	115.3	± 79.0*[a]	57.6	± 28.8
Cholesterol	193.1	± 36.2	173.4	± 25.5
HDL cholesterol	47.5	± 8.3**	54.8	± 17.2
LDL cholesterol	121.9	± 32.8	104.8	± 28.1
VLDL cholesterol	23.0	± 15.8*	12.7	± 7.5
Apo A-I	140.0	± 15.4	151.3	± 30.4
Apo A-II	78.2	± 12.4	72.1	± 10.9
Apo B	96.7	± 29.7	84.2	± 29.6
Apo C-III	11.6	± 4.7**	9.6	± 2.3
Apo E	15.4	± 4.7	13.7	± 3.8
Apo C III-HS[b]	6.1	± 1.8	5.8	± 2.2
Apo C III-HP[c]	4.5	± 3.6***	3.0	± 1.5
Apo A-I/apo B	1.8	± 1.8	1.9	± 0.6
Apo A-I/apo C-III	13.8	± 5.2	16.7	± 3.8
Apo A-I/apo A-II	1.8	± 0.3**	2.1	± 0.4
Apo C-III/apo E	0.77	± 0.25	0.77	± 0.24
LDL cholesterol/apo BB	1.4	± 0.94	1.2	± 0.2
HDL cholesterol/apo A-I	0.34	± 0.05	0.38	± 0.08
LDL cholesterol/HDL cholesterol	1.7	± 0.9***	1.9	± 1.0
Cholesterol/HDL cholesterol	4.2	± 1.2	3.2	± 1.1

From Wild et al., ref. 16.
[a]Values are in mg/dL, mean ± SD.
[b]In heparin-Mn^{++} supernate.
[c]In heparin-Mn^{++} precipitate.
*$p > 0.001$; **$p > 0.01$ ***$p > 0.05$

endogenous androgen and the beneficial effects of endogenous estrogen in determining apolipoprotein profiles of predominantly obese women with hirsutism and hyperandrogenism (16,17). A decrease in HDL cholesterol and an increase in LDL cholesterol are well-established risk factors for CAD in both nondiabetic and diabetic subjects. Although less commonly appreciated, evidence is mounting that elevated VLDL levels are a risk factor for the development of CAD in both nondiabetic and diabetic (non–insulin dependent) women. The decrease in HDL cholesterol is intimately related to the defect in VLDL metabolism and impaired lipoprotein lipase activity.

Hyperinsulinemia is implicated in the etiology of various lipid abnormalities [increased VLDL, intermediate-density lipoproteins (IDL), and LDL levels and decreased HDL levels] (Fig. 2) that are known risk factors for CAD and other macrovascular complications. Insulin resistance by itself or more likely in combination with hyperinsulinemia, is responsible for the elevated VLDL and decreased HDL cholesterol levels in nondiabetic individuals with normal weight and insulin resistance and in individuals with NIDDM and obesity (18). Patients with PCOS may present with any of these states of altered insulin sensitivity. Hypertriglyceridemia with or without hypercholesterolemia occurs more frequently in patients with premature coronary disease than does hypercholesterolemia. Recent prospective epidemiological studies have shown that in some subsets of patient populations, increased concentrations of triglycerides represent an independent risk factor for CAD (19,20). A number of clinical and metabolic studies have suggested that partially degraded, triglyceride-rich lipoproteins of hepatic and intestinal origin (remnant lipoproteins) may have atherogenic action almost equal to that of cholesterol-rich LDL particles. Substantial evidence indicates that individuals with smaller LDL

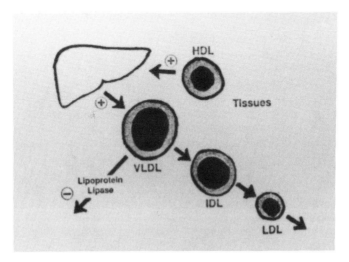

FIG. 2. The effects of insulin (+) and insulin resistance (−) on lipoprotein lipid metabolism in the insulin resistance syndrome. (Adapted from ref. 5.)

particles are at increased risk of developing coronary heart disease. Small, dense LDL (Subclass B) have higher triglyceride and lower HDL concentrations. Intermediate and pattern B LDL particle size is associated with insulin resistance (21).

Insulin Resistance and Hypertension

A number of prospective and cross-sectional studies have demonstrated a relationship between insulin resistance, hyperinsulinemia, and elevated blood pressure (5). Essential hypertension, like obesity and NIDDM, is characterized by insulin resistance that primarily affects muscle and involves a defect in glycogen synthesis. Essential hypertension should be considered a metabolic disease. These metabolic abnormalities may contribute to the development of hypertension. Several mechanisms have been postulated, including insulin-mediated sodium retention, direct stimulation of the sympathetic drive through norepinephrine-mediated responses, and the growth-promoting effects of insulin. Women with PCOS have higher blood pressure than normal, weight-matched controls, and they are more likely to develop hypertension over time (9,16). Recent studies have questioned whether a causal relationship between insulin and hypertension really exists. Population-based studies have raised questions about ethnic differences in the relationship between insulin, insulin resistance, and hypertension (Pima Indians, Pacific Islanders, Mexican-Americans, and blacks) (22,23). Because of the prevalence of hypertension and because of its established risk implications for both CAD and stroke, its study in different ethnic groups of patients with PCOS deserves further intensive investigation.

Central Obesity

Patients with PCOS frequently have an increase in abdominal girth as measured by the waist/hip ratio (16). In obese women, when the waist/hip ratio exceeds 0.76, menstrual abnormalities and hirsutism are more prevalent (24). Women with upper body obesity have increased production of testosterone (25). In classic studies from Goteborg, Sweden (26), longitudinal evaluation demonstrated that the ratio of waist to hip circumference is significantly positively associated with a 12-year incidence of myocardial infarction, angina pectoris, stroke, and death in women. This association is independent of age, body mass index, smoking habit, serum cholesterol concentration, serum triglyceride concentration, and systolic blood pressure. Although general indices of obesity such as body mass index (BMI) or sum of skinfold measurements predicted myocardial infarction in women, the ratio of waist/hip circumference is stronger in this respect. Insulin resistance in obese women, as assessed by the hyperinsulinemic, euglycemic clamp technique, is associated with upper abdominal region localization of fat. This visceral fat accumulation is accompanied by impaired glucose disposal to insulin, impaired capacity of insulin to stimulate glycogen synthetase in skeletal muscle, and higher circulating nonesterified

Hirsutism in women with Coronary Artery
Disease (CAD): Implications for the cardiovascular
risk of androgen excess

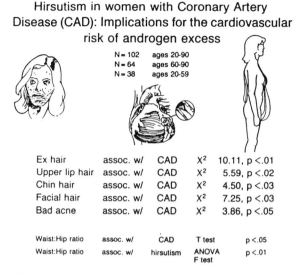

N = 102	ages 20-90
N = 64	ages 60-90
N = 38	ages 20-59

Ex hair	assoc. w/	CAD	X^2	10.11, p <.01
Upper lip hair	assoc. w/	CAD	X^2	5.59, p <.02
Chin hair	assoc. w/	CAD	X^2	4.50, p <.03
Facial hair	assoc. w/	CAD	X^2	7.25, p <.03
Bad acne	assoc. w/	CAD	X^2	3.86, p <.05
Waist:Hip ratio	assoc. w/	CAD	T test	p <.05
Waist:Hip ratio	assoc. w/	hirsutism	ANOVA F test	p <.01

FIG. 3. Hirsutism in women with coronary artery disease (CAD): Implications for the cardiovascular risk of androgen excess. (From ref. 28, with permission.)

fatty acids (27). Among consecutive women coming to coronary artery catheterization, confirmed CAD was found more commonly in those reporting problems earlier in life with extra upper lip, chin, and facial hair and bad acne than those who did not recall these abnormalities. This was found in older women. For women, CAD is of greatest magnitude in older ages. In this angiographic study, the associations of waist/hip ratio with CAD was reconfirmed and the associations of waist/hip ratio with complaints of hirsutism and bad acne were established (28) (Fig. 3). In older women the waist/hip circumference ratio is a better marker for risk of death than BMI.

Clustered Risk Factors and the Effects of Aging, Diet, and Inactivity

Women with hirsutism often have insulin resistance, hyperinsulinemia, obesity, impaired glucose tolerance, NIDDM, hypertension, and dyslipidemia. All components of cardiovascular risk factors for patients with PCOS occur with increasing frequency with advancing age (Table 3). Insulin resistance has been suggested as a characteristic feature of the normal aging process. Insulin resistance, however, may be clustered with other abnormalities in aging and may not be a characteristic feature of the normal aging process per se (29). Insulin resistance may be related to age-related increase in atherosclerotic coronary vascular disease (ASCVD), NIDDM, obesity, hypertension, and dyslipidemia. Inactivity, characteristic in patients with PCOS (16), is manifested by a decline in maximum oxygen capacity (Vo_2 max) and is also characteristic of aging. It is well established that a reduction

TABLE 3. *Overall and age-related prevalences of cardiovascular risk factors in the general population*

	Overall prevalence (%)	Age-related prevalence (%)	
		20 yr	70 yr
Non–insulin dependent diabetes mellitus	7[a]	<1	10
Obesity	30	5	50
Essential hypertension	20	5	50
Atherosclerotic cardiovascular disease	25	<1	50

Adapted from ref. 5.
[a]All figures are approximate values.

in physical activity and exercise tolerance is associated with impaired insulin sensitivity (30), ASCVD, dyslipidemia, diabetes mellitus, and hypertension (31). In several studies (9,32), the prevalence of each risk factor in its isolated form, free of other factors with the exception of obesity, is quite low. Insulin resistance has been implicated directly in the development of obesity, NIDDM, impaired glucose tolerance, hypertension, hypertriglyceridemia, hypercholesterolemia, and reduced HDL cholesterol (5,33). It is likely that hyperinsulinemia and insulin resistance found in PCOS, by acting both directly on blood vessels and indirectly by promoting a more atherogenic cardiovascular risk profile (in an industrialized lifestyle setting), foster the development of atherosclerosis (Fig. 4). Some patients with PCOS consume diets high in saturated fats (16). A high saturated-fat diet is an unequivocal risk factor for coronary vascular disease (CVD). The consequences of aging, diet, clustering of risk factors, and associated alterations of insulin resistance need to be understood when understanding cardiovascular risk and when developing strategies for prevention of this disorder in patients with androgen disorders.

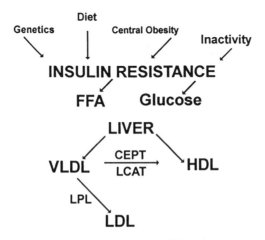

FIG. 4. Multiple factors aggravating insulin resistance. FFA, free fatty acids; LCAT, lecithin cholesterol acyltransferase deficiency; LPL, lipoprotein lipase CEPT, cholesterol ester transfer protein.

SIGNS AND SYMPTOMS

Commonly, patients with androgen disorders seek out medical assistance for cosmetic concerns of hirsutism, acne, menstrual aberration, or infertility without a real awareness of their clustered risk factors. As physicians become more aware of the increasing importance for preventive medicine of screening and providing for assessment of risk factors, and as the wider understanding of the public health importance of androgen disorders become recognized, the reasons patients with these disorders present to the health care system will increase. The majority give a history of menstrual aberration (gross or subtle) beginning at puberty, but a number are troubled with significant hirsutism in the abscence of menstrual abnormalities or with prolonged use of an oral contraceptive agent that masks the development of aberrant menstrual function with time. Family histories of patients with PCOS are frequently clustered with overt cardiovascular disease (including diabetes and/or hypertension with or without obesity) or cardiovascular disease risk factors, breast cancer, and endometrial cancer (1). Family history of breast cancer should be recorded as to its pre- or postmenopausal status. Clustering of familial body habitus and timing of the adolescent growth spurt is sometimes useful and a history of breast cancer prompts the query for body type in the relative of interest. There are familial clusters of patients with PCOS with premature CVD on both the paternal and maternal sides (Fig. 5). Patients with androgen excess can present with acne alone, hirsutism alone, androgenic alopecia, or more commonly, a combination. Menstrual disturbances of all types are seen; these are usually an expression of anovulation. All degrees of hirsutism and virilization can be seen. No correlation exists between the circulating concentrations of testosterone and the grade of hirsutism. Temporal balding and clitoromegaly may be seen. Androgenic alopecia is not infrequent (see Chapter 11). Acanthosis nigricans (AN) (Fig. 6) commonly has been found. While AN is found on multiple body sites (Table 4), it is most commonly encountered on the vulva. Central obesity is common in patients with PCOS (16). Many patients present with thickened acral parts not unlike patients with acromegaly.

DIAGNOSIS

History and Physical

History and physical exam are of utmost importance in the differential diagnosis and the assessment of risk factors for metabolic diseases (1). Because presentations may differ and because the patient herself may be unaware of her risk status for certain disorders, a clear understanding of the reason the patient is seeking help is essential. A careful questioning of menstrual function, as well as the need for and understanding of birth control risks and benefits will help in deciding the need for endometrial sampling and deciding upon appropriate strategies for therapy (1). Varying degrees of amenorrhea, oligomenorrhea, and hirsutism may be encountered (Fig. 7). One year of anovulation associated with unopposed estrogen stimulation of

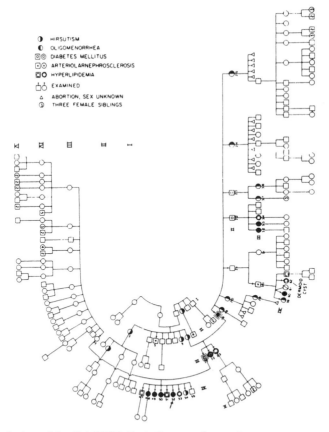

FIG. 5. Family tree of familial PCOS illustrating prevalence of premature coronary vascular disease and carbohydrate abnormalities. (From ref. 41, with permission.)

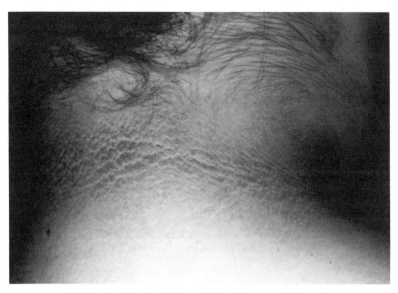

FIG. 6. Acanthosis nigricans (*AN*) at the nape of the neck.

TABLE 4. *Frequency of distribution of AN by body site*

Body site	No. of patients (%) (n = 43)
Axilla	14 (32.6)
Neck	13 (30.2)
Breast	7 (16.3)
Thigh	7 (16.3)
Waist	3 (7.0)
Knee	1 (2.3)
Elbow	4 (9.3)
Vulva	24 (55.8)

From ref. 39, with permission.

the uterus suggests the need for endometrial sampling. Fertility desires and priority of these needs in relation to desire to control cosmetic complications help dictate treatment strategies.

A search for overt cardiovascular disease and risk factors in the family, including gynecological disorders such as breast and endometrial disease, is important, with particular attention to age of onset of the disorders. Careful questioning for clues to altered lipid and carbohydrate metabolism is often rewarding. Questions concerning diet (including amount of saturated fat and protein intake, as well as intake of fruits, vegetables, and grain products), extent, type, and tolerance of physical activity, stress encountered in daily living, smoking habits, and current and past use of medications are important and should be incorporated into daily office practice (34). The physical examination includes blood pressure assessment; it is critical that it be measured in a quiet, restful atmosphere with a large cuff if the arm is large. It should be taken in both arms, when the patient is lying down, sitting up, and standing erect. Sometimes it is important to measure it in the legs as well if there is a suspicion of blockage of flow in the arterial system to the lower parts of the body. A reading of 140/90 or greater on three separate visits demands evaluation and probable intervention.

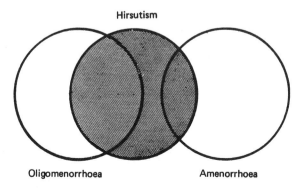

FIG. 7. Varying degrees of amenorrhea, oligomenorrhea, and hirsutism in women with polycystic ovaries.

The physical examination emphasizes evaluation for extent and type of androgenization, striae, fat distribution, estrogenization, stigmata of insulin resistance (type and degree of obesity, and site and extent of AN), and stigmata of hyperlipidemia including arcus senilis, papillomata, and diabetic sequelae (retinopathy and neuropathy).

Procedures

Vaginal ultrasound can reveal distinct ovarian morphology characteristic of PCO. A string of pearls morphology at the periphery of the ovary surrounding an enlarged central ovarian stroma is common (Fig. 8). Alternatively, follicles may be found throughout the stroma, but the picture is distinct from the multifollicular ovary where the stroma compartment is sparse in comparison. Waist/hip ratio is easily measured with a tape measure and is performed as a seamstress would measure for a fitting. Three valid measures at the largest diameter above the umbilicus and three valid measures at the hip area are performed. The minimum waist measure is divided by the maximum hip measurement. Values greater than 0.76 indicate increased risk for CVD (Fig. 9).

Scoring of the hirsutism is most frequently accomplished with the use of the Ferriman Gallwey Scoring system (35). A more objective measure is to determine microscopically the presence of the medulla in the hair shaft for a number of hairs in a defined area on the body (36). However, due to the cumbersome nature of this technique, it has not achieved wide acceptance.

Laboratory

If the history and physical examination indicate the need to rule out Cushing's syndrome, overnight dexamethasone suppression test and the 24-hour urinary free cortisol determination are useful. Congenital adrenal hyperplasia of the most common variety (21-hydroxylase deficiency) can be screened with the use of 0800-hr 17α-hydroxyprogesterone or adrenocorticotropic hormone (ACTH) stimulation testing if necessary to detect abnormality in mild cases. Serum testosterone (T) or markedly elevated dehydroepiandrosterone (DHEA) concentrations suggest the need to rule out an ovarian or adrenal androgen-secreting tumor.

A complete lipoprotein lipid profile is indicated in this population because of the frequency and probably atherogenicity of altered triglyceride particles. Normal limits for gynecoid women are given in Table 5.

Before therapy, it is wise to confirm the profile to determine variability. Random serum glucose of greater than 200 mg/dL is diagnostic of diabetes mellitus. By usual definitions, fasting serum glucose between 115 mg/dL and 140 mg/dL is diagnostic of carbohydrate intolerance. A fasting value of greater than 140 mg/dL is diagnostic of overt diabetes. However, the probability of mild but actual diabetes is

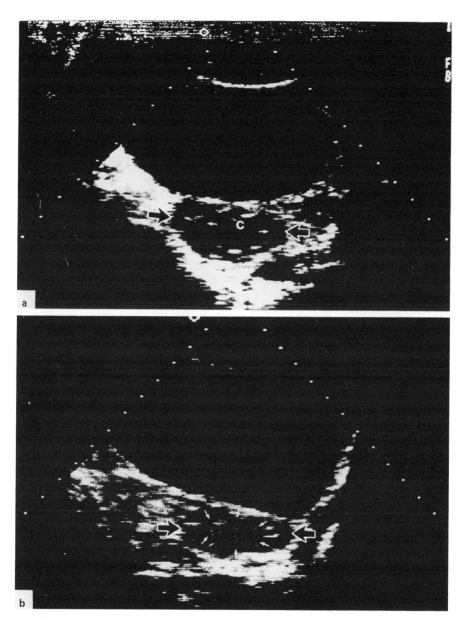

FIG. 8. Characteristic string of pearls morphology by vaginal ultrasound; concurrent follicular cyst (note *arrows*).

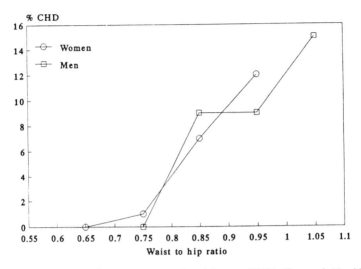

FIG. 9. Waist-to-hip ratio and percent coronary heart disease (CHD). (From ref. 42, with permission.)

high with any elevation of fasting serum glucose. Fasting insulin concentrations are a reasonable but not a perfect indicator of presence of insulin resistance. Normal levels should be known from the laboratory of reference; they are usually less than 10 μU/ml.

METABOLIC

Lipoprotein Lipid Alterations

The target lipoprotein lipid profiles are shown in Table 5. Once an aberrant value is confirmed, the first line of therapy is lifestyle alteration if indicated by risk factor assessment. This is best accomplished by behavior modification tailored to individual patient needs. Multiple risk factors cluster; the most serious should be targeted first. For instance, smoking cessation can be addressed in a support-group behavior-modification setting. The use of the nicotine patch is not recommended without coupling to a behavior modification program. Because targeting obesity affects so

TABLE 5. *Normal lipid profiles (gynecoid women)*

Cholesterol	<200 mg/dL
LDL-Cholesterol	<130 mg/dL
HDL-Cholesterol	> 35 mg/dL
Triglycerides	<135 mg/dL
Cholesterol/HDL ratio	<3.5

From ref. 1, with permission.

many other risk factors, it is worthwhile to effect weight loss through a combination of exercise, counseling (behavior modification), and diet to limit saturated fats. American Heart Association Guidelines are available to all physicians, and Step I guidelines do not require the services of a dietician. If lipoprotein lipid values do not respond on repeat testing in 3 months, prescribing an American Heart Association Step II diet is in order. This usually requires the assistance of a knowledgeable dietician. If at the 6-month follow-up visit the lipid parameters are still not under control, pharmaceutical control of the lipids in conjunction with more lifestyle alteration therapy is important to pursue. Isolated low HDL cholesterol is increasingly recognized as a risk factor for CVD and intervention is indicated. The advantages and side effects of all the lipid-lowering agents should be understood. They should be used if lifestyle alterations fail. When they are used, lifestyle alteration therapy should be encouraged.

Insulin Resistance

Hyperinsulinemia and insulin resistance are treatable. The optimal therapy is exercise. Because limiting saturated fats affects weight loss, and because exercise improves insulin resistance, targeting the obesity through a combination of diet and exercise is most effective. Exercise can improve insulin resistance and lipoprotein lipid profiles even if weight loss is not affected.

Hypertension

If blood pressure is borderline, it often responds to lifestyle alteration. When weight reduction was found to decrease blood pressure, it was hailed as a causative factor. This association may be secondary to a correlation between diet-induced metabolic change and the sympathetic nervous system. A select group such as overweight hypertensives may have a genetic predisposition for such a correlation. In overweight hypertensive patients, low caloric, especially very low caloric, diets correlate with improved glucose metabolism, a decrease in plasma insulin concentration, and altered norepinephrine concentrations and thus sympathetic nervous system activity. Medication is indicated to keep blood pressure under 140/90. This silent killer (hypertension) is very common. Blood pressure nonresponsive to lifestyle alteration requires pharmaceutical intervention to keep it under control. Antihypertensive agents that do not aggravate lipoprotein lipid metabolism have been increasingly utilized.

Diabetes

Overt carbohydrate intolerance requires control with oral agents and/or insulin if indicated after change in lifestyle is targeted and coupled with behavior modification. Requirements can be reduced for pharmacological therapy, and deterioration of carbohydrate tolerance can be prevented for as long as a decade by vigorous preventive lifestyle alterations.

Obesity

Targeting obesity is the most efficient way to address multiple clustered risk factors. Fortunately, the abdominal fat that is responsible for the increased waist/hip ratio is the type of fat that is most easily mobilized. An excellent simple technique to monitor effectiveness of therapy is to monitor serial changes of the waist/hip ratio.

PROGNOSIS

Because the etiologies of most cases of polycystic ovaries are unknown, prognosis of cure is unlikely at the current stage of our knowledge. Both patient and physician need to understand that these disorders are chronic. However, the ability to control the manifestations of the disease process is quite good (37). Control of skin and hair abnormalities, although laborious, can be achieved in most instances. Long-term prognosis for weight control in the population at large has been guarded. However, realistic and culturally specific behavior modification techniques for living in the 1990s are not widely utilized. Newer methodologies have been successful in other populations. Long-term evaluations of risk reduction strategies in populations of patients with PCOS have not been completed, but are ongoing (R. A. Wild, *unpublished data*). Most patients with these disorders have been ignored and are affected by psychosocial factors that affect body image, and they welcome interest and understanding regarding their medical needs. We have encountered highly motivated individuals quite eager to deal with their disorders. A positive preventive approach, coupled with sensitivity to major concerns for seeking medical assistance and a thorough explanation of the chronicity of their condition, has been quite rewarding. The success of any preventive strategy is linked to success of behavior modification leading to meaningful permanent lifestyle alteration.

AN EYE TO THE FUTURE

The high prevalence of these disorders will become widely recognized. Studies focusing on women and cardiovascular disease will move from the erroneous concept that all women are biologically equal to a better understanding of risk associated with large subpopulations, such as hirsute women, etc., to better define individual risk. As the pathophysiologies of the disorders become more understood, treatment strategies will include a more scientific rationale for complete care. Newer agents for control with respect to their long-term metabolic implications will be discovered and developed. The physiological implications of the disorder will be focused away from a specific organ system orientation (i.e., ovarian only [PCOS], adrenal only, pancreas only, brain only, etc.) to the realization that these complex disorders do not occur with organ isolation but instead are influenced by multiple genetic and environmental interactive factors.

REFERENCES

1. Wild RA. Hyperandrogenism: implications for cardiovascular, endometrial, and breast disease. In: Adashi E, Rock J, Rosenwaks Z, eds. *Reproductive endocrinology, surgery and technology*. New York: Raven Press; (*in press*).
2. Chang RJ, Nakamura RM, Judd FK. Insulin resistance in nonobese patients with polycystic ovarian disease. *J Clin Endocrinol Metab* 1983;57:356
3. Lo Dico G, Alongi G, Savatteri L, et al. Polycystic ovary syndrome: obesity, insulin resistance, hyperandrogenism. *Acta Eur Fertil* 1989;20:309–313.
4. Wajchenberg BL, Giannella-Neto D, Lerario AC, Marcondes JA, Ohnuma LY. Role of obesity and hyperinsulinemia in the insulin resistance of obese subjects with the clinical triad of polycystic ovaries, hirsutism and acanthosis nigricans. *Horm Res* 1988;29:7–13.
5. DeFronzo RA. Insulin resistance, hyperinsulinemia, and coronary artery disease: a complex metabolic web. *Curr Sci* 1992;3:11–25.
6. McKeigue PM, Marriot MG, Syndercombe Court YD, Rehman S, Tiemersma RA. Diabetes, hyperinsulinemia, and coronary risk factors in Bangladeshis in East London. *Br Heart J* 1988;60:390–396.
7. Benerji MA, Lebovita HE. Coronary heart disease risk factor profiles in black patients with non-insulin-dependent diabetes mellitus: paradoxic patterns. *Am J Med* 1991;91:51–58.
8. Dahlgren E, Johansson S, Linstedt G, et al. Women with polycystic ovary syndrome wedge resected in 1956 to 1965: a long-term follow-up focusing on natural history and circulating hormones. *Fertil Steril* 1992;57(3):505–513.
9. Dunaif A, Graf M, Mandeli T, Laumas V, Dobrjansky A. Characteristics of groups of hyperandrogenic women with acanthosis nigricans, impaired glucose tolerance, and/or hyperinsulinemia. *J Clin Endocrinol Metab* 1987;65(3):499–507.
10. Dunaif A, Segal KR, Futterweit W, Dobrjansky A. Profound peripheral insulin resistance, independent of obesity, in polycystic ovary syndrome. *Diabetes* 1989;38(9):1165–1174.
11. Ling L, Lithell H, Pollare T. Is it hyperinsulinemia or insulin resistance that is related to hypertension and other metabolic cardiovascular risk factors? *J Hypertens Suppl* 1993;11(4):S11–16.
12. Jahan-Vague I, Thompson SG, Jespersen J. Involvement of the hemostatic system in the insulin resistance syndrome: a study of 1500 patients with angina pectoris. The ECAT Angina Pectoris Study. *Arterioscler Thromb* 1993;13(K):1865–1873.
13. Sasson Z, Rasooly Y, Bhesania T, Rasooly I. Insulin resistance is an important determinant of left ventricular function in the obese. *Circulation* 1993;88(4pti):1431–1436.
14. Wild RA, Bartholomew MJ. The influence of body weight on lipoprotein lipids in patients with polycystic ovary syndrome. *Am J Obstet Gynecol* 1988;159:423–427.
15. Laasko M, Sarlund H, Mykkanen L. Insulin resistance is associated with lipid lipoprotein abnormalities in subjects with varying degrees of glucose tolerance. *Arteriosclerosis* 1990;10:223–231.
16. Wild RA, Alaupovic P, Parker IJ. Lipid and apolipoprotein abnormalities in hirsute women I: The association with insulin resistance. *Am J Obstet Gynecol* 1992;166:1191–1197.
17. Wild RA. Role of endogenous estrogen: *effects on lipoprotein lipid alterations* in the hirsutism paradigm. *J Reprod Med* 39(4):273–276.
18. Lapidus L, Bengtsson C, Lindquist O, Sigurdsson JA, Rybo E. Triglycerides: main lipid risk factor for cardiovascular disease in women? *Acta Med Scand* 1985;217:481–489.
19. Blankendorn DH, Alaupovic P, Wickham E, Chin HP, Azen SP. Prediction of angiographic change in native human coronary arteries and aortocoronary bypass grafts: lipid and nonlipid factors. *Circulation* 1990;81:470–476.
20. Reaven GM. Banting lecture: role of insulin resistance in human disease. *Diabetes* 1988;37:1595–1607.
21. Reaven GM, Chen YD, Teppesen J, Maheux P, Krauss RM. Insulin resistance and hyperinsulinemia in individuals with small, dense low density lipoprotein particles. *J Clin Invest* 1993;92(1):1416.

22. Saad MJ, Lillioja S, Nyomba BL, et al. Racial differences in the relation between blood pressure and insulin resistance. *N Engl J Med* 1991;324:733–739.

23. Falkner B, Hulman S, Tannenbaum J, Kushner H. Insulin resistance and blood pressure in young black men. *Hypertension* 1990;16:706–711.

24. Hartz AJ, Rupley DC, Rimm AA. The association of girth measurements with disease in 93,856 women. *Am J Epidemiol* 1984;119(1):71–80.

25. Kirschner MA, Samojlik E, Szmal E, Schneider G, Ertel N. Androgen-estrogen metabolism in women with upper body versus lower body obesity. *J Clin Endocrinol Metab* 1990;70:473.

26. Lapidus K, Bengtsson C, Larsson B, Kjell P, Rybo E, Sjostrom L. Distribution of adipose tissue and risk of cardiovascular disease and death: a 12 year follow up of participants in the population study of women in Gothenburg, Sweden. *Brit Med J* 1984;289:1257–1261.

27. Pedersen SB, Borglum JD, Schmitz O, Bak JF, Richelsen B, Sorensen NS. Abdominal obesity is associated with insulin resistance and reduced glycogen synthetase activity in skeletal muscle. *Metabolism* 1993; 42(8):998–1005.

28. Wild RA, Grubb B, Hartz A, Van Nort JJ, Bachman W, Bartholomew M. Clinical signs of androgen excess as risk factors for coronary artery disease. *Fertil Steril* 1991;54:255–259.

29. Coon PJ, Rogus EM, Drinkwater D, Muller DC, Goldberg AP. Role of body fat distribution in the decline in insulin sensitivity and glucose tolerance with age. *J Clin Endocrinol Metab* 1992;75 (40):1125–1132.

30. Koivisto V, DeFronzo RA. Physical training and insulin sensitivity. *Diabetes Metab Rev* 1986;1: 445–481.

31. Schneider SH, Vitug A, Ruderman N. Atherosclerosis and physical activity. *Diabetes Metab Rev* 1986;1:513–553.

32. Zavaroni I, Bonora E, Pagliara M, et al. Risk factors for coronary artery disease in healthy persons with hyperinsulinemia and normal glucose tolerance. *N Engl J Med* 1989;320:702–706.

33. Modan M, Halkin H, Almog S, et al. Hyperinsulinemia: a link between hypertension, obesity and glucose intolerance. *J Clin Invest* 1985;75:809–817.

34. Pommerenke FA, Dietrich A. Improving and maintaining preventive services Part 1: applying the patient model. *J Fam Prac* 1992;34:86–97.

35. Ferriman D, Gallwey JD. Clinical assessment of body hair growth in women. *J Clin Endocrinol Metab* 1961;21:1440.

36. Madanes AE, Novotny M. The vellus index: a new method of assessing hair growth. *Fertil Steril* 1987;48:1064–1066.

37. Loriaux DL, Wild RA. Contraceptive choices for women with endocrine complications. *Am J Obst Gynecol* 1993;168(2):2021–2026.

38. Kannel WB, McGee DL, *Circulation* 1979;59:8–13.

39. Grasinger C, Wild RA, Parker IJ et al. Vulvar acanthosis nigricans: A marker for insulin resistance in hirsute women. *Fertil Steril* 1993;59:583–586.

40. Wild RA. Hyperandrogenism in the adolescent. *Obstet Gynecol Clin North Am* 1992;19:71–89.

41. Givens JR. Historical overview of the polycystic ovary. In: Dunaif A, Givens JR, Haseltine F, Merriam GR, eds. *Current issues in endocrinology and polycystic ovary syndrome*. Boston: Blackwell Scientific; 1992:3–12.

42. Bjorntorp P. Abdominal fat distribution and disease: An overview of epidemiological data. *Ann Med* 1992;24:15–18.

Androgenic Disorders,
edited by G. P. Redmond.
Raven Press, Ltd., New York © 1995.

13

Treatment of Androgenic Disorders

Geoffrey P. Redmond

Foundation for Developmental Endocrinology, Inc., Department of Endocrinology, Cleveland, Ohio 44122.

WHAT NEEDS TREATMENT IN ANDROGENIC DISORDERS?

Androgenic disorders are the result of increased androgen action on a woman's body. The increased action may be due to increased secretion or to increased end-organ responsiveness, or, in probably the most common situation, both factors may contribute. There are also associated abnormalities, notably glucose intolerance, whose relationship to androgen action is apparently indirect. Some androgen actions are dynamic in that they are closely correlated in the short term with the effect. Sebum secretion with the acne that may result from it is an example. Others result from long-term tissue exposure to androgens and may be only slowly and incompletely reversible. Hirsutism and, especially, alopecia fit into this category. It follows that the less dynamically related manifestations will respond more slowly and incompletely to treatment.

To the extent that androgenic disorders are due to increased androgen secretion and action, the cause is treatable by reducing secretion or by blocking action. However the causes of the increased secretion and action are themselves incompletely understood and not directly treatable. Thus the abnormal hypothalamic–pituitary–ovarian interaction that constitutes the polycystic ovary syndrome (PCOS) cannot be corrected by presently available modalities.

Despite these limitations of present day therapy, most women with androgenic disorders can be significantly helped by the therapeutic approach discussed in this chapter. Physicians are usually more pessimistic than they need to be about the chances of success. While response is usually slow in coming and usually does not totally reverse the androgenic changes, it does come and is perceived as beneficial by most women who are properly treated. This chapter will describe a rational approach to the treatment of the woman with an androgenic disorder and indicate what treatment can and cannot accomplish.

In order to plan treatment, clinical evaluation must include determining which androgenic changes are present, identification of which, if any, androgens are elevated and their source (adrenal or ovarian or mixed), success of local measures, associated or intercurrent medical conditions such as diabetes mellitus or abnormal menstrual pattern (regarding possible anovulation), and the concerns of the patient. Treatment falls into several separate modalities:

1. Antagonism of androgen action
2. Suppression of elevated androgens
3. Local measures
4. Fertility considerations
5. Progestin therapy for anovulation, if present
6. Hormone replacement for menopause, if present
7. Associated metabolic abnormalities

All of these issues must be considered although not all will be pertinent for any given patient.

RELATION OF CLINICAL AND BIOCHEMICAL FINDINGS TO CHOICE OF TREATMENT

Androgenic action is the major causative factor in female acne, hirsutism, and androgenic alopecia. While there are specific treatments for each of these conditions (which will be addressed below), the choice of treatment will depend less on the skin or hair manifestation than on the underlying endocrine factors. These are worked out with the help of the laboratory, as described in Chapters 3 and 5. As androgen action is involved in all women with these conditions, prescription of an antiandrogen is necessary for a good result, with only infrequent exceptions. Endocrinologists more often think of suppressive treatment because they regard excessive secretion as the primary etiologic factor. However receptor sensitivity is probably a bigger factor in a majority of patients. Furthermore, it is usually not possible to reduce androgens to prepubertal, that is, negligible, levels. For these reasons, selection of an antiandrogen is usually necessary for a good result.

Suppressive treatment is indicated when one or more androgens are elevated to a clinically significant degree. In general, this is a total testosterone level above 50 ng/dL, a free testosterone at the upper end of or above the reference range (which may vary between laboratories depending on their methodology), an androstenedione level above 225 to 250 ng/dL, and a dihydroepiandrosterone sulfate (DHEA-S) level above 350 to 400 μg/dL. The last is least certain. DHEA-S does seem to be often elevated in women with acne and possibly those with alopecia, but its effect as an androgen is unclear. If no other androgen is elevated and if other modalities are being employed, adrenal suppression to lower DHEA-S is probably unnecessary with values below 450 μg/dL.

If androgen levels are normal, then addition of suppressive therapy to antiandrogen therapy is unnecessary and will not increase the effectiveness of treatment. Conversely, suppressive therapy alone with glucocorticoids or oral contraceptives (OCs) is unlikely to give much benefit. Acne is an exception as it often responds to OCs alone; presence or absence of androgen elevation does not seem to predict the response of acne to OCs.

A combination of increased DHEA-S, regular menses, lack of obesity, and older age make an adrenal source for increased testosterone or androstenedione more likely but not certain (1). It is possible for a woman to have elevated testosterone and DHEA-S levels with the source of the testosterone being the ovary, not the adrenal. Dexamethasone suppression testing is the only way to determine relative ovarian and adrenal contributions.

ANTIANDROGENS

Until recently, available antiandrogens were compounds introduced for other actions and found to have antiandrogenic activity as a side effect. The most useful and established compound in this category is spironolactone. This agent was introduced as an aldosterone antagonist and found to have antiandrogenic activity as well. It is registered for treatment of hirsutism in Australia but not the United States. However, numerous studies confirm its efficacy (2–7) and it is widely used for this purpose. It will be discussed in more detail. A variety of other available drugs have some degree of antiandrogenic activity (8). Cimetidine, an H_2 blocker, seems to have some antiandrogenic activity (9), but recent studies have not confirmed earlier ones suggesting it can reduce hirsutism. My own experience has been disappointing even with high doses up to 800 mg t.i.d. Ketoconazole, introduced as an antifungal, is quite effective as an antiandrogen. Unfortunately, it can cause serious liver toxicity and so does not seem an appropriate long-term treatment for a benign condition. It may have some use however in its topical cream form for acne, sebaceous dermatitis, or acne rosacea. A general problem with topical formulations of antiandrogens, though they would seem theoretically to be ideal for androgenic changes in skin or hair, is that they probably do not penetrate deeply enough into the pilosebaceous unit to be effective. Development of topical antiandrogens is a promising area for further research however. Use of topical spironolactone has been reported (10).

Cyproterone acetate (CPA), a potent progestin with antiandrogenic activity, has been widely used in Europe for over twenty years for hirsutism and acne (11,12) but is not registered in the United States. It is usually given in the so-called reverse Hammerstein regimen, that is, for the first 11 days of the cycle in a dose of 50 or 100 mg daily. Ethinyl estradiol in a dose of 50 μg is given on days 1 to 21. No hormone is given on days 22 to 28, which is when menses occur. Because of the lipid solubility of CPA, blood levels persist for several days beyond the 11-day period when the patient takes it. While of established efficacy, CPA in these high doses has side effects not unlike the related progestin medroxyprogesterone acetate: mood changes, fluid retention, and weight gain. Complaints of decreased libido are common from women on CPA. While a direct comparison with spironolactone has not been done, to my knowledge, it appears the latter is as effective or almost as effective and has far fewer deleterious effects on well-being. Nonetheless, for the many women who do tolerate it, CPA can be very effective. CPA is also available in the form of two combination OCs, Diane and Diane-35 (Schering AG), which have 50 and 35 μg of ethinyl estradiol respectively with 2 mg of CPA. Dianette has 1 mg of CPA. There are reports that Diane is effective for mild hirsutism (13). These are available in Europe and Canada but not the United States. It is unclear that they are more effective than other OCs for androgenic disorders. Some studies have shown greater efficacy for CPA containing OCs (14) but others have not (15).

Recently, compounds have been introduced that were designed specifically as antiandrogens for treatment of prostate disease. Flutamide is labeled in the United States for treatment of advanced prostatic cancer but has been extensively studied in hirsutism and is quite effective (16,17). Its drawbacks are being quite expensive and a potential risk of hepatotoxicity (18,19). Its main side effects are abdominal distress and diarrhea, possibly because it is compounded with lactose. These occur in a minority of patients. The hepatotoxicity is not well understood. It manifests with jaundice, hyperbilirubinemia, and extreme elevation of transaminases. It can be fatal, although the symptoms apparently resolve if the flutamide is discontinued immediately. One reported case occurred in a 20-year-old woman, but all others have been in elderly men with prostate cancer. Hepatotoxicity has not been known to occur in children. If it occurs in healthy women under treatment for androgenic disorders, it must be exceedingly rare. However, in the present state of knowledge, flutamide should be used only as a last resort and with full explanation to the patient of the potential for liver disease and an explanation of symptoms to watch for: jaundice, vomiting, fatigue, dark urine, and light stool. Flutamide is probably the most effective antiandrogen currently available, but its disadvantages limit its use.

Finasteride was developed as an inhibitor of 5α-reductase as a treatment for benign prostatic hypertrophy (20). Because men with inherited deficiency of the 5α-hydroxylase enzyme do not develop balding and do have decreased body hair, it has been thought that finasteride might be useful for alopecia and hirsutism. Studies are in early stages but suggest the agent may have some effectiveness for hirsutism. Trials are also in progress to determine its efficacy in halting male balding. More recently, it has been discovered that there are two 5α-reductase enzymes. Type 2, which is best inhibited by finasteride is more plentiful in the prostate than in hair follicles (20a). It is possible that a more specific inhibitor for type 1 5α-reductase will be developed for treatment of hirsutism and alopecia.

At least in studies in older men with benign prostatic hypertrophy, finasteride has few side effects. In women, however, there is considerable reason to worry about teratogenicity. Genital formation in a male fetus occurs as a result of high levels of androgens secreted by the testes. Anything that interferes with androgen response can result in incomplete virilization and some degree of genital ambiguity. Genetic males born with inherited deficiency of 5α-reductase have a condition known as pseudovaginal perineoscrotal hypospadias (PVPH) (21). Usually they are thought to be girls at birth but change gender role at puberty when further genital virilization occurs.

Any agent that interferes with androgen secretion or action must be regarded as potentially teratogenic to a male fetus. Finasteride is most worrisome in this regard because of the known effects of 5α-reductase lack in man or inhibition in animals. To my knowledge, there have not been reports of ambiguous genitalia in infants born to women on other antiandrogens. However, this should not be taken as evidence of safety, and scrupulous care must be taken to inform women of childbearing age of this possible risk of antiandrogens, and contraceptive counseling must be given. Young women and others who seem casual about contraception should not be placed on antiandrogens unless they clearly agree to use OCs or other equally reliable methods. Another group who may be more likely to inadvertently become pregnant are those with long-term infertility who have given up using contraception. Whether because of unvoiced yearning for a pregnancy or because they are convinced pregnancy is impossible for them, women in this group frequently do not use contraception in spite of promising to do so. Anecdotal experience suggests that antiandrogens may restore ovulation in some previously infertile women so that previous lack of conception does not guarantee future lack of conception in women who go on these agents. OC regimens are more likely to be complied with than methods that require positive measures to be taken with each act of intercourse.

Spironolactone was widely used in the prethalidomide era when medication use in pregnancy was much more casual. It seems likely, though unproven, that it was taken in many pregnancies for hypertension or diuresis and yet no cases of ambiguous genitalia have been reported with its use, to my knowledge. I have heard anecdotal reports of its efficacy in reversing infertility in women with PCOS. While it should not be casually concluded that spironolactone is safe during pregnancy, it is likely that it has less teratogenic potential than finasteride and flutamide.

The possibility of interfering with the development of male genitalia is the main factor limiting not only use but development of antiandrogens. However, industry and regulators are becoming more aware that avoiding development of medications for women of childbearing age because of worry about teratogenicity amounts to a form of gender discrimination, and policies in this area are being rethought. In the meantime, given the lack of safety data, it is essential that antiandrogens be prescribed only for women who will not become pregnant while taking them.

Spironolactone is the most generally useful antiandrogen. While side effects while taking it are common, they tend to be inconvenient or uncomfortable rather than serious. Because it is a diuretic, spironolactone can cause very mild hypovolemia. Symptoms are lethargy and dizziness or light-headedness. Some women complain of polyuria while taking spironolactone but they are a small minority. The entire dose may be taken in the morning to minimize this effect, but even with this measure, a very few women have more nocturia or polyuria than they can accept and discontinue the drug. Women beginning spironolactone should be advised to drink six to eight glasses of water daily; when this advice is followed, problems related to the diuretic effect are rare. Those who are physically active in hot weather may need to drink more in conjunction with their exercise.

A slightly less common but more troublesome side effect with spironolactone is polymenorrhea. Many women on the drug develop cycles which are shorter by only one or a few days but some have periods as close together as every two weeks, a situation which is most unwelcome. The likelihood of this is dose related and is more common with a dose of 200 mg than 100 mg per day. Polymenorrhea often but not invariably resolves spontaneously. OCs are virtually invariably successful in controlling the cycle, but monthly progestins are less so. If polymenorrhea occurs on spironolactone, it is best to wait a few cycles to see if cyclicity reverts to a more normal interval. If it does not, dose reduction or prescription of an OC or a progestin may be tried. For young women, simultaneous prescription of an OC has the advantage of also ensuring that pregnancy will not occur on the antiandrogen. For older women, those with pill contraindications, or those who cannot tolerate OCs, there is more of a problem. Usually a solution can be worked out, however.

The cause of polymenorrhea with spironolactone is unknown, but it is possibly progestinlike effect on the endometrium. It is also unclear if the polymenorrhea is a sign of anovulation. In the present limited state of knowledge, it is better to assume that ovulation may not be occurring and institute therapy that would prevent endometrial pathology from developing if ovulation is not occurring. However, a few months of polymenorrhea on spironolactone does not seem to be harmful, so it is best to wait a few cycles before instituting therapy since the problem often resolves by itself.

Doses of spironolactone range from 25 to 200 mg daily but those below 75 mg daily are rarely effective. The main factor that limits the use of higher doses is the greater incidence of polymenorrhea. An appropriate starting dose for most patients is 100 mg daily which can be raised to 150 or 200 mg daily in the event of incomplete response. Timing of dose increments is based on the duration of therapy required for response to become apparent. For patients with very severe manifestations or who show marked distress at the androgenic changes, starting at 200 mg daily may be appropriate. One such situation is cystic acne, to limit scarring. With use of maximal doses of spironolactone, simultaneous prescribing of an OC is desirable.

Although spironolactone was introduced as a potassium-sparing diuretic, significant hyperkalemia does not occur in healthy women on the drug. Simultaneous use of other potassium-sparing diuretics or fixed dose combinations with them should be avoided as should angiotensin converting enzyme (ACE) inhibitors unless potassium levels are monitored initially.

Spironolactone also appears to be safe in children although it is rare that treatment for androgenic disorders is necessary before menarche.

ADRENAL SUPPRESSION

When elevated androgens have been demonstrated by dexamethasone suppression testing to be of adrenal origin, adrenal suppression may be a useful adjunct to antiandrogen therapy. As stated previously, clinical criteria for adrenal origin are not reliable enough to justify use of glucocorticoids without testing. The exception is the patient in whom DHEA-S, but no other androgen, is elevated. Since this sulfated steroid is virtually exclusively of adrenal origin, it always decreases with appropriate glucocorticoid suppression, unless its source is neoplastic, an exceedingly rare situation. It is not necessary to belabor the point that glucocorticoids can have extremely deleterious effects on appearance and metabolism. Used with care, they are helpful and quite safe; in even slightly excessive doses they are potentially harmful.

The adrenal is most active under ACTH stimulation in the early morning hours prior to awakening. Maximal suppression with a given dose will be obtained when it is given at bedtime. The goal is to suppress ACTH when most of its secretory activity occurs, *not* to imitate the diurnal cortisol rhythm. If the dose is taken in the morning upon awakening, it is too late to suppress ACTH, and adrenal suppression will be far less effective. In order to have maximum activity remaining some hours after bedtime to suppress ACTH secretion by the pituitary, the longest-acting agent is the most logical one to select. For a given total glucocorticoid activity, the greatest effect will be several hours after absorption. A short-acting version will have to be given in a relatively larger dose in order to have sufficient activity remaining several hours later. For these reasons, dexamethasone is the agent of choice. Concern about greater side effects of this glucocorticoid are a result of failure to allow for its marked potency when making dosage decisions.

We have done detailed dose–response studies using dexamethasone to suppress DHEA-S levels in women with androgenic disorders (22). About 25% of such women show suppression to normal levels with a dose of 0.125 mg nightly, and 50% show suppression with the next step up at 0.25 mg h.s. At most, 25% require 0.375 mg and virtually none require as much as 0.5 mg. Yet recommendations for doses of 0.5 to 0.75 mg are not unusual. Starting doses this high are unjustified with the possible exception of short-term use for infertility in which adrenal hyperandrogenism is a factor. Even at doses like these that are only slightly higher than the physiological replacement level, weight gain and striae are common. Women who begin to take the medication to improve their appearance are not pleased by such changes. Although striae fade, they do leave permanent residua. These problems can be completely avoided by careful dose titration. Our approach has been to start everyone at a dose of 0.125 mg nightly which is one-half of the smallest available tablet size. After one month, the level of the elevated androgen is measured again and the dose is increased if the level has not fallen into the mid-normal range. This titration approach was adapted from that reported by Marynick et al. (23). Useful target levels are 40 ng/dL for total testosterone, 150 ng/dL for androstenedione and 200 μg/dL for DHEA-S. However a further increase is not indicated if values are only slightly above those given. If the dose is increased, levels are repeated in an additional month and a further increase made if target levels are not reached. However, increases above 0.25 mg should be made only upon careful consideration; they are rarely necessary. Once the target level is reached, further testing is unnecessary; adrenal androgens rarely escape from suppression. Similar dosing and titration can be used for adult women with congenital or acquired adrenal hyperplasia.

Titration not only avoids cushingoid side effects, it seems to reduce the possible dangers that would occur if adrenal suppression were more complete. Androgens are suppressed to normal rather than to low levels. This appears to preserve adrenal reserve. While it is prudent to give steroid coverage for general anesthesia, high fever, or other physical stress, we have never observed an episode of adrenal crisis in the several hundred women we have treated with small doses of dexamethasone titrated in this fashion.

Alternate-day steroid therapy was devised to reduce side effects when given for suppression of inflammation. Its use for adrenal suppression is not rational. It is better to use a daily but minimum dose. Similarly, prednisone, because it is shorter acting than dexamethasone, may have to be given in a larger equivalent total dose to get the same degree of ACTH suppression.

OVARIAN SUPPRESSION

Oral Contraceptives

Oral contraceptives have an important but limited place in the treatment of androgenic disorders. OCs suppress ovarian androgen production and increase sex hormone–binding globulin (SHBG) levels. However in the absence of an antiandrogen, these effects may be insufficient to greatly improve androgenic hair changes. By themselves OCs are most effective for acne which often clears almost completely. While there are reports that growth rate of the hair shaft is reduced in hirsutism, the change is small and growth rates remain above those of nonhirsute women. There is little information about the effects of OCs alone on androgenic alopecia. Since estrogen prolongs the length of the hair cycle, OCs would be expected to be helpful. However, hair may shed after a fall in estrogen levels (for example, a few weeks after childbirth), so discontinuation of an OC may exacerbate alopecia or unmask it, but here too data are sparse.

There are several indications for OCs in androgenic disorders. Ovarian suppression is logical when dexamethasone testing has indicated an apparent ovarian source for elevated androgen levels. When the origin is mixed, OCs may also be useful alone or in combination with dexamethasone. When contraception or cycle control is required, OCs are also appropriate. The details of prescribing and monitoring OCs are discussed elsewhere (24,25).

There is a temptation to use a higher than minimal dose of OC for ovarian suppression in androgenic disorders, but the literature suggests that 35 μg ethinyl estradiol pills are as effective for acne as those with 50 μg (26). With 50 μg, however, estrogenic side effects such as nausea and mastalgia are more common.

The choice of progestin has received much attention. It is evident that one of low androgenicity should be chosen, but how great a difference this makes has not been established. Most of the data on androgenicity of the older pills were derived from animal testing. However there are limited human data suggesting some advantage of low androgenicity progestins in androgenic disorders. For example an OC with desogestrel produced a greater rise in SHBG than one with levonorgestrel, although the degrees of suppression of free testosterone itself were similar at about 60% (27). The desogestrel pill was also more effective in suppressing acne. However, there is another compelling reason to select a nonandrogenic progestin and this is the avoidance of androgenic effects on serum lipids. While the older progestins tend to lower high-density lipoprotein (HDL)-cholesterol, or at best to leave it unaffected, the newer ones have been reported to elevate it (28,29). Despite the lack of definitive data on the significance of androgenicity with OCs, no one has come up with a rational reason why, given a choice, one should prescribe a more androgenic pill.

Appropriate choices include OCs with the new progestins norgestimate (Ortho-Cyclen and OrthoTriCyclen) and desogestrel (Desogen and OrthoCept). These have desirable side-effect profiles with minimal changes in weight and blood pressure and a low incidence of spotting. Norgestrel and levonorgestrel are thought to be more androgenic than other currently available progestins and seem to be less desirable choices for women with androgenic disorders; however, the androgenicity is minimized in the phasic preparations (Triphasyl and Trilevulen). An alternative to the newer progestins are those with very low doses of norethindrone such as Ovcon 35 which has 0.4 mg and Modicon which has 0.5 mg. These are sometimes tolerated by women who are sensitive to progestin side effects such as premenstrual mood changes. The progestin ethynodiol diacetate contained in Demulen 35 has long been preferred for women with androgenic disorders because of its reputation for low androgenicity. Its advantages are less clear with the availability of norgestimate and desogestrel which were specifically designed to have minimal androgenicity. OCs with gestodene have been widely used in Europe, but safety concerns have emerged which are not yet resolved.

Our experience indicates that OCs are most effective when combined with an antiandrogen such as spironolactone. However, they are often used alone to treat women with androgenic disorders. For acne, numerous studies demonstrate the effectiveness of OCs (30–32). In the case of hirsutism, there is evidence for a decrease in hair growth (33) but it is usually not sufficient to satisfy the patient. Sometimes hirsutism emerges after OCs are withdrawn, suggesting that they had been suppressing an unsuspected androgenic disorder. The great advantages of using OCs alone are simplicity and their familiarity to many physicians and patients.

The norethindrone implant (Norplant) has achieved some popularity as a long-acting hormonal contraceptive. There are anecdotes of the norethindrone implant increasing acne and hirsutism, and it does not seem in the present state of knowledge to be the best choice for women with androgenic disorders, compared to combination OCs.

GnRH Analogues

These agents are widely used in gynecology in any situation in which there may be therapeutic benefit from cessation of ovarian function. They return the pituitary to a prepubertal state by down-regulating the receptors for GnRH. For myomata and endometriosis they achieve their benefits by lowering ovarian estrogen production. Simultaneously, androgen secretion decreases, hence their potential use in androgenic disorders. Several studies show them to be effective in this situation (34).

There are drawbacks of GnRH analogues that limit their use for androgenic disorders, however. The first is cost, which is problematic for long-term treatment. Monthly intramuscular injections or t.i.d. use of a nose spray become quickly tiresome to most patients. Finally, GnRH analogues suppress all ovarian hormone production, so that the endocrine abnormalities of PCOS are replaced by a state of estrogen deficiency. Cyclic estrogen and progestins need to be taken, further increasing the level of cost and inconvenience. For all these reasons, GnRH analogues have so far had limited use in ovarian androgen excess. They may be helpful when used for a period of a few months to see if a decrease in ovarian androgen production will produce clinical improvement in the patient's androgenic changes. If so, surgical ovariectomy can be considered. However, this is appropriate only for the very few women with severe PCOS or hyperthecosis in which androgen levels are very high (a testosterone level of 150 ng/mL or greater) and who cannot take OCs or do not respond to them.

RESPONSE TO ENDOCRINE THERAPY

Androgen-related skin and hair changes develop slowly, and accordingly they resolve slowly. Acne is quickest to respond because without androgen stimulation the sebaceous glands become much less active. However, existing lesions do not seem to heal much faster and so improvement of the complexion is limited by the rate of healing. There seems to be a progressive decrement in appearance of new lesions. Facial skin becomes less oily within several weeks. Acne is usually noticeably improved by 2 months of treatment and further improved by 4 months. While antiandrogenic treatment probably does not affect scarring directly, it seems that when the skin is no longer chronically inflamed, scarring, although it does not totally disappear, becomes much less noticeable. Pitting seems to level out and areas of erythema become fainter. Many women who were considering dermatologic surgery before antiandrogenic therapy decide that they do not need it after 6 to 12 months of endocrine treatment. There are exceptions, of course, but usually the improvement of the complexion is considerable. Of all the androgenic skin changes, acne responds most completely to treatment. This makes it particularly unfortunate that the endocrine nature of acne is not more widely recognized.

Hirsutism does improve with the treatment as outlined, but it does so gradually. It is essential that both patient and physician be aware that improvement does not come at once, so that they do not become discouraged and discontinue treatment before it has had time to work. The first change, which appears no sooner than 3 to 4 months after initiation of treatment, is slowing of growth of the hair shaft. At this point the hairs are no lighter or finer, and area coverage has not changed, but the growth rate of the shaft is slower. This is most noticeable for women with more marked hirsutism because they remove hair daily and can see that less needs to be removed each morning. Those who remove only infrequently may not notice a change at this point. Beginning during the second 6 months of treatment and continuing sometimes into the second year, there is progressive change in the hairs so that they are lighter, finer, and softer. Area covered by terminal hairs also decreases. Some women even see further improvement during the third year on medication.

The main effect of hormonal treatment on hirsutism is on the individual hairs. It is not clear that the number of hairs changes but the individual hairs become less noticeable. The area covered by visible hair often decreases, especially on the body. Many women notice that they do not have to shave their legs nearly as often. Frequency may decrease from every 2 days to once a week. Forearm hair, bothersome to some women because it is revealed by short-sleeved summer clothing, is variable in its response, sometimes quickly decreasing, other times hardly changing.

Generally, treatment of hirsutism does not eliminate the need for local removal. However, removal is often less time-consuming (for some women a major burden of hirsutism is the need to spend a half hour or more each morning removing hairs) and the result of removal is better because the skin looks more normal and is softer. Some hirsute women become apprehensive in the late afternoon that the hair will become noticeable. Antiandrogenic treatment often slows hair growth in addition to lightening it so that this worry goes away.

The final judge of success of treatment must be the woman herself. Many women are happy with a result that seems too limited to their physician. Physicians, especially those inexperienced with treatment, may think that unless all extra hair is eliminated, the treatment has not accomplished anything. However reduction of the burden of removal and improving its result is a major benefit for the affected woman.

Androgenic alopecia has been less studied. The impression among physicians who have interested themselves in this problem is that antiandrogenic treatment does help (35) but controlled studies are limited. One reason for this is the extreme difficulty of quantitating scalp hair. The majority of women given antiandrogenic therapy for androgenic alopecia do feel it has helped, though not always as much as they would have liked.

Alopecia shows itself to affected women in two ways. First, shedding may be excessive and more hair is noticed on clothes, on combs, and covering the bathtub drain. Second, there is less hair on the scalp and thinning is evident when the patient looks in her mirror. It is important to separate these in order to get an accurate impression of the effects of treatment.

Usually the first change with antiandrogenic treatment is that the shedding slows down. This is often noticed within only a few weeks. In the same time frame, the scalp hair becomes livelier and healthier looking. This is admittedly subjective, but so many women spontaneously comment on it that it seems to be a real change. It may be due to the hair becoming less oily, but other factors may be involved since women often comment that their hair is less brittle after a few weeks of anti-androgenic treatment.

Regrowth does not always occur, and when it does, it may not be noticeable until the second year of treatment. Only rarely does the hair return to its fullest state before treatment. This is especially true if the hair loss has been long-standing or severe. Androgenic alopecia of recent onset seems to be more readily reversed. Interruptions of treatment are often followed by a shed.

DURATION OF TREATMENT

The chronic nature of androgenic disorders and the slowness of response to treatment mean that medication must be taken for a prolonged period to be beneficial. The time required for response is long, as described. Generally it is not worth embarking on antiandrogenic therapy unless the patient can be on it a minimum of 9 months. A shorter duration may show response but it will be limited, except for acne. Our practice is to have the patient satisfied with the result for a minimum of 1 to 2 years before attempting to taper. Of course, treatment can be discontinued before that if adverse effects occur, because pregnancy is desired or for other reasons.

While some women can discontinue antiandrogenic treatment after 2 or more years without recurrence of the unwanted changes, it must be admitted that many women cannot. In such cases, control of the condition requires that medication be maintained for many years. However, it is often possible to taper gradually so that the dose or number of medications can be reduced. In particular, adrenal androgen hypersecretion rarely returns when dexamethasone is discontinued after 2 or more years of adrenal suppression. This can be verified by measuring the previously elevated androgen, but this is not necessary unless the condition escapes from control. Similarly it is unusual to have an androgenic change worsen if OCs are discontinued after a similar interval. However, previously existent menstrual abnormalities may reemerge, including polymenorrhea from spironolactone.

Tapering spironolactone is more difficult because androgenic manifestations are more likely to return to a higher level of severity. If spironolactone is tapered at a rate of about 50 mg every 6 months, any reemergence will be mild and the patient can return to her previous dose level without too much increase in severity of acne, hirsutism, or alopecia. Acne is most likely to go into permanent remission. It appears that hair follicles, once they have been exposed to long-term androgen action, remain more sensitive to it. This is seen, for example, in hypogonadal males who do not have rapid beard growth but do not return to a prepubertal beardless state.

If pregnancy is desired, antiandrogenic therapy must be discontinued due to the potential for teratogenicity discussed before. OCs must be stopped for obvious reasons. Dexamethasone, however, is best continued until pregnancy is established, at which time it is discontinued. This is because it increases the chance of ovulation. A conservative practice is to have women off OCs and other unnecessary medication for three cycles before they try to conceive.

There does not seem to be any rebound of acne or hirsutism if antiandrogenic therapy is abruptly discontinued. However, there may be with alopecia. For this reason, it is best to taper especially slowly in the latter condition, over six or more months before trying to conceive and longer before permanent discontinuation.

ANDROGENIC DISORDERS AND INFERTILITY

Anovulation is one of the classic features described by Stein and Leventhal in the PCOS. It is a common cause of infertility. Ovulation induction in women with PCOS has reached a high state of development and is covered in texts on infertility. Only a few points will be made here. First, infertility does not invariably accompany androgenic disorders. Slender women with normal cycles who have hirsutism or other androgenic features are usually normally ovulatory. Presumably they have adrenal androgen excess which affects ovarian function less than when the increased androgen synthesis occurs in the latter organ. When anovulation occurs in association with androgen excess, adrenal suppression with dexamethasone may increase the likelihood of conception. Use of clomiphene citrate together with dexamethasone is also a reasonable approach. If this is not successful after several cycles, more complete evaluation is needed. However, many women with mild androgenic disorders will conceive on this simple regimen, avoiding the expense and effort of a full-scale infertility workup. Whether dexamethasone is effective as an adjunct to other means of stimulating ovulation when androgen excess is ovarian in origin is not clear. It is possible that some ovarian androgen synthesis and secretion is ACTH dependant and that suppression with dexamethasone will lower intraovarian androgen levels. Anecdotally, this approach works, but this is hardly definitive since in any group of infertile women a few will conceive spontaneously over time. However, adrenal suppression, when used with care, is safe and is worth trying as an adjunct when clomiphene or menopausal gonadotropins have been unsuccessful.

When used for infertility, dexamethasone can be given in the slightly higher dose of 0.5 mg at bedtime. However this should not be continued for more than a few cycles and should be lowered or discontinued if weight gain or cushingoid changes such as facial rounding or striae appear. It is discontinued when a positive pregnancy test is obtained, although it is unlikely that low doses are fetotoxic.

NONHORMONAL TREATMENTS FOR ANDROGENIC SKIN AND HAIR CHANGES

Most women with androgenic disorders do not receive endocrine evaluation or treatment. A variety of other treatments have been developed, with varying efficacies. These are most fully developed in the case of acne and are discussed in

Chapter 10. The sort of treatment a teenager or woman with acne receives depends to a great degree on what sort of specialist she consults. For most acne patients, oral antibiotics together with topicals such as antibacterials or tretinoin produce good results. When acne is severe or resistant to these measures, however, systemic treatment must be considered. There have been no direct comparisons of oral isotretinoin to antiandrogenic therapy, but both are usually effective in severe cases. Antiandrogenic therapy is generally better tolerated and can be continued for several years until acne becomes inactive. Isotretinoin can be used for only a few months, although such a course sometimes, but by no means always, induces a lasting remission. Further advantages of antiandrogenic therapy are its beneficial effect on other androgenic manifestations that often accompany severe acne and an improvement in the tone or appearance of the skin, giving it a more glowing or healthily feminine appearance. Neither approach avoids concern about teratogenicity; simultaneous use of oral contraceptives is desirable unless a contraindication is present.

Women have removed unwanted hair for centuries and a variety of methods have evolved. These are described in Chapter 15. Unless hirsutism is mild or restricted to a small area, women are usually not fully satisfied with the results of local removal; it is not a substitute for antiandrogenic therapy. Electrolysis in combination with antiandrogenic medication is often helpful. The medication reduces the rate of growth and the amount of hair to the point that what remains can be removed with a reasonable amount of electrolysis. If a patient is not currently receiving electrolysis, it is often a good idea for her to wait several months until the antiandrogenic therapy begins to show benefit. She can then decide if she still wants electrolysis and, if she does, she will get a much better result for the time and money she spends.

Remedies for hair loss are, if anything, even more ancient than those for hair removal. Miraculous cures are regularly announced in advertisements in publications ranging from supermarket newspapers to fashion magazines. Some are extremely expensive, costing thousands of dollars. Because of the desperation felt by many women who are losing their hair, they are easily preyed upon. There do not seem to be any scientifically validated nonprescription treatments for androgenic alopecia. A variety of hair addition methods are available, but for most women using artificial hair is not the same as having their own, however convincingly natural it may appear to others. Decisions about using hair additions can be made by the patient, but the physician should try to protect patients from exploitation by unscrupulous makers of ineffective scalp treatments.

Women with alopecia often ask if their hair-care products might be causing or exacerbating the hair loss. Modern hair-care products are almost universally safe; although some women develop hypersensitivity reactions, these do not manifest as hair loss. The most damaging hair treatment is bleaching or, for black women, using lye as a hair straightener, although most available commercial hair straighteners do not use this. Dying hair a lighter color requires initial bleaching. Bleaching is best avoided by women with alopecia; even though it does not damage hair at the level of the follicle, it may make hair more brittle and make thinning more apparent. Mechanical stress on hair such as tight rolling and twisting can avulse it or break it off, again giving a thinner look to the hair. Perms will not exacerbate alopecia if they are gentle and avoid tight rolling. Heat makes hair more fragile, so when a blow dryer is used it is best to turn the heat off. Pomades, which are often used by black women, make the hair stickier and therefore more likely to be pulled out during styling. Mechanical injury to hair is discussed in Chapter 2. It is rare for hair-care products or methods to be a significant factor in alopecia.

Recently, hair sprays have been introduced that temporarily darken the scalp, diminishing the contrast between it and the hair. These may be useful, but like other styling methods such as the use of blow drying and mousses, they do not completely satisfy the patient who wants her hair back. Physicians are not particularly qualified to advise their female patients on hair styling, but most women with alopecia are able to discover styling methods which work for them.

MEDICAL COMPLICATIONS OF ANDROGENIC DISORDERS

Because androgenic disorders are so common, it is not unusual to find them in women with other medical problems or situations that must be taken into account when making therapeutic decisions. Several of these will be briefly discussed here. In general, other medical conditions do not prevent treatment of the hair and skin manifestations of androgenic disorders, but they may give it a lower priority.

The association of androgen excess with android obesity, insulin resistant diabetes, and dyslipidemia has been discussed in Chapters 2 and 13. It is not unusual for a woman who comes for help with an androgenic disorder to be found to have diabetes, unfavorable lipids, and hypertension. Often she was unaware of these conditions or perhaps denied their significance. One must then begin to treat these more urgent conditions without losing sight of the patient's distress at the hirsutism or alopecia that brought her to the physician. While detailed discussion of treatment of these common medical illnesses is beyond the scope of this book, those aspects pertinent to the treatment of women with androgenic disorders will be briefly discussed.

In general the treatment for these conditions does not fundamentally differ because an androgenic disorder is present, but there some implications for choice of therapy. Unfortunately, treatment of the androgenic disorder itself with androgen antagonists and suppression does not alter the metabolic complications. Treatment for them must be directed at the specific abnormality using standard methods.

Obesity

The special implications of obesity for women have been discussed in detail elsewhere (36). There is no question but that obesity and androgenization are associated. However, it is unclear which is causative. It seems most likely that weight gain somehow causes expression of a tendency to androgen excess, especially ovarian, but how it does so remains to be elucidated. The alternate theory, that androgens stimulate weight gain, seems less plausible since this is clearly not the case in men. Weight reduction is at least as difficult for women with androgenic disorders as for other obese women. Some women with androgen excess and marked obesity seem to be particularly passive and do not acknowledge the seriousness of their condition. They show no interest in weight reduction and may be resistant to taking pills for diabetes, hypercholesterolemia, or hypertension. This is a difficult group to work with, but patience and demonstration of sympathy and concern frequently result in eventual compliance. It is important to give attention to the androgenic problem since that may be what interests the patient.

There is no need to enumerate the various approaches to weight reduction. Most obese people do not achieve long-term weight control. However, some do achieve it, so motivated patients should be given help or appropriate referral to a medically based obesity program.

The best treatment for the associated metabolic abnormalities of androgenic disorders is weight reduction. This is not a moral but a medical statement. Especially for non–insulin dependant diabetes mellitus (NIDDM), weight reduction may achieve attenuation or even permanent cure of the diabetes. A common mistake, however, is to withhold medication for too long in the hope that weight reduction will be accomplished. Unless there is actual weight loss within a period of a few months, medication should be initiated. This does not prevent the patient from losing weight and medication can always be withdrawn if she does.

Diabetes Mellitus

The diabetes associated with androgenic disorders is of the non–insulin dependant variety. The glucose intolerance is caused by resistance to insulin action. Early in the course, insulin levels are actually elevated. Giving insulin tends to exacerbate receptor down-regulation and also causes weight gain. For these reasons, oral agents are to be preferred to insulin until the advanced stage is reached when pancreatic reserve is diminished and relative insulin deficiency is present. It is not always clear what stage a patient is at. More than trace to mild ketonuria suggests insulin deficiency. Usually, the need for insulin becomes apparent when even a maximum dose of an oral agent is found to be ineffective in lowering blood glucose to desirable levels.

Standard treatment for NIDDM is one of the second generation sulfonylureas, glipizide or glyburide. Recently, sustained release forms have been introduced, which may be slightly more effective. The dose range is broad and a period of titration of several weeks is necessary to find the effective dose. It is only a slight exaggeration to say that patients either respond to the minimum dose or do not respond at all. Both agents should be initiated as a single morning dose of 2.5 mg and upward adjustments made at about 2-week intervals until normoglycemia has been obtained or at least approximated. The maximum dose is 20 mg divided into two doses for the short-acting forms.

Self–blood testing, although not usually covered by insurance for NIDDM, is a necessity for achieving an adequate level of control. There are several meters on the market designed for NIDDM patients that are quite inexpensive but give acceptable accuracy. In NIDDM, blood glucose levels are excessive but relatively stable. The wide swings so frustrating in insulin dependant diabetes do not occur. A practical regimen is to test 3 days a week before and again 2 hours after breakfast. This indicates the fasting and postprandial levels. The desirable range is less than 100 to 105 mg/dL fasting and less than 140 mg/dL 1 hour after eating.

Dietary therapy of diabetes is widely misunderstood. While avoiding refined carbohydrates that may elevate blood glucose levels is desirable, it is also important to try to limit calories as well as saturated fat and cholesterol. The single most important goal however is prevention of hypoglycemia. While severe symptomatic hypoglycemia is rare with oral agents, mild reactions are common and often distressing to the patient, who may be led to discontinue medication because of them. Because the oral agents stimulate insulin release, prolonged periods of fasting may lead to glucose levels falling sufficiently to provoke epinephrine release and resulting subjective symptoms of anxiety and shakiness. This can be prevented by inclusion of snacks in the meal plan, especially one before retiring to bed since this is the longest normal period of fasting. Use of snacks should be taught before the patient begins taking oral agents.

Hemoglobin A_{1c} is a useful measure of long-term control; however, it may be high-normal in early NIDDM. If the patient conscientiously does self-monitoring, the level of control will be evident to her and her physician.

Lipid Abnormalities

Except for the rare severe forms, unfavorable lipid patterns give no symptoms or warning signs. Women with androgenic disorders who have android obesity should have a fasting lipid profile. Indeed all adults should have a fasting lipid profile every few years, but it is particularly important for those at risk.

There are two common unfavorable lipid patterns which arouse concern. The most straightforward is in the individual with elevated total and low-density lipoprotein (LDL)-cholesterol levels. Treatment with a 3-hydroxy-3-methylglutaryl (HMG) coenzyme A reductase inhibitor usually successfully lowers these parameters into the desirable range. While use of low doses is sometimes urged, it seems more important whenever possible to bring LDL-cholesterol down to the desirable level of 100 mg/dL, or at least close to it. More difficult is the situation in which the most conspicuous feature is a low HDL-cholesterol that may or may not be accompanied by high triglycerides. Elevated triglycerides may be due to diabetes or excessive alcohol intake with obvious implications for treatment. Reduction of obesity also lowers triglycerides. When other measures are ineffective, gemfibrozil may be used. It does elevate HDL modestly but mainly in situations in which there is hypertriglyceridemia. Exercise is effective in raising HDL in sedentary women, but it is not always carried out by the patient.

Currently, many lipid experts recommend lowering LDL-cholesterol in prefer-ence to raising HDL-cholesterol, because the former is more readily accomplished. Use of an HMG CoA reductase inhibitor in combination with gemfibrozil creates a risk of rhabdomyolysis and so is reserved for severe situations, although the risk may not be as great as originally supposed. Older agents such as nicotinic acid or bile-sequestering resins are poorly accepted by patients because of side effects and have a very limited role in modern lipid-lowering therapy.

Hypertension

Considerable evidence now links hypertension with insulin resistance which is in turn linked to androgenic disorders, especially when android obesity is present. Treatment of hypertension in women with androgenic disorders does not greatly differ from that in other patients, but there are a few special considerations. If the patient is receiving spironolactone, use of another potassium-sparing diuretic, such as one of those often contained in popular combinations should usually be avoided. There also may be risk of hyperkalemia with ACE inhibitors. When there is reason for preferential use of an ACE inhibitor, such as diabetes, in which ACE inhibitors have been shown to substantially slow progression of diabetic nephropathy, then potassium levels should be monitored when spironolactone is used. The combination should be avoided when renal ability to excrete potassium is compromised.

Combination of a beta blocker with spironolactone can result in exaggeration of orthostatic symptoms, but it can be used cautiously. However, a beta blocker is not generally the first choice in this group of women. In general, calcium channel blockers followed by thiazide diuretics are the most useful antihypertensives in women with androgenic disorders because they are unlikely to have unfavorable interactions. For the same reason, calcium channel blockers are preferred over beta blockers for migraine prophylaxis in women on spironolactone.

THE ADOLESCENT WITH AN ANDROGENIC DISORDER

Although often thought of as adult conditions, androgenic disorders usually have their onset in adolescence. It is even possible that they begin in infancy since hirsute mothers sometimes note hypertrichosis in their daughters prior to puberty. The pituitary–gonadal axis is active in the first several weeks of life; it can be speculated that hyperandrogenism may sometimes be present in infancy, sensitizing hair follicles that later respond further when androgen levels rise again with the onset of puberty. It is important that androgenic disorders be recognized when they occur in adolescence (37).

It should be remembered that hirsutism and alopecia develop gradually. Whatever degree exists in the early adolescent years is likely to increase before stabilizing. Thus even a mild degree raises concern that there will be worsening with further maturation. Prevention of progression is more effective than attempting later to reverse hair changes. When acne has more than mild inflammatory lesions, scarring occurs and there is gradual accumulation of injury to the skin, which can eventually lead to a pock-marked appearance that is difficult to conceal and a major source of embarrassment.

All of these factors favor early treatment when an adolescent girl has noticeable androgenic changes. Sometimes there is concern on the part of mother or physician that too-early hormonal treatment will have adverse effects on pubertal development. There is no evidence or theoretical reason to believe that this occurs. While OCs might accelerate epiphyseal closure if initiated too early, by 2 years after menarche growth is virtually complete. Prior to this age, OCs might be best avoided, but some girls do receive them for contraception not long after beginning to menstruate without evident adverse effect. When menarche does not occur because of PCOS however, OCs may be appropriate. Except for those who are sexually active, OCs are probably best avoided in girls less than 2 years postmenarchal. Only infrequently do girls need treatment for androgenic disorders prior to this point in their development. There do not seem to be special problems associated with the use of spironolactone or dexamethasone in adolescents even prior to menarche.

This is not to say that any adolescent with a slight amount of facial hair or minimal acne needs antiandrogenic treatment. In many, perhaps most, cases, it is sufficient to observe at regular follow-up visits, since not everyone will show progression. Local removal and conventional acne treatments can be used, and if skin or hair changes further increase, hormonal therapy can be instituted before the changes become marked. However, age alone is not a reason to withhold therapy for an androgenic disorder.

CONCLUSIONS

A variety of effective treatments for androgenic disorders exist. A rational approach to treatment selection and titration has been presented in this chapter. It is true that these treatments are somewhat complex to initiate. Once chosen and adjusted, however, they are relatively simple and well tolerated. In my experience, the degree of improvement that results can be a great relief to the patient. Furthermore there is the opportunity to intervene early in conditions which predispose to later serious disease. Treatment of androgenic disorders can be highly rewarding to patient and physician alike.

REFERENCES

1. Redmond GP, Gidwani G, Bergfeld W, Skibinksi C, Gupta M, Parker R, Bedocs N. Regulation of excessive androgen secretion in women: role of ACTH responsive endocrine tissue. *Fertil Steril Program Suppl* 1987:83.
2. Boisselle A, Tremblay RR. New therapeutic approach to the hirsute patient. *Fertil Steril* 1979;32: 276–279.
3. Shapiro G, Evron S. A novel use of spironolactone: treatment of hirsutism. *J Clin Endocrinol Metab* 1980;51:429–432.
4. Cumming DC, Yang JC, Rebar RW, Yen SC. Treatment of hirsutism with spironolactone. *JAMA* 1982;247:1295–1298.
5. Tremblay RR. Treatment of hirsutism with spironolactone. *Clin Endocrinol Metab* 1986;15:363–371.

6. Pittaway DE, Maxon WS, Wentz AC. Spironolactone in combination drug therapy for unresponsive hirsutism. *Fertil Steril* 1985;43:878–882.
7. Muhlemann MF, Carter GD, Cram JJ, Wise P. Oral spironolactone: an effective treatment for acne vulgaris in women. *Br J Dermatol* 1986;115:227–232.
8. Sciarra F, Toscano V, Concolino G, DiSilverio F. Antiandrogens: clinical applications. *J Steroid Biochem Mol Biol* 1990;37:349–362.
9. Vigersky RA, Mehlman I, Glass AR, Smith CE. Treatment of hirsute women with cimetidine. *N Engl J Med* 1980;303:1042.
10. Messina M, Manieri C, Rizzi G, Gentile L, Milani P. Treating acne with antiandrogens: the confirmation of the validity of a percutaneous treatment with spironolactone. *Curr Ther Res* 1985;38:269–282.
11. Hammerstein J, Meckies J, Leo-Rossberg I, Moltz L, Zielske F. Use of cyproterone acetate (CPA) in the treatment of acne, hirsutism and virilism. *J Steroid Biochem* 1975;6:827–836.
12. Belisle S, Love EJ. Clinical efficacy and safety of cyproterone acetate in severe hirsutism: results in a multicentered Canadian study. *Fertil Steril* 1986;46:1015–1020.
13. Lachnit-Fixon U. The development and evaluation of an ovulation inhibitor (Diane) containing an antiandrogen. *Acta Obstet Gynecol Scand* 1979;58:33–42.
14. Carlborg L. Cyproterone acetate versus levonorgestrel combined with ethinyl estradiol in the treatment of acne. Results of a multicenter study. *Acta Obstet Gynecol Scand Suppl* 1986;134:29–32.
15. Wishart JM. An open study of Triphasyl and Diane 50 in the treatment of acne. *Australas J Dermatol* 1991;32:51–54.
16. Cusan L, Dupont A, Berlanger A, Tremblay RR, Manhes G, Labrie R. Treatment of hirsutism with the pure antiandrogen flutamide. *J Am Acad Dermatol* 1990;23:462–469.
17. Marconides JA, Minnani SL, Luthold WW, et al. Treatment of hirsutism in women on flutamide. *Fertil Steril* 1992;57:543–547.
18. Wysowski DK, Freiman JP, Tourtelot JB, Horton ML. Fatal and nonfatal hepatoxicity associated with flutamide. *Ann Int Med* 1993;118:860–864.
19. Wallace C, Lalor EA, Chik CL. Hepatotoxicity complicating flutamide treatment of hirsutism [Letter]. *Ann Int Med* 1993;110:1150.
20. Stoner E. The clinical development of a 5 alpha-reductase inhibitor, finasteride. *J Steroid Biochem Mol Biol* 1990;20:375–378.
20a. Imperato-McGinley J, Geautier T, Cail-Q, Yee B, Epstein J. Pochi P: The androgen control of sebum P reduction. Studies of subjects with dihydrotestosterone deficiency and complete androgen insensitivity. *J Clin Endocrinol Metab* 1993;76:524–528.
21. Thigpen AE, Davis DL, Gautier T, Imperato-McGinley J, Russell DW. Brief report: the molecular basis of steroid 5 alpha-reductase deficiency in a large dominican kindred. *N Engl J Med* 1992;327:1216–1219.
22. Redmond GP, Gidwani GP, Gupta MK, Bedocs NM, Parker R, Skibinski C, Bergfeld W. Treatment of androgenic disorders with dexamethasone: dose–response relationship for suppression of dehydroepiandrosterone sulfate. *J Am Acad Dermatol* 1990;22:91–93.
23. Marynick SP, Chakmakjian ZH, McCaffree DL, Herndon JH. Androgen excess in cystic acne. *N Engl J Med* 1983;308:981–986.
24. Dickey RP. *Managing contraceptive pill patients.* 7th ed. Durant, OK: Essential Medical Information System Inc.
25. Speroff L, Darney P, eds. *A clinical guide for contraception.* Baltimore: Williams & Wilkins; 1992.
26. Vermeulen A, Rubens R. Effects of cyproterone acetate plus ethinylestradiol low dose on plasma androgens and lipids in mildly hirsute or acneic young women. *Contraception* 1988;38:419–428.
27. Palasti R, Hirvensalo E, Liukko P, Malmiharju T, Mattila L, Riihiluoma P, Ylostalo P. Serum total and unbound testosterone and sex hormone binding globulin (SHBG) in female acne patients treated with two different oral contraceptives. *Acta Derm Venereol (Stockh)* 1984;64:517–523.
28. Janaud A, Rouffy J, Upmalis D, Dain M-P. A comparison study of lipid and androgen metabolism with triphasic oral contraceptive formulations containing norgestimate or levonorgestrel. *Acta Obstet Gynecol Scand Suppl* 1992;71:33–38.
29. Van der Vange N, Blankenstein MA, Kloosterboer HJ, Haspels AA, Thijssen JHH. Effects of several low-dose oral contraceptives on sex hormone binding globulin, corticosteroid binding globulin, total and free testosterone. *Contraception* 1990;41:345–352.
30. Wishart JM. An open study of Triphasil and Diane 50 in the treatment of acne. *Australas J Dermatol* 1991;32(1):51–54.
31. Berg M. Desogestrel: using a selective progestogen in a combined oral contraceptive. *Adv Contracept* 1991;7(2–3):241–250.

32. Anderson FD. Selectivity and minimal androgenicity of norgestimate in monophasic and triphasic oral contraceptives. *Acta Obstet Gynecol Scand Suppl* 1992;156:15–21.
33. Cullberg G, Hamberger L, Mattson LA, Mobacken H, Samisoe G. Effects of a low dose desogestrel–ethinylestradiol combination on hirsutism, androgens and sex hormone binding globulin in women with a polycystic ovary syndrome. *Acta Obstet Gynecol Scand* 1985;64:195–202.
34. Adashi EY. Potential utility of gonadotropin-releasing hormone antagonists in the management of ovarian hyperandrogenism. *Fertil Steril* 1990;53:765–769.
35. Bergfeld WF, Redmond GP. Androgenic alopecia. *Dermatol Clin* 1986;5:491–500.
36. Redmond GP. Obesity in women. In: Redmond GP, ed. *Lipids and Women's Health*. New York: Springer-Verlag; 1991:119–131.
37. Wild RA. Hyperandrogenism in the adolescent. *Obstet Gynecol Clin North Am* 1992;19:71–89.

Androgenic Disorders,
edited by G. P. Redmond.
Raven Press, Ltd., New York © 1995.

14

Androgens and Oral Contraception

Richard J. Derman

*Department of Obstetrics and Gynecology, University of Illinois School of Medicine,
Chicago, Illinois 10952.*

More than 80% of women in the United States use oral contraceptives (OCs) at some time during their childbearing years (1). Although the average duration of OC use is relatively short (e.g., about 5 years) (1), many women use this form of contraception for a decade or more. Because of the potentially protracted and continuous nature of this contraceptive commitment, there is often concern on the part of both the patient and physician regarding short- and long-term side effects related to pill use. This is especially true in the case of potential alterations in lipoprotein and carbohydrate metabolism, which may have a profound impact on a woman's health and longevity. The following chapter addresses these issues and provides a perspective on how the 19-nortestosterone-derived agents incorporated into today's combination OCs play a key role in the metabolic and clinical effects of these compounds.

The evolution of the pill has been largely determined by an emerging awareness of the vascular side effects of OCs, leading to a progressive modification of the two key elements of such formulations: their dosage (and dosing regimen) and their steroidal component(s). The prototypic OC was Enovid, which first became available in the United States in the early 1960s and contained what is now known to be high doses of both estrogen (i.e., 150 μg mestranol) and progestin (i.e., 9.85 mg norethynodrel). Initially hailed as a milestone in modern day medicine, it and other new OCs were soon plagued by reports of associated thromboembolic complications, such as simple thrombophlebitis, frank deep venous thrombosis, and even fatal pulmonary embolism. Of particular note were the results of several retrospective, case-control studies demonstrating a significantly higher incidence of thromboembolic-related morbidity and mortality among users of OCs as compared with nonusers (2–5).

It was soon determined that the adverse thromboembolic effects of combination OCs were related to the estrogen, rather than the progestin component of the pill (6). Namely, the potentially life-threatening vascular events associated with the use of OCs appeared to result from the detrimental effects of estrogen on the venous system, presumably due to an elevation of certain blood clotting factors. The results of several long-term, prospective studies, such as the Royal College of General Practitioners study, the Oxford Family Planning Association study, and the Walnut

Creek Contraceptive Drug study, showed that these effects were dose related (7–9). As a result, there was a progressive decline in the dosage of estrogen used in combination OCs.

In 1969, the Committee on Safety of Drugs in the United Kingdom recommended that all OCs should contain no more than 50 μg of estrogen. By 1976, the estrogen dosage had been reduced to the standard low of 30 or 35 μg. This new, low dose was based on the findings of investigators such as Meade et al. (10), who showed a dramatically higher incidence of venous and nonvenous deaths, stroke, and ischemic heart disease in users of an OC containing 50 μg of ethinyl estradiol as compared with one containing 30 μg. Dosages lower than 30 μg proved unacceptable because of higher rates of pregnancy and breakthrough bleeding. Ultimately, this change has had an ongoing, favorable impact on the incidence of thromboembolic disease among OC users (11).

Even after the dosage of estrogen had been reduced to its lowest effective level, however, there were still reports of presumed arterially-mediated side effects associated with the use of OCs, including hypertension, ischemic heart disease, and cerebrovascular accident. Since it appeared that these adverse events were not solely related to the estrogen component of OCs, researchers shifted their focus to the progestin component. This reevaluation of the steroidal content of these compounds was galvanized by convergent data from diverse sources directly or indirectly implicating progestins in the etiology of OC-related arterial side effects. First, a series of epidemiologic studies demonstrated a higher incidence of ischemic heart disease in users of OCs than in nonusers, a phenomenon that appeared to be directly related to progestin dosage (12–16). This association pertained primarily to women over the age of 35 and to those who smoked. A separate series of population studies not related to contraceptive use revealed that individuals with high levels of low-density lipoprotein (LDL) cholesterol and/or low levels of high-density lipoprotein (HDL) cholesterol were at higher risk of coronary heart disease (CHD) than were those with relatively low levels of LDL cholesterol and/or high levels of HDL cholesterol (17). This was a pivotal finding, because metabolic studies indicated that monophasic pills containing the original, more androgenic progestins (e.g., levonorgestrel) appeared to induce adverse effects on these lipid fractions (18,19).

As discussed in depth later in this chapter, these and other data led to progressive refinements in the progestin component of OCs—most notably, a reduction in dosage and the introduction of new and more selective (i.e., less androgenic) progestational agents. Today, the goal of research in the area of oral contraception is to develop compounds that offer all the many reproductive and nonreproductive health benefits associated with this class of drugs, with a minimal risk of adverse metabolic and clinical effects potentially related to an OC's androgenicity.

ASSESSING THE ANDROGENIC ACTIVITY OF PROGESTINS

The term progestin derives from the predominantly progestational biologic activity of these synthetic steroids. However, each progestin has a constellation of biologic effects. Some compounds are markedly androgenic, while others produce minimal androgenic effects. Given the adverse clinical effects (e.g., acne, weight gain, hirsutism) and metabolic effects (e.g., long-term alterations in lipid and carbohydrate metabolism) associated with the androgenic activity of a progestin, there has been a concerted effort to improve the selectivity of the progestins used in OCs.

The pharmacologic concept of selectivity was first used more than two decades ago to describe certain cardiovascular drugs (e.g., those with beta$_1$-adrenergic activity) and histamine antagonists (e.g., those with H_2-blocking activity). In the case of progestins, selectivity is technically defined as the ratio of the affinity of the progestin to the progesterone receptor, to its affinity to the androgen receptor. However, the more widespread, clinical interpretation of this term is based on the assumption that a selective progestin is one that will produce its desired, pharmacologic effects in the absence of ancillary (in this case, androgenic) effects. In other words, an ideal progestin is one that exerts a progestational effect at low doses and is androgenic only at high concentrations. Given that the antiovulatory (i.e., contraceptive) effects of a progestin may be achieved at low doses (20), there is no clinical rationale for using higher doses of these steroids.

All of the synthetic progestins currently contained in OCs available in the United States are 19-nortestosterone derivatives (testosterone-derived), which are classified as either estranes [e.g., norethindrone, (norethisterone in Europe)] or gonanes (e.g., levonorgestrel, norgestimate, and desogestrel). Both are characterized by the absence of a methyl group between rings A and B and by the presence of an ethinyl group in position 17a. However, the gonanes also have a methyl group in position 18, which increases their progestogenic activity. All 19-nortestosterone derivatives are rapidly absorbed following oral administration and bind actively to plasma proteins.

Several paradigms have been used to evaluate the progestational versus the androgenic activity of progestins used in OCs. However, it is important to note that the concept of potency is an ambiguous one that has proven difficult to quantify. This is in large part because a progestin's potency varies not only as a function of the test used, but also in terms of the parameter measured, the route of administration, and the species studied. Ultimately, a progestin's potency must be determined clinically in relation to the estrogen component of an OC. Hence, the degree to which the in vitro or in vivo potency of a progestin can be extrapolated to the effects of a combination OC in clinical practice has yet to be fully elucidated. Nevertheless, the following models are useful in establishing the *relative* potencies of progestins within the context of preclinical or experimental testing.

Animal Testing

Classic bioassays in various animal models were traditionally used to characterize progestins according to their progestational, estrogenic, and androgenic, and their antiestrogenic, antiandrogenic, and antigonadotropic activity or potency (21). For example, transformation of the estrogen-primed endometrium (e.g., Clauberg or

McPhail assays) and maintenance of pregnancy were considered evidence of progestational activity, cornification of the vaginal epithelium was thought to demonstrate estrogenic activity, and an increase in prostate weight and fetal masculinization was believed to signify androgenic activity. Numerous other such measures were used to establish the predominant biologic activity of the older progestins in animal models.

Today, these tests are used primarily to determine the progestational activity of new and emerging progestins. For instance, it has been widely shown that all three new progestins (i.e., norgestimate, desogestrel, and gestodene) are highly progestational on the basis of endometrial stimulation, inhibition of ovulation, and maintenance of pregnancy (22). In addition, both desogestrel and gestodene produce a delay in menstruation at relatively lower doses than, for example, norethindrone. The relative progestational potency of the new progestins is significantly greater than that contained in the older combined OC formulations. According to several of the above indices, desogestrel and gestodene have slightly more progestational activity than norgestimate (22). In another assay, however, norgestimate was more potent than desogestrel on the basis of pregnancy maintenance in ovariectomized rats (23).

Progesterone Receptor Binding

Further evidence of the relative progestational potency of the new versus the old progestins has been derived from studies designed to evaluate their in vitro binding to progesterone receptors. While the results of these tests vary according to the methodology used, an assay based on displacement of radiolabeled progesterone from rabbit uterine progesterone receptors showed that the relative binding affinity (RBA) of norgestimate was similar to that of progesterone itself (RBA = 1.24 vs. 1.00, respectively) (Fig. 1) (24–26). In contrast, the relative receptor binding affinities of levonorgestrel (RBA = 5.41), the major metabolite of desogestrel, 3-keto desogestrel (RBA = 8.59), and gestodene (RBA = 9.21) were markedly greater than that of progesterone. These findings indicate that all three new progestins bind avidly to progesterone receptors and that their relative affinities are gestodene >3-keto desogestrel>levonorgestrel>norgestimate.

Androgen Receptor Binding Studies

Studies of androgen receptor binding are a widely accepted preclinical standard of a progestin's androgenicity. Since all 19-nortestosterone progestins are testosterone derivatives, they all have some residual androgenic effects that may be measured according to androgen receptor studies (27). However, there are marked differences between them. For example, the IC_{50} (e.g., the concentration at which there is 50% displacement of radiolabeled dihydrotestosterone from androgen receptors) of a new progestin such as norgestimate is extremely high, even in com-

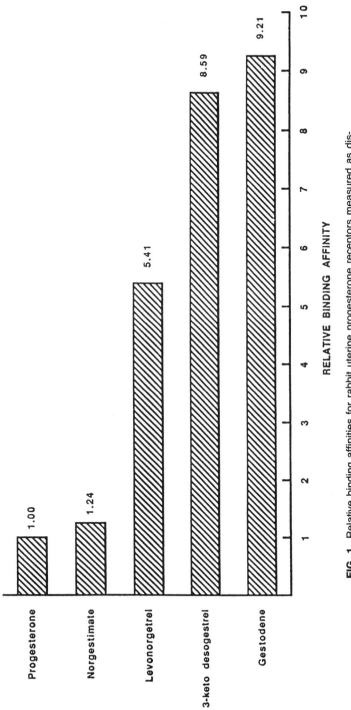

FIG. 1. Relative binding affinities for rabbit uterine progesterone receptors measured as displacement of ^{3}H-R5020 (25, 26).

parison with progesterone (764 nM vs. 401 nM, respectively), indicating an almost undetectable level of androgen receptor binding (28). While relatively lower, the IC_{50} values for both 3-keto desogestrel and gestodene (17 and 13 nM, respectively) are still higher than those of levonorgestrel (9 nM) or dihydrotestosterone (2 nM) (28).

These findings are reflected in the relative binding affinities of these progestins for rat prostatic androgen receptors. As shown in Fig. 2, the RBA of norgestimate is only 0.003 times that of dihydrotestosterone itself (1.000). The RBAs of 3-keto desogestrel and gestodene (0.118 and 0.154, respectively) are also considerably lower than that of dihydrotestosterone (25,26,29).

Selectivity Index

Receptor binding studies can also be used to calculate the selectivity index (i.e., the ratio of androgen receptor binding affinity to progestin receptor binding affinity) of various progestins on the basis of their binding affinities for androgen versus progestin receptors. According to IC_{50} data, the new progestins are considerably more selective than their more androgenic predecessors (Fig. 3). For example, the selectivity index of norgestimate is considerably higher than that of even progesterone itself (219 vs. 93, respectively), and is almost 20 times that of levonorgestrel (219 vs. 11, respectively) (26). The selectivity indices of 3-keto desogestrel and gestodene are approximately three times higher than that of levonorgestrel (33 and 28 vs. 11, respectively), but lower than that of progesterone (26). Thus, the relative selectivity of these various progestins (from high to low) is norgestimate>progesterone>3-keto desogestrel>gestodene>levonorgestrel.

Role of SHBG in the Assessment of Androgenicity

Another approach that may be used to evaluate a progestin's androgenicity is based on its interaction with the steroid-binding plasma glycoprotein, sex hormone–binding globulin (SHBG). SHBG binds reversibly and with high affinity to the main biologically active circulating androgen, testosterone, and to a lesser extent to the active estrogen, estradiol (E_2) (30). Estrogens (particularly those that are synthetic) may cause an increase in SHBG levels, while androgens may reduce plasma SHBG levels (30,31). Certain progestins (e.g., those with high androgenic activity) may also *indirectly* cause androgenic side effects by lowering serum levels of SHBG or by binding to SHBG, thereby displacing testosterone and leading to elevated levels of free testosterone (32).

Effects of Combination OCs on Serum SHBG Levels

While progesterone and the synthetic, hydroxyprogesterone-derived pregnanes have virtually no independent impact on SHBG levels, many of the earlier and more

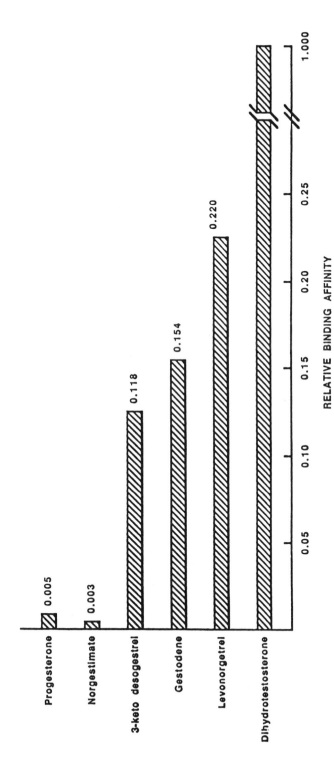

FIG. 2. Relative binding affinities for rat prostatic androgen receptors measured as displacement of ^{3}H-dihydrotestosterone (25, 26).

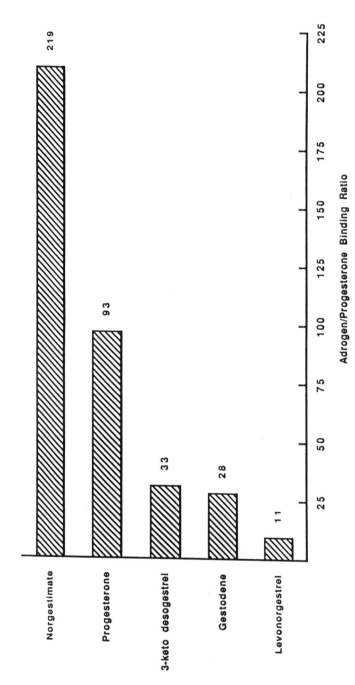

FIG. 3. Selectivity of various progestins as expressed by the ratio of the IC_{50} concentration for androgen binding divided by the IC_{50} concentration for progestin binding (26).

androgenic 19-nortestosterone derivatives (e.g., levonorgestrel) decrease serum SHBG levels (33,34). However, it may be of little clinical utility to view the androgenic effects of a progestin as an independent variable, since most OCs in use today are combination products containing different dosages of both a progestin and an estrogen (e.g., ethinyl estradiol). Therefore, it is customary to evaluate the combined effects of both components of an OC on SHBG in order to determine a pill's estrogenic:androgenic ratio (34). The *net* effect of an OC on SHBG is a function of the dose of ethinyl estradiol and the type and dose of progestin (35).

As would be expected, the question of whether a specific combination OC is estrogen or androgen dominant (as determined by its effects on SHBG) is a function of the dosage and type of steroids used. For example, a low-dose pill containing 1 mg of norethindrone and 0.035 mg of ethinyl estradiol has been shown to produce an increase in SHBG, whereas a high-dose pill containing 3 mg of norethindrone and 0.05 mg of ethinyl estradiol had virtually no effect on SHBG (36). Likewise, a pill containing different dosages and types of steroids—namely, 0.5 mg of norgestrel and 2 mg of estradiol valerate—has been found to have little impact on serum SHBG (37). It is also recognized now that the androgenic effects of a progestin, as measured by circulating levels of SHBG, vary as a function of the dosing form (38).

A substantial body of data accumulated over more than a decade have confirmed the relative nonandrogenicity of the new progestins vis-à-vis their forerunners as measured by OC-induced changes in SHBG levels. Reports appearing in the early 1980s offered some of the first evidence that levonorgestrel-containing OCs elevated, or did not alter, SHBG levels, whereas desogestrel-containing pills produced a dramatic increase in plasma levels of SHBG (39–41). This pattern has been consistently supported by subsequent studies, virtually all of which have demonstrated a significant elevation in SHBG associated with the use of all three new progestin-containing OCs (35,42–46).

Binding Affinity of Progestins for SHBG

Because SHBG serves as a transport protein for testosterone and other androgens, the relative binding affinities of progestins for SHBG are thought to reflect their relative binding affinities for cellular androgen receptors. Thus, another way of assessing androgenicity is to evaluate the affinity of progestins for human SHBG by assessing their ability to displace [3H]testosterone from the binding globulin. Generally, the more potent the androgen (and, inferentially, the more androgenic the progestin), the greater its binding affinity for SHBG (47).

Although all 19-nortestosterone derivatives can bind to testosterone receptors on SHBG, their binding affinities vary markedly. Bergink et al. have shown that the binding affinity of levonorgestrel for SHBG is more than five times that of norethindrone (48), and that the binding affinity of norgestrel is twice that of norethindrone (27). Gestodene has been shown to have the highest binding affinity human SHBG of the new progestins (28,49), a finding consistent with other evidence of androgenicity provided by the animal and other receptor binding studies discussed above. In fact, Phillips et al. (28) report that the binding affinity of gestodene for SHBG exceeds that of levonorgestrel or testosterone. Desogestrel binds slightly (i.e., 0.51), while norgestimate (in common with progesterone) has demonstrated virtually no (i.e., <0.005) binding affinity for SHBG (28,29). It is interesting to note that these relative binding affinities for SHBG parallel those previously described for rat prostatic androgen receptors (28).

ADVERSE METABOLIC EFFECTS OF ANDROGENS IN OCs

The preceding discussion has illustrated that certain progestins can be considered more androgenic than others according to various animal and experimental test models. However, the relative androgenicity of the progestins, ipso facto, lacks predictive value. It is only within the larger context of clinical practice that the biologic effects of progestins gain significance. In particular, the key question that must be addressed is how the concept of selectivity translates into health-related benefits and risks when a progestin is co-administered with an estrogen as a component of an OC. The following section addresses this issue with respect to the most potentially serious, progestin-related side effect: an increased risk of CHD associated with alterations in lipid and carbohydrate metabolism.

Effects on Lipid Metabolism

It is now well established that CHD is the leading cause of mortality in women (50), as well as in men (51,52), resulting in more than twice the number of deaths in women as all cancers combined (Fig. 4) (53,54). In fact, it is estimated that approx-

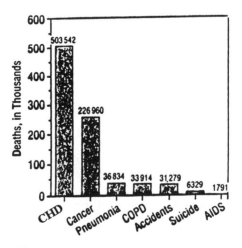

FIG. 4. Leading causes of death in women (53).

imately one out of every two women will die as a result of a cardiovascular event (e.g., an MI or a stroke) (53). Several risk factors for CHD have been identified in women, including alterations in lipids and lipoproteins, smoking, hypertension, diabetes mellitus, android obesity, and family history. The present discussion focuses on the association of lipid and lipoprotein abnormalities and CHD risk in women, since these parameters are particularly sensitive to the androgenicity of progestins. Additionally, androgens have been shown to adversely affect the prostacyclin/thromboxane ratio favoring platelet aggregation and vasoconstriction (55–57).

Dyslipidemias as Risk Factors for CHD in Women

Several epidemiologic studies have shown that hypercholesterolemia is an important risk factor for CHD in women (58–60). In the case of the Framingham Study (59), a direct correlation was found between the level of total cholesterol and the annual incidence of CHD. The risk of CHD in women with high total cholesterol levels (e.g., >265 mg/dL) was approximately twice that of normocholesterolemic women. Other studies have reported an increase in risk ranging from threefold (the Donolo–Tel Aviv study) (61) to as high as sevenfold (the Lipid Research Clinics trial) (62). Similar findings have been reported for LDL cholesterol. Consequently, the National Cholesterol Education Program (NCEP) (63) has recommended that both men and women maintain LDL levels below 130 mg/dL.

Data generated by the Framingham study (54,59) and the Lipid Research Clinics follow-up study (64,65) indicate that a low level of HDL cholesterol is a stronger and more consistent independent risk factor for CHD in women than an elevation in LDL. Indeed, an alteration in this lipoprotein has a greater predictive value in women than in men (59). According to the Framingham study (51,59), each 10 mg/dL change in HDL is associated with a 40% to 50% change in CHD risk. Furthermore, a subfraction of HDL, HDL_2, is considered to be an even more accurate risk discriminator than HDL itself. (66,67). In fact, it has been shown that variations in HDL cholesterol concentrations are largely determined by variations in HDL_2, which, when elevated, is considered to play a key cardioprotective role in the development of CHD (68,69). The serum levels of the main protein of HDL, apolipoprotein A_1, are also inversely correlated with CHD risk (70,71). A growing body of data suggest that an elevation in serum triglycerides is another independent risk factor for CHD in women, particularly in those with low HDL levels. (65,72,73).

Effects of Progestins on Lipoprotein Moieties

It is well-known that exogenous steroids have an important effect on lipid and lipoprotein metabolism. For example, the two hormones contained in an OC have fundamentally opposing effects on lipoproteins when administered separately. Estrogens increase HDL cholesterol and triglycerides and reduce LDL cholesterol, while progestins increase LDL cholesterol and decrease HDL cholesterol, including

TABLE 1. *Effects of OCs containing new progestins on HDL cholesterol and apo A_1*

Progestin	N	Change from baseline (%)	
		HDL-C	Apo A_1
Desogestrel	608	+12.9	+11.3
Norgestimate	>2550	+9.9	+7.3
Gestodene	296	+8.1	+7.1

Apo A_1, apolipoprotein A_1; HDL-C, high-density lipoprotein cholesterol.

both HDL_2 and apolipoprotein A_1 (Table 1) (74–78). Overall, the net effect of most combination OCs is to increase levels of cholesterol and triglycerides, while the effects on LDL cholesterol and HDL cholesterol (as well as on HDL subfractions and carrier lipoproteins) are more variable (69,79–84). Since almost all combination OCs available today contain 30 or 35 μg of estrogen, however, any differences between the effects of these various preparations on lipoprotein metabolism must be attributed to the dosage and/or type of progestin, rather than to the estrogen component of the OC.

The adverse effects of a progestin on serum lipoproteins are known to be dose-related (33,85,86). Therefore, the present focus of interest is on the growing body of data which indicate that the more androgenic progestins generally have a greater impact on serum lipoproteins than do their less androgenic counterparts (87,88). The following discussion reviews some of the key findings that support this observation. However, the reader must be cautioned that the statements presented here are generalizations that do not (because of the limitations of space) take into account the marked variability in metabolic outcome that can be influenced by such factors as OC formulation (e.g., fixed-dose vs. multiphasic), duration of follow-up, and even the time during the menstrual cycle when blood samples are obtained.

Most information suggests that OCs containing the older progestins tend to cause a greater and more consistent elevation in total cholesterol than do those containing the newer (and less androgenic) progestins (e.g., desogestrel, gestodene, or nor-gestimate) (82,84,89–92). In addition, the older and more androgenic progestins tend to produce an increase in LDL cholesterol, whereas the new progestin-containing OCs have a negligible effect on this lipoprotein. Namely, desogestrel produces a 2% overall decrease, gestodene causes virtually no change, and norgestimate induces a slight (3.4%) overall increase (76,84,91–94). All combination OCs appear to cause variable increases in triglycerides, although this effect is quite modest in the case of the new progestin-containing monophasic compounds (76,84,91,92). Of particular note is recent evidence suggesting that the transient rise in triglycerides associated with the use of a norgestimate-containing OC resolves with continued therapy (95).

Numerous studies have shown that even the low doses of the more androgenic progestins (e.g., norgestrel, norethindrone acetate, and levonorgestrel) contained in currently available combination OCs produce a significant reduction in HDL cholesterol (93,94,96–98), whereas relatively nonandrogenic progestins usually *in-*

crease levels of HDL cholesterol (84,93). Overall, desogestrel and norgestimate have been shown to produce the greatest increases in HDL (84). A similar, although less pronounced, trend has been observed for apolipoprotein A_1 (84,99,100). Consistent with the above findings, levonorgestrel and norethindrone and its derivatives also reduce levels of HDL_2 (69,101,102), whereas OCs containing the new progestins either elevate, or have a neutral effect, on this lipoprotein subfraction (35,46,100,103). Lipoprotein(a) or Lp(a) is an atherogenic lipoprotein. Estrogens tend to lower Lp(a). The impact of androgens is less clear (17,104,105).

Effects on Carbohydrate Metabolism

Almost 30 years ago, Wynn and colleagues (106) first reported alterations in carbohydrate metabolism (e.g., elevations in plasma glucose and insulin levels) among OC users. It was independently observed that both insulin-dependent and non–insulin-dependent diabetics—precisely that population which exemplifies the potential complications of hyperinsulinemia—are at increased risk for CHD (107, 108), and that the potential for morbidity related to impaired glucose tolerance is greater in women than in men (109). Although the relationship between the effects of OCs on carbohydrate metabolism and CHD risk has not been as fully elucidated as have the lipid effects of OCs, several noncontraceptive studies have shown that even a minimal impairment of glucose tolerance increases the incidence of CHD (99,110–112), and that hyperinsulinemia is a significant and independent risk factor for CHD (99,113–115).

Since the estrogen component of an OC has been shown to have a minimal effect on carbohydrate metabolism (116,117), it appears that the progestin component alone or in combination with an estrogen is responsible for any adverse effects on insulin or glucose levels. This is presumably due to a decrease in insulin-binding affinity and the number of insulin receptors, leading to an increase in peripheral insulin resistance (77,118). As was the case with the effects of OCs on lipid metabolism, a progestin's effects on carbohydrate metabolism seem to be related to its dosage and type (i.e., potency), as well as to the duration of use (69,117,119–121). While the Royal College of General Practitioners study (122) and the Oxford Family Planning study (123) failed to demonstrate that even the long-term use of OCs had a diabetogenic effect, low-dose compounds containing progestins with minimal androgenicity appear to have the greatest overall insulin-sparing effect. However, the study outcomes in this area are notoriously difficult to interpret because of methodologic limitations, such as small sample size, insufficient follow-up, and within-individual variability (84,92).

Although the results of the initial studies with OCs containing the older and more androgenic progestins were often conflicting, the net conclusion that can be drawn from the data is that many of these preparations alter carbohydrate metabolism, usually based on increased glucose and/or insulin levels during an oral glucose tolerance test. In one study, levonorgestrel produced a marked increase in both metabolic indices, while norethindrone increased peripheral insulin resistance but did not affect glucose tolerance (124). In another investigation, norgestrel altered both parameters, whereas the less androgenic norethindrone did not significantly alter either (125). It also has been noted that fixed-dose combination OCs containing levonorgestrel or norethindrone acetate reduce glucose tolerance, independent of the dose of estrogen used (90,126). The results of two studies have shown that even triphasic formulations of levonorgestrel had an adverse effect on glucose tolerance, whereas a triphasic form of norethindrone did not (127).

In many cases, low-dose OC formulations containing the new progestins have been associated with minimal changes in glucose tolerance (100,128–130), even in women with a prior history of gestational diabetes (131). In fact, numerous studies have shown that low-dose norethindrone and the new progestins have a more favorable effect on carbohydrate metabolism than do the more androgenic progestins (90, 92,108,126,132). However, some investigators have reported a minimal change (117,133–136), or a decline (137), in glucose tolerance with OCS containing a variety of progestins (including the new progestins as well as levonorgestrel), while others have cited marked increases in both plasma insulin and glucose levels during an oral glucose tolerance test with a comparable spectrum of agents (42,69,138). The only progestin that has, as of this time, consistently demonstrated an absence of adverse effects on serum glucose or insulin levels is norgestimate (84,95). This may be particularly important in patients with polycystic ovary syndrome who are already at increased risk for insulin resistance and cardiovascular disease (139).

OBJECTIVE CLINICAL MARKERS OF OC ANDROGENICITY

The progestins contained in OCs may also cause adverse clinical effects, such as acne, weight gain, and hirsutism. While none of these side effects poses any great risk with respect to patient morbidity or mortality, they play a key role in patient compliance and ultimately determine a patient's overall satisfaction with OC use. Indeed, the fact that as many as 50% of women discontinue OC use during the first year (77) reflects the frustration many patients feel about unsightly and highly visible physical changes. Weight gain has been identified as the leading physical reason for patient discontinuation of OC use (140), and acne and other "nuisance-type" side effects are also important deterrents to long-term use.

As previously discussed, progestins administered alone induce a decrease in SHBG as a function of their androgenic properties. Since there is an inverse correlation between circulating concentrations of SHBG and free testosterone, it would appear that a progestin with low androgenic activity would be less likely to cause clinical side effects than a highly androgenic one. Numerous studies have shown that the new progestins are generally neutral with respect to clinically objective manifestations of androgenicity and may actually have a positive impact on certain clinical parameters. For example, several investigators have shown that pills containing desogestrel improve acne in women with a pre-existing condition (141–143), and a large-scale study comparing a levonorgestrel- versus a desogestrel-containing pill showed significantly greater improvement in acne with the desogestrel formulation (144). Norgestimate also has been shown to have a neutral or a salutary effect on acne (145,146), and it is associated with a lower incidence of acne than norgestrel when both are administered as components of OCs (147). The findings with regard to gestodene are less clear-cut (148).

Similar observations have been made with respect to changes in body weight. In the case of desogestrel, most studies have demonstrated that OCs containing this new progestin cause either no change, or a slight (<1 kg) increase, in weight (44,149). In fact, one group of investigators reported no change in weight after 24 cycles of treatment with a desogestrel-containing OC in 70% of study participants, and a decrease in weight of 2 or more kg in 12% of women (149). Likewise, multicenter studies conducted in Europe in more than 40,000 women who used a norgestimate-containing OC for six cycles revealed a mean increase in weight of only 0.6% at the end of the study (145). Other investigators have reported that norgestimate has no effect on body weight (145,150,151). According to two studies, weight gain has resulted in study discontinuation in 1% or fewer women using a norgestimate-containing pill, as compared with 1.4% or more of those using a norgestrel-containing compound (147,152). Gestodene-containing OCs also appear to have a minimal effect on body weight (148).

The new progestins also appear to have a favorable impact on hirsutism. A study in 20 hirsute women with polycystic ovary syndrome (PCO) treated for 8 months with a desogestrel-containing pill revealed a significant reduction in hirsutism, based on both hair diameter and the semiquantitative hair score, which was apparent as early as 3 months after the onset of treatment (Fig. 5) (153). In addition, acne resolved in those patients with this condition and obese women experienced a reduction in body weight. Similar findings have been reported in other studies in women with pre-existing hirsutism (143,154). In addition, a recent report suggests that monthly treatment with a desogestrel-containing OC can be used to maintain remission of hirsutism in patients whose hirsutism has been controlled with a desogestrel-containing OC (155).

CONCLUSIONS

A substantial body of data generated by more than three decades of clinical experience has demonstrated that there are marked differences in the metabolic and clinical effects of combination OCs. Given that all currently available combination OCs contain equivalent amounts of estrogen, it is now recognized that it is the characteristics of the progestational constituent that ultimately determine the metabolic profile in OC users and, in large measure, impact on compliance. In particu-

Total testosterone ↓

Total testosterone ↓

Androstenedione ↔

SHBG ↑ (5x)

Body weight ↓

Hair growth ↓

Hair coarseness ↓

Depilation interval ↑

Acne ↓

BP ↔

FIG. 5. PCOS women on desogestrel plus ethinyl estradiol for 8 months.

lar, the more selective a progestin—in other words, the greater the ratio of its progestational activity to its androgenic activity—the more favorable the overall therapeutic outcome.

This finding has had important implications for the prescribing of OCs. Clearly, certain contraindications to pill use remain in effect, independent of an OC's steroidal composition or dosage (156–158). However, even in apparently healthy women, there appears to be a rationale for selecting low-dose combination OCs containing progestins with the least androgenic activity. For example, androgens and the androgenic progestins contained in OCs have been shown to have an HDL cholesterol–lowering effect (18,130,159). Given the protective role of HD cholesterol in the development of CHD (66,160–162), it would seem prudent to avoid using combination OCs that lower HDL and its subfractions (67). This is especially true in light of the fact that combination OCs containing progestins with high androgenic activity can counteract the HDL-elevating effects of estrogen, a change that is compounded by the low doses of estrogen contained in current OCs (33,85).

Another factor to consider when prescribing a combination OC is its impact on carbohydrate metabolism. The early clinical experience with combination OCs revealed that these high-dose compounds increased plasma glucose and insulin levels (106). Subsequent studies have shown that an elevation in plasma insulin levels is a significant, independent risk factor for the development of CHD (113–115), and that even minor alterations in glucose tolerance place patients at increased risk (110–112). The evidence suggests that pills containing androgenic progestins can adversely affect carbohydrate metabolism (117,163), while those containing the new and less androgenic progestins appear to have a more neutral effect (69,108,132).

A subgroup of women who already manifest clinical signs of androgen excess (perhaps 10% to 15% of reproductive-age women) are likely at already increased risk for diabetes and cardiovascular disease. Use of an OC containing a non-androgenic progestin such as norgestimate may be particularly appropriate.

Nonetheless, it is important to recognize that there exists minimal randomized data on pill type related to subsequent relative morbidity and mortality. There is, in fact, evidence to suggest that the estrogen component contained in OCs may provide cardioprotection, offsetting adverse lipid and carbohydrate effects, and that 10 years of clinical use of OCs has not yielded statistically significant cardiovascular outcomes among non-smokers using OCs compared to controls.

In conclusion, a number of factors must be taken into consideration when prescribing an OC. The progressive reduction in the steroid content of OCs has led to a reduced incidence of adverse effects, while the growing awareness of risk factors and patient selection has significantly reduced the incidence of OC-related mortality. Nevertheless, there remains a segment of women for whom OC use is absolutely contraindicated, as well as a population in whom the use of OCs may theoretically be associated with an increased risk of cardiovascular disease. The latter group includes women over the age of 35 who smoke and those with hypertension, hyperlipidemia, significant android obesity, diabetes, PCO, or a family history of coronary artery disease. For women with known risk factors, as well as for patients who contemplate long-term use of OCs, the use of one of the less androgenic progestin compounds would be a reasonable choice.

REFERENCES

1. Ortho Birth Control Survey, 1992.
2. Royal College of General Practitioners. Oral contraception and thromboembolic disease. *J Royal Coll Gen Pract* 1967;13:267–279.
3. Inman WHW, Vessey MP. Investigation of deaths from pulmonary, coronary and cerebral thrombosis and embolism in women of child-bearing age. *Br Med J* 1968;2:193–199.
4. Vessey MP, Doll R. Investigation of relation between use of oral contraceptives and thromboembolic disease. *Br Med J* 1968;2:199–205.
5. Sartwell PE, Masi AT, Arthes PG, et al. Thromboembolism and oral contraceptives: an epidemiologic case-control study. *Am J Epidemiol* 1969;90:365–380.
6. Inman WHW, Vessey MP, Westerholm B, et al. Thromboembolic disease and the steroidal content of oral contraceptives: a report to the Committee on Safety of Drugs. *Br Med J* 1970;2:203–209.
7. Royal College of General Practitioners. *Oral contraceptives and health: an interim report.* London: Pitman; 1974:1–100.
8. Vessey MP, Doll R, Peto R, et al. A long-term follow-up of women using different methods of contraception: an interim report. *J Biosoc Sci* 1976;8:373–427.
9. Petitti DB, Wingerd J, Pellegrin E, et al. Oral contraceptives, smoking, and other risk factors in relation to risk of venous thromboembolic disease. *Am J Epidemiol* 1978;108:480–485.
10. Meade TW, Greenberg G, Thompson SG. Progestogens and cardiovascular reactions associated

with oral contraceptives and a comparison of the safety of the 50 and 30 mcg estrogen preparations. *Br Med J* 1980;280:1157–1161.

11. Bottinger LE, Bowman G, Eklund G, et al. Oral contraceptives and thromboembolic disease. *Lancet* 1980;i:1097–1101.

12. Mann JI, Vessey MP, Thorogood M, et al. Myocardial infarction in young women with special reference to oral contraceptive practice. *Br Med J* 1975;2:441–445.

13. Mann JI, Inman WHW, Thorogood M. Oral contraceptive use in older women and fatal myocardial infarction. *Br Med J* 1976;2:445–447.

14. Jick H, Dinan B, Rothman KJ. Oral contraceptives and nonfatal myocardial infarction. *JAMA* 1978;239:1403–1406.

15. Kay CR. Progestogens and arterial disease. Evidence from the Royal Colleage of General Practitioners study. *Am J Obstet Gynecol* 1982;142:762–776.

16. Frank P. Oral contraceptives and arterial disease: recent evidence from the Royal College of General Practitioners Oral Contraceptive Study. *Singapore J Obstet Gynecol* 1984;15:14–21.

17. Gordon DJ, Knoke J, Probstfield JL, et al. High-density lipoprotein cholesterol and coronary heart disease in hypercholesterolemic men: The Lipid Research Clinic's coronary primary prevention trial. *Circulation* 1986;74:1217–1225.

18. Fotherby K. Oral contraceptives, lipids and cardiovascular disease. *Contraception* 1985;31:367–394.

19. Silfverstolpe G, Gustafson A, Samsioe G, et al. Lipid metabolic effects in oophorectomized women: effects of three different progestagens. *Acta Obstet Gynecol Scand* 1979;99(suppl):89–95.

20. Upton GV, Corbin A. The relevance of the pharmacologic properties of a progestational agent to its clinical effects as a combination oral contraceptive. *Yale J Biol Med* 1989;62:445–457.

21. Kistner RW. Steroid compounds with progestational activity. *Postgrad Med* 1964:35:225–229.

22. Rebar RW, Zeserson K. Characteristics of the new progestogens in combination oral contraceptives. *Contraception* 1991;44:1–10.

23. Phillips A, Hahn DW, Klimek S, et al. A comparison of the potencies and activities of progestogens used in contraceptives. *Contraception* 1987;36:181–192.

24. Anderson FD. Selectivity and minimal androgenicity of norgestimate in monophasic and triphasic oral contraceptives. *Acta Obstet Gynecol Scand* 1992;71(suppl):15–21.

25. Phillips A, Hahn DW, McGuire JL. Preclinical evaluation of norgestimate, a progestin with minimal androgenic activity. *Am J Obstet Gynecol* 1992;167:1191–1196.

26. Phillips A. The selectivity of a new progestin. *Acta Obstet Gynecol Scand* 1990;152(suppl):21–24.

27. Bergink EW. Binding of contraceptive progestogen to receptor proteins in human myometrium and MCF-7 cells. *Br J Fam Plann* 1984;10:33–38.

28. Phillips A, Hahn DW, McGuire JL. Relative binding affinity of norgestimate and other progestins for human sex hormone–binding globulin. *Steroids* 1990;55:373–375.

29. Collins D. Selectivity information on desogestrel. *Am J Obstet Gynecol* 1993;168:1010–1016.

30. Anderson DC. Sex-hormone–binding globulin. *Clin Endocrinol* 1974;3:69–96.

31. Lobl TJ. Androgen transport proteins: physical properties, hormonal regulation, and possible mechanism of T, CBG and ABP action. *Arch Androl* 1981;7:133–151.

32. Nilsson B, Schoultz V. Binding of levonorgestrel, norethisterone and desogestrel to human sex hormone binding globulin and influence on free testosterone levels. *Gynecol Obstet Invest* 1989;27:151–154.

33. Bergink EW, Kloosterboer HJ, Lund L, et al. Effects of levonorgestrel and desogestrel in low-dose oral contraceptive combinations on serum lipids, apolipoproteins A-I and B, and glycosylated proteins. *Contraception* 1984;30:61–72.

34. El Makhzangy MN, Wynn V, Lawrence DM. Sex hormone binding globulin capacity as an index of oestrogenicity or androgenicity in women on oral contraceptive steroids. *Clin Endocrinol* 1979;10:39–45.

35. van der Vange N, Blankenstein MA, Kloosterboer HJ, et al. Effects of seven low-dose combined oral contraceptives on sex hormone binding globulin, corticosteroid binding globulin, total and free testosterone. *Contraception* 1990;41:345–352.

36. Odlind V, Weiner E, Victor A, et al. Effects on sex hormone binding globulin of different oral contraceptives containing norethisterone and lynestrenol. *Br J Obstet Gynaecol* 1980;87:416–421.

37. Hagstad A, Damber J, Janson PE, et al. Effects of two estradiol/norgestrel combinations on the ovulatory pattern and on sex hormone binding globulin capacity in women around forty years of age. *Acta Obstet Gynecol Scand* 1984;63:321–324.

38. Granger LR, Roy S, Mishell DR Jr. Changes in unbound sex steroids and sex hormone binding globulin binding capacity during oral and vaginal progestogen administration. *Am J Obstet Gynecol* 1982;144:578–504.

39. Bergink EW, Holma P, Pyorala T. Effects of oral contraceptive combinations containing levonorgestrel or desogestrel on serum proteins and androgen binding. *Scand J Clin Lab Invest* 1981; 41:663–668.

40. Cullberg G, Dovre P-A, Lindstedt G, et al. On the use of plasma proteins as indicators of the metabolic effects of combined oral contraceptives. *Acta Obstet Gynecol Scand* 1982;111(suppl): 47–54.

41. Hammond GL, Langley MS, Robinson PA, et al. Serum steroid binding protein concentrations, distribution of progestogens, and bioavailability of testosterone during treatment with contraceptives containing desogestrel or levonorgestrel. *Fertil Steril* 1984;42:44–51.

42. Liukko P, Erkkola R, Lammintausta R, et al. Blood glucose, serum insulin, serum growth hormone and serum glycosylated proteins during two years' oral contraception with low-estrogen combinations. *Ann Chir Gynaecol* 1987;76(suppl 202):45–49.

43. Kauppien-Makelin R, Kuusi T, Ylikorkala O, et al. Contraceptives containing desogestrel or levonorgestrel have different effects on serum lipoproteins and post-heparin plasma lipase activities. *Clin Endocrinol* 1992;36:203–209.

44. Ball MJ, Ashwell E, Jackson M, et al. Comparison of two triphasic contraceptives with different progestogens: effects on metabolism and coagulation proteins. *Contraception* 1990;41:363–375.

45. London RS, Chapdelaine A, Upmalis D, et al. Comparative contraceptive efficacy and mechanism of action of the norgestimate-containing triphasic oral contraceptive. *Acta Obstet Gynecol Scand* 1992;71(suppl):9–14.

46. Janaud A, Rouffy J, Upmalis D, et al. A comparison study of lipid and androgen metabolism with triphasic oral contraceptive formulations containing norgestimate or levonorgestrel. *Acta Obstet Gynecol Scand* 1992;156(suppl):33–38.

47. Dickey RP, Stone SC. Progestational potency of oral contraceptives. *Obstet Gynecol* 1976;47:106–112.

48. Bergink EW, Hamburger AD, De Jager E, et al. Binding of a contraceptive progestogen ORG 2969 and its metabolites to receptor proteins and human sex hormone binding globulin. *J Steroid Biochem* 1981;14:175–183.

49. Bergink W, Assendorp R, Kloosterboer L, et al. Serum pharmacokinetics of orally administered desogestrel and binding of contraceptive progestogens to sex hormone-binding globulin. *Am J Obstet Gynecol* 1990;163:2132–2137.

50. Kuhn FE, Rackley CE. Coronary artery disease in women: risk factors, evaluation, treatment, and prevention. *Arch Intern Med* 1993;153:2626–2636.

51. Castelli WP. Cardiovascular disease in women. *Am J Obstet Gynecol* 1988;158:1552–1560.

52. Lerner DJ, Kannel WB. Patterns in coronary heart disease—morbidity and mortality in the sexes: a 26-year follow-up of the Framingham population. *Am Heart J* 1986;111:383–390.

53. American Heart Association. *1992 Heart and stroke facts*. Dallas, Texas: American Heart Association; 1992.

54. Stadel BV. Oral contraceptives and cardiovascular disease. *N Engl J Med* 1981;305:612–618.

55. Weyrich AS, Rejeski WJ, et al. The effects of testosterone on lipids and eicosanoids in cynomolgus monkeys. *Med Sci Sports Exerc* 1992;24:333–338.

56. Makao J, Change WC, et al. Testosterone inhibits prostacyclin productin by rat aortic smooth muscle cells in culture. *Atherosclerosis* 1981;39:203–209.

57. Jouve, et al. *Am Heart J* 1984.

58. Mann JI, Doll R, Thorogood M, et al. Risk factors for myocardial infarction in young women. *Br J Prev Soc Med* 1976;30:94–100.

59. Kannel WB. Metabolic risk factors for coronary heart disease in women: perspective from the Framingham Study. *Am Heart J* 1987;114:413–419.

60. Castelli WP, Garrison RJ, Wilson PWF, et al. Incidence of coronary heart disease and lipoprotein cholesterol levels: the Framingham Study. *JAMA* 1986;256:2835–2838.

61. Brunner D, Weisbort J, Meshulam N, et al. Relation of serum total cholesterol and high-density lipoprotein cholesterol percentage to the incidence of definite coronary events: twenty-year follow-up of the Donolo-Tel Aviv prospective coronary artery disease study. *Am J Cardiol* 1987;59:1271–1276.

62. Bush TL, Criqui MH, Cowan LD, et al. Cardiovascular disease mortality in women: results from

the Lipid Research Clinics follow-up study. In: Eaker ED, Packard B, Wenger NK, et al., eds. *Coronary heart disease in women: proceedings of an NIH workshop.* New York: Haymarker Dayma, Inc; 1987:106–111.

63. Expert Panel. Report of the National Cholesterol Education Program Expert Panel on detection, evaluation, and treatment of high blood cholesterol in adults. *Arch Intern Med* 1988;148:36–69.

64. Crouse JR III. Gender, lipoproteins, diet and cardiovascular disease. *Lancet* 1989;1;318–320.

65. Bass KM, Newschaffer CJ, Klag MH, et al. Plasma lipoprotein levels as predictors of cardiovascular death in women. *Arch Intern Med* 1993;153:2209–2216.

66. Miller NE, Forde OH, Thelle DS, et al. The Tromso Heart Study. High-density lipoprotein and coronary heart disease: a prospective case-control study. *Lancet* 1977;1:965–968.

67. Miller GJ. Progesterone and progestins. Paris; International Symposium; May 7–9, 1981.

68. Godsland IF, Wynn V. Progestogens and high-density lipoprotein. *Lancet* 1984;ii:1406.

69. Godsland I, Crook D, Simpson R, et al. The effects of different formulations of oral contraceptive agents on lipid and carbohydrate metabolism. *N Engl J Med* 1990;323:1375–1381.

70. Avogaro P, Bittolo Bon G, Cassolato G, et al. Are apolipoproteins better discriminators than lipids for atherosclerosis? *Lancet* 1979;1:901–903.

71. Miller NE. Association of high-density subclasses and apolipoproteins with ischemic heart disease and coronary atherosclerosis. *Am Heart J* 1987;113:589–597.

72. Lapidus L, Bengtsson C. Lindquist O, et al. Triglycerides: main risk for cardiovascular disease in women. *Acta Med Scand* 1985;217:481–489.

73. Castelli WP. The triglyceride issue: a view from Framingham. *Am Heart J* 1986;112:432–437.

74. Bush TL, Barrett-Connor E. Noncontraceptive estrogen use and cardiovascular disease. *Epidemiol Rev* 1985;7:80–104.

75. Knopp RH, Walden CE, Wahl PE, et al. Oral contraceptive and postmenopausal estrogen effects on lipoprotein triglyceride and cholesterol in an adult female population: relationships to estrogen and progestin potency. *J Clin Endocrinol Metab* 1981;53:1123–1132.

76. Wahl PW, Walden CE, Knopp RH, et al. Effect of estrogen/progestin potency on lipid/lipoprotein cholesterol. *N Engl J Med* 1983;308:862–867.

77. Fotherby K. Desogestrel and gestodene in oral contraception: a review of European experience. *J Drug Dev* 1991;4:101–111.

78. Hirvonen E, Malkonen M, Manninen V. Effects of different progestins on lipoproteins during postmenopausal replacement therapy. *N Engl J Med* 1981;304:560–563.

79. Vaziri SM, Evans JC, Larson MG, et al. The impact of female hormone usage on the lipid profile. *Arch Intern Med* 1993; 153:2200–2206.

80. Robinson GE, Bounds W, Mackie IJ, et al. Changes in metabolism induced by oral contraceptives containing desogestrel and gestodene in older women. *Contraception* 1990;42:263–273.

81. Wallace RB, Hoover JJ, Sandler D, et al. Altered plasma-lipids associated with oral contraceptive or oestrogen consumption: the Lipid Research Clinics Program. *Lancet* 1977;2:11–14.

82. Wallace RB, Hoover J, Barrett-Connor E, et al. Altered plasma lipid and lipoprotein levels associated with oral contraceptive and oestrogen use. *Lancet* 1979;2:111–115.

83. Heiss G, Tamir I, Davis CE, et al. Lipoprotein-cholesterol distribution in selected North American populations: the Lipid Research Clinics Program Prevalence Study. *Circulation* 1980;61:302–315.

84. Speroff L, DeCherney A, and the Advisory Board for the New Progestins. Evaluation of a new generation of oral contraceptives. *Obstet Gynecol* 1993;81:1034–1047.

85. Bradley DD, Wingerd J, Petitti DB, et al. Serum high-density lipoprotein cholesterol in women using oral contraceptives, estrogens, and progestins. *N Engl J Med* 1978;299:17–20.

86. Wingrave SJ. Progestogen effects and their relationship to lipoprotein changes: a report from the oral contraception study of the Royal College of General Practitioners. *Acta Obstet Gynecol Scand* 1982;105(suppl):33–36.

87. Derman RJ. Oral contraceptives and cardiovascular risk. Taking a safe course of action. *Postgrad Med* 1990;88:119–122.

88. Derman RJ. Oral contraceptives and cardiovascular risk. Current perspectives. *J Reprod Med* 1989;34:747–765.

89. Hennekens C, Evans D, Castelli W, et al. Oral contraceptive use and fasting triglyceride, plasma cholesterol and HDL cholesterol. *Circulation* 1979;60:486–489.

90. Wynn V, Adams PW, Godsland I, et al. Comparison of effects of different combined oral-contraceptive formulations on carbohydrate and lipid metabolism. *Lancet* 1979;1:1045–1049.

91. LaRosa JC. Effects of oral contraceptives on circulating lipids and lipoproteins: maximizing benefit, minimizing risk. *Int J Fertil* 1989;34(suppl):71–84.
92. Krauss RM, Burkman RT. The metabolic impact of oral contraceptives. *Am J Obstet Gynecol* 1992;167:1177–1184.
93. Kloosterboer HJ, Rekers H. Effects of three combined oral contraceptive preparations containing desogestrel plus ethinyl estradiol on lipid metabolism in comparison with two levonorgestrel preparations. *Am J Obstet Gynecol* 1990;163:370–373.
94. Knopp RH. Cardiovascular effects of endogenous and exogenous sex hormones over a woman's lifetime. *Am J Obstet Gynecol* 1988;158:1630–1643.
95. Kafrissen ME. A norgestimate-containing oral contraceptive: review of clinical studies. *Am J Obstet Gynecol* 1992;167:1196–1202.
96. Sassolas A, Lagarde M, Guichardant M, et al. Plasma lipoproteins and fatty acid composition after "minipill." *Contraception* 1983;28:357–368.
97. Larsson-Cohn U, Fahraeus L, Wallentin L, et al. Effects of the estrogenicity of levonorgestrel/ ethinylestradiol combinations on the lipoprotein status. *Acta Obstet Gynecol Scand* 1982:105 (suppl):37–40.
98. Refn H, Kjaer A, Lebech A-M, et al. Metabolic changes during treatment with two different progestins. *Am J Obstet Gynecol* 1990;163:374–377.
99. Fotherby K. Clinical experience and pharmacological effects of an oral contraceptive containing 20 micrograms oestrogen. *Contraception* 1992;46:477–488.
100. Kuhl H, Marz W, Jung-Hoffmann C, et al. Time-dependent alterations in lipid metabolism during treament with low-dose oral contraceptives. *Am J Obstet Gynecol* 1990;163:363–369.
101. Wynn V, Niththyananthan R. The effect of progestins in combined oral contraceptives on serum lipids. *Am J Obstet Gynecol* 1982;142:766–771.
102. Kjaer A, Lebech A-M, Borggaard B, et al. Lipid metabolism and coagulation of two contraceptives: correlation to serum concentrations of levonorgestrel and gestodene. *Contraception* 1989; 40:665–673.
103. Burkman RT. Lipid metabolism effects with desogestrel-containing oral contraceptives. *Am J Obstet Gynecol* 1993;168:1033–1040.
104. Abbott RD, Wilson PWF, Kannel WB, et al. High density lipoprotein-cholesterol, total cholesterol screening and myocardial infarction. The Framingham Heart Study. *Arteriosclerosis* 1988;8:207–213.
105. Lawn RM. Lipoprotein(a) in heart disease. *Sci Am* 1992;266:54.
106. Wynn V, Doar JW. Some effects of oral contraceptives on carbohydrate metabolism. *Lancet* 1966;ii:715–719.
107. Jarrett RJ. The epidemiology of coronary heart disease and related factors in the context of diabetes mellitus and impaired glucose tolerance. In: Jarrett RJ, ed. *Diabetes and heart disease*. Amsterdam: Elsevier Science; 1984:1–23.
108. Gaspard UJ, Lefebvre PJ. Clinical aspects of the relationship between oral contraceptives, abnormalities in carbohydrate metabolism, and the development of cardiovascular disease. *Am J Obstet Gynecol* 1990;163:334–343.
109. Skouby SO. Oral contraception with a triphasic combination of gestodene and ethinyl estradiol: results of a multicenter study. *Int J Fertil* 1987;32:45–49.
110. Pyorala K, Savolainen E, Lehtovirta E, et al. Glucose tolerance and coronary heart disease: Helsinki policeman study. *J Chron Dis* 1979;32:729–745.
111. Fuller JH, Shipley MJ, Rose G, et al. Mortality from coronary heart disease and stroke in relation to degree of glycemia: The Whitehall Study. *Br Med J* 1983;287:867–870.
112. Donahue RP, Abbott RD, Reed DM, et al. Postchallenge glucose concentration and coronary heart disease in men of Japanese ancestry. Honolulu Heart Program. *Diabetes* 1987;36:689–692.
113. Welborn TA, Wearne K. Coronary heart disease in incidence and cardiovascular mortality in Busselton with reference to glucose and insulin concentrations. *Diabetes Care* 1979;2:154–160.
114. Ducimetiere P, Eschwege E, Papoz L, et al. Relationship of plasma insulin levels to the incidence of myocardial infarction and coronary heart disease mortality in a middle-aged population. *Diabetologia* 1980;19:205–210.
115. Pyorala K, Savolainen E, Kaukola S, et al. Plasma insulin as coronary heart disease risk factor: relationship to other risk factors and predictive value during 9-1/2 year follow-up of the Helsinki Policemen Study population. *Acta Med Scand* 1985;701:38–52.
116. Spellacy WN, Buhi WC, Birk SA. The effect of estrogens on carbohydrate metabolism: glucose

insulin and growth hormone studies in one hundred seventy-one women ingesting Premarin, Mestranol and ethinylestradiol for six months. *Am J Obstet Gynecol* 1972;114:378–390.

117. Spellacy WN. Carbohydrate metabolism during treatment with estrogen, progestogen, and low-dose oral contraceptives. *Am J Obstet Gynecol* 1982;142:732–739.

118. Skouby SO, Andersen O, Petersen KR, et al. Mechanism of action of oral contraceptives on carbohydrate metabolism at the cellular level. *Am J Obstet Gynecol* 1990;163:343–348.

119. Perlman JA, Russell-Briefel R, Ezzati T, et al. Oral glucose tolerance and the potency of contraceptive progestins. *J Chronic Dis* 1985;38:857–864.

120. Kalkoff RK. Effects of oral contraceptive agents on carbohydrate metabolism. *J Steroid Biochem* 1975;6:949–956.

121. Ramcharan S, Pelligrin FA, Ray R, et al. *The Walnut Creek Contraceptive Drug Study: a prospective study of the side effects of oral contraceptives.* Washington, DC: Government Printing Office, 1981.

122. Hannford PC, Kay CR. Oral contraceptives and diabetes mellitus. *Br Med J* 1989;299:1315–1316.

123. Grice D, Villard-MacKintosh L, Yeates D, et al. Oral contraceptives and diabetes mellitus. *Br J Fam Plann* 1991;17:39–40.

124. Spellacy WN. Carbohydrate metabolism in male infertility and female fertility-control patients. *Fertil Steril* 1976;27:1132–1141.

125. Spellacy WN, Buhi WC, Birk SA. Carbohydrate metabolism prospective studied in women using low-estrogen oral contraceptives for six months. *Contraception* 1979;20:137–147.

126. Wynn V, Godsland IF. Effects of oral contraceptives on carbohydrate metabolism. *J Reprod Med* 1986;31:892–897.

127. Spellacy WN, Ellingson AB, Tsibris JCM. Glucose and insulin levels after six months of treatment with a triphasic oral contraceptive containing ethinyl estradiol and norethindrone. *J Reprod Med* 1989;34:540–542.

128. Runnebaum B, Rabe T. New progestogens in oral contraceptives. *Am J Obstet Gynecol* 1987; 1059–1063.

129. Lepot MR, Gaspard UJ. Metabolic effects of two low-dose triphasic oral contraceptives containing ethinyl estradiol and levonorgestrel or gestodene. *Int J Fertil* 1987;32(suppl):15–20.

130. Gaspard UJ. Metabolic effects of oral contraceptives. *Am J Obstet Gynecol* 1987;157:1029–1041.

131. Skouby SO, Kuhl C, Molsted-Pedersen L, et al. Triphasic oral contraception: metabolic effects in normal women and those with previous gestational diabetes. *Am J Obstet Gynecol* 1985;153:495–500.

132. Chez R. Clinical aspects of three new progestogens: desogestrel, gestodene and norgestimate. *Am J Obstet Gynecol* 1989;160:1296–1300.

133. Kuhl H, Gahn G, Romberg G, et al. A randomized cross-over comparison of two low-dose oral contraceptives upon hormonal and metabolic serum parameters: II. Effects upon thyroid function, gastrin, STH, and glucose tolerance. *Contraception* 1985;32:97–107.

134. van der Vange N, Kloosterboer HJ, Haspels AA. Effect of seven low-dose combined oral contraceptive preparations on carbohydrate metabolism. *Am J Obstet Gynecol* 1987;156:918–922.

135. Luyckx AS, Gaspard UJ, Romus MA, et al. Carbohydrate metabolism in women who used oral contraceptives containing levonorgestrel or desogestrel: a 6-month prospective study. *Fertil Steril* 1986;45:635–642.

136. Barsivala VM, Virkar K, Kulkarni RD. Carbohydrate metabolism of Indian women taking steroid contraceptives. *Fertil Steril* 1976;27:87–91.

137. Gaspard UJ, Romus MA, Luyckx AS. Carbohydrate metabolism alterations with monophasic, sequential and triphasic oral contraceptives containing ethinyl-oestradiol plus levonorgestrel or desogestrel. In: Rolland R, Harrison RF, Bonnar J, Thompson W, eds. *Advances in fertility control and the treatment of sterility.* Hingham, MA: MTP Press Limited; 1984:107–111.

138. Petersen KR, Skouby SO, Dreisler A, et al. Comparative trial of the effects on glucose tolerance and lipoprotein metabolism of two new oral contraceptives containing gestodene and desogestrel. *Acta Obstet Gynecol Scand* 1988;67:37–41.

139. Wild RA, Painter PC, Coulson PB, et al. Lipoprotein lipid concentrations and cardiovascular risk in women with polycystic ovary syndrome. *J Clin Endocrinol Metab* 1985;61(5):946–951.

140. Pratt WF, Bachrach CA. What do women use when they stop using the pill? *Fam Plann Perspect* 1987;19:257–266.

141. Erkkola R, Hirvonen EE, Luikka J, et al. Ovulation inhibitors containing cyproterone acetate or desogestrel in the treatment of hyperandrogenic symptoms. *Acta Obstet Gynecol Scand* 1990;69: 61–65.

142. Venturoli S, Porcu E, Gammi L, et al. The effects of desogestrel and ethinyl estradiol combination in normal and hyperandrogenic young girls: speculations on contraception in adolescence. *Acta Eur Fertil* 1988;19:19.
143. Bilotta P, Favilli S. Clinical evaluation of a monophasic ethinyl estradiol/desogestrel-containing oral contraceptive. *Drug Res* 1988;38:932–934.
144. Palatsi R, Hirvensalo E, Liukko P, et al. Serum total and unbound testosterone and sex hormone binding globulin (SHBG) in female acne patients treated with two different oral contraceptives. *Acta Derm Venereol (Stockh)* 1984;64:517–523.
145. Grunwald K, Rabe T, Runnenbaum. Clinical tolerance of a low-dose norgestimate-containing combination oral contraceptive (Cilest) in a West German multicenter study (Heidelberg Multicenter Oral Contraceptive Study). In: Keller PJ, ed. *Aktuelle Aspekte der Hormonalen Kontraception*. Basel: Karger; 1991:67–78.
146. Runnebaum B, Grunwald K, Rabe T. The efficacy and tolerability of norgestimate/ethinyl estradiol (250 micrograms of norgestimate/35 micrograms of ethinyl estradiol): results of an open, multicenter study of 59,701 women. *Am J Obstet Gynecol* 1992;166:1963–1968.
147. Chapdelaine A, Desmarais J-L, Derman RJ. Clinical evidence of the minimal androgenic activity of norgestimate. *Int J Fertil* 1989;34:347–352.
148. Loudon NB, Kirkman RJE, Dewsbury JA. A double-blind comparison of the efficacy and acceptability of Femodene and Microgynon-30. *Eur J Obstet Gynecol Reprod Biol* 1990;34:257–266.
149. Rekers H. Multicenter trial of a monophasic oral contraceptive containing ethinyl estradiol and desogestrel. *Acta Obstet Gynecol Scand* 1988;67:171–174.
150. Gauthier A, Upmalis D, Dain M-P. Clinical evaluation of a new triphasic oral contraceptive: norgestimate and ethinyl estradiol. *Acta Obstet Gynecol Scand* 1992;71(suppl):27–32.
151. Becker H. Supportive European data on a new oral contraceptive containing norgestimate. *Acta Obstet Gynecol Scand* 1990;152(suppl):33–39.
152. Corson SL. Efficacy and clinical profile of a new oral contraceptive containing norgestimate. U.S. clinical trials. *Acta Obstet Gynecol Scand* 1990;152(suppl):25–31.
153. Cullberg G, Hamberger L, Mattson LA, et al. Effects of a low-dose desogestrel-ethinyl estradiol combination on hirsutism, androgens and sex hormone-binding globulin in women with polycystic ovary syndrome. *Acta Obstet Gynecol Scand* 1985;64:195–202.
154. Ruutiainen K. The effect of an oral contraceptive containing ethinyl estradiol and desogestrel on hair growth and hormonal parameters of hirsute women. *Int J Gynaecol Obstet* 1986;24:361–368.
155. Porcile A, Gallardo E. Oral contraceptive containing desogestrel in the maintenance of the remission of hirsutism: monthly versus bimonthly treatment. *Contraception* 1991;44:533–540.
156. Kubba A, Guillebaud J. Combined oral contraceptives: acceptability and effective use. *Br Med Bull* 1993;49:140–157.
157. Thorogood M, Vessey M. Oral contraceptive prescribing in the presence of risk factors. *Br J Fam Plann* 1991;17:2–3.
158. Derman RD. Oral contraceptives: a reassessment. *Obstet Gynecol Surv* 1989;44:662–668.
159. Taggert HM, Applebaum-Bowden D, Haffner S, et al. Reduction in high density lipoprotein by anabolic steroid (Stanozolol) therapy for postmenopausal osteoporosis. *Metabolism* 1982;31:1147–1152.
160. Lipid Research Clinics Program: The Lipid Research Clinics Primary Prevention Trial Results: I. Reduction in incidence of coronary heart disease. *JAMA* 1984;251:351–358.
161. Castelli WP, Doyle JT, Gordon T. HDL cholesterol and other lipids in coronary heart disease. The cooperative lipoprotein phenotyping study. *Circulation* 1977;55:767–772.
162. Gordon T, Castelli WP, Hjortland MC, et al. High density lipoprotein as a protective factor against coronary heart disease. *Am J Med* 1977;62:707–714.
163. Simon D, Senan C, Garnier P, et al. Effects of oral contraceptives on carbohydrate and lipid metabolism in a healthy population: the Telecom Study. *Am J Obstet Gynecol* 1990;163:382–387.

Androgenic Disorders,
edited by G. P. Redmond.
Raven Press, Ltd., New York © 1995.

15

Local Removal of Facial and Body Hair

Richard F. Wagner, Jr.

Department of Dermatology, The University of Texas Medical Branch, Galveston, Texas 77555.

Historically, many cultures across the globe have used various techniques to disguise or eliminate unwanted facial and body hair. Ancient techniques such as shaving and waxing continue to be used into the modern day, albeit modified by technological advancements. The modern era for hair removal dawned in 1875 when Charles Michel, a St. Louis ophthalmologist, reported that abnormal eyelashes (trichiasis) could be successfully treated through electrolysis, an electrochemical destructive technique (1). Dermatologists of the era were quick to apply electrolysis to unwanted hair on other parts of the body (1). The technique lent its name to its practitioners, who became known as electrologists.

In 1924, the French physician Bordier first reported his experience with thermolysis, an electrothermal destructive technique (1). Thermolysis has become the most frequently used technique for permanent hair removal because of its temporal efficiency over the older electrochemical technique. Interestingly, the medical community, consumers, and the electrologists themselves never widely adopted the new title "thermologist" in recognition of the popular technique.

Ionizing radiation is effective but should not be used for hair removal due to the later risk of cancer (2).

CHRONIC NATURE OF HIRSUTISM

There are usually no quick and easy cures for unwanted hair, and patients should be so informed before engaging in electrolysis or thermolysis treatment. Systemic intervention should be considered, especially when an underlying hormonal abnormality can be identified (3). Permanent destruction of unwanted hair usually is approached one hair at a time, and regrowth of unsuccessfully treated hair should be anticipated and explained to the patient. If the hormonal milieu has been controlled, electrolysis treatments typically become less frequent, but nonetheless they are usually required on a periodic basis.

METHODS OF HAIR REMOVAL

Hair removal techniques can be characterized as temporary or permanent with regard to future hair growth from the hair follicle. Temporary techniques (depilation) are of two types: partial removal of hair close to the skin surface (i.e., shaving) and attempted avulsion (epilation) of the entire hair from the hair follicle (plucking and waxing). Although an occasional avulsed hair may not regrow due to permanent damage to the hair follicle, the vast majority of these hairs reappear.

In accepted techniques of permanent hair removal (electrolysis and thermolysis), successful destruction of the germinative area within a hair follicle prevents any more hairs from developing there.

Shaving

Although shaving will neither increase the rate of growth nor the diameter of hair, widespread cultural myth to the contrary continues to abound. Controlling facial hair growth through shaving remains unacceptable to many women because of its masculine connotation. If this cultural obstacle can be surmounted, shaving frequency will relate to the variables of growth rate, diameter, and color, just as it does on skin where shaving is acceptable (4). Shaving is typically done dry with an electric razor or wet with shaving cream or gel (5). Wetting hair causes it to hydrate and soften. Surfactant in shaving preparations facilitates hydration through sebum removal, and alkalinity results in hair swelling (5). Shaving gels have been reported superior to foam preparations because of greater lubrication (comfort) and efficacy (closer shave) (6).

Manual and Automated Hair Avulsion Techniques

Hair plucking is commonly practiced and is usually accomplished with tweezers on a few undesired hairs. In the Middle East and Asia, a teethheld rotating string entraps and avulses multiple hairs as it is moved along the skin surface (7). A case of skin telangiectasia was reported following mechanical hair removal (8).

In waxing hairy areas, the wax is warmed and spread on the treatment site. Once wax hardens it is pulled off in sheets, taking the trapped hair along with it. Thermal burns are a potential hazard if care is not used in applying hot wax, and contact dermatitis may result due to sensitizers (beeswax, rosin, fragrance, and benzocaine) (4). Pretesting small inconspicuous areas of skin (anterior wrist and a postauricular region) before undergoing full waxing is wise in order to attempt detection of a potential allergy (4). Although such steps will not prevent all instances of irritant or contact dermatitis, they increase the probability that sensitive individuals will be identified early so that they may avoid further exposure.

Chemical Depilatories

The common mechanism of action of chemical depilatories is reduction of disulfide bonds in cysteine-rich hair through reducing agents (5). Less irritating thioglycollates are widely preferred over more rapidly acting sulfides because of the unpleasant odor of hydrogen sulfide with the latter (5). The combination of calcium thioglycollate with calcium hydroxide facilitates hair destruction because alkalinity causes hair to swell (5). Enzymatic depilatories containing keratinase from *Streptomyces fradiae* are reported to be less effective (5). Following chemical depilation, a low potency topical steroid has been suggested in order to prevent subsequent irritant dermatitis (4). Allergic contact dermatitis has also been reported to be due to fragrances and mercaptans (4). For this reason, testing small areas of skin (anterior wrist and postauricular region) as previously advised for waxing is advised prior to treating the face or other hairy skin with a depilatory (4).

Electrolysis and Thermolysis

Successful electrolysis and thermolysis are surgical techniques that destroy the germinative hair follicle cells such that no further hair ever develops from that follicle. The combined approach of electrolysis and thermolysis is known as the blend. In both techniques, a probe or needle is inserted into the hair follicle, and a subcutaneous microscar is created that is not visible on the surface of the skin (1). It is a blind procedure because the electrologist cannot directly visualize the probe tip once it enters the hair follicle. The treated hair is then removed with a forceps. Insulated disposable probes are in widespread use for decreased risk of infectious disease and more targeted destruction of the hair follicle (3).

The destruction (via direct current) of a hair follicle during electrolysis occurs because of the generation of lye around the probe (a negative electrode) (1). A current of 0.2 to 2 mA is typically required, and 30 to 60 seconds is a typical treatment time for each hair (1). A positive electrode is required during electrolysis, and it is usually hand-held by the patient (1). Efficiency may be improved by using electrolysis devices that permit multiple probe insertions. Tattooing may occur if the leads are reversed (1). Self-use electrolysis devices are often unsatisfactory (1).

During thermolysis (diathermy), current quickly heats water around the probe, and thermally destroys the hair follicle (1). The most popular thermolysis technique (uniterminal) does not require a grounding electrode. Modern thermolysis equipment allows the operator to select the intensity and duration of settings, which are individualized according to patient pain tolerance and hair characteristics. Flash thermolysis uses high intensity and short duration, and it is the technique most widely used. Promotion of electronic tweezers by manufacturers led Willis to declare that such equipment is "no better than nonelectrified household tweezers" (9).

Complications of electrolysis and thermolysis include viral (warts and herpes simplex) and bacterial (folliculitis) infections. Blood-born infectious disease remains a potential risk if equipment is not sterile (3). Diphtheroid endocarditis has also been reported (10). Noninfectious complications are remarkably similar to other types of surgery and include pain, swelling, erythema, scarring, and pigmentary change (1). Changed sensory perception at the treatment site is also known and is presumptively due to damaged cutaneous nerves after repetitive treatments. A 5% lidocaine/prilocaine eutectic mixture (EMLA cream, Astra Pharmaceutical Products, Inc., Westborough, MA) significantly decreased pain reported by subjects undergoing thermolysis on the upper lip (11).

Surgical Approaches to Unwanted Hair

A much more invasive approach to hirsutism involves surgical incision into the area of unwanted hair growth. The skin is undermined up to 4 cm in all directions and the hair follicles are visualized and removed with a serrated scissor (12). Bouman termed this operation "surgical (subcutaneous) depilation" (12). Continued hair growth in the treatment site is likely due to untreated cycling telogen hairs and vellus hairs that undergo later terminal transformation (12). Surgical (subcutaneous) depilation is not currently a frequent treatment method for hirsutism in the United States. If considered a treatment option in selected instances, careful preoperative planning would be necessary to maximize incision site disguise.

Lasers

Although the argon laser has been used successfully to treat recurrent trichiasis, its advantages for eyelid surgery are liabilities for the treatment of hirsutism. Eyelash follicle destruction by laser creates a small crater that has depth of 2 to 3 mm (13). However, future laser research may be successful in creating technologies that selectively destroy critical elements of the hair follicle that are necessary for hair production without causing visible skin surface damage.

PSEUDOFOLLICULITIS BARBAE

Pseudofolliculitis barbae (PB) is caused by hair piercing the skin in a transfollicular or an extrafollicular manner and results in a foreign body reaction that is initially clinically manifested by papules and pustules (14,15). Black men are predominantly affected in the beard region, but since PB is aggravated by standard shaving techniques and plucking, women attempting to remove unwanted hair may also experience PB (14).

While beard growth is a viable solution for men with PB, this strategy will be rejected by most women. Men who must avoid facial hair typically adopt modified shaving techniques in conjunction with antibiotic therapy that leaves a longer stubble than conventional shaving techniques, but this approach is also unsatisfactory to women who desire complete hair removal. Chemical depilatories may be helpful, and any resulting irritation may be managed through thorough posttreatment rinsing, immediately applied cool compresses, and a low-potency topical corticosteroid (15). The medical literature is divided about the usefulness of electrolysis for PB (14,15).

REFERENCES

1. Wagner RF Jr, Tornich JM, Grande DJ. Electrolysis and thermolysis for permanent hair removal. *J Am Acad Dermatol* 1985;12:441–449.
2. Martin H, Strong E, Spior RH. Radiation-induced skin cancer of the head and neck. *Cancer* 1970;25:61–71.
3. Wagner RF Jr. Medical and technical issues in office electrolysis and thermolysis. *J Dermatol Surg Oncol* 1993;19:575–577.
4. Wagner RF Jr. Physical methods for the management of hirsutism. *Cutis* 1990;45:319–326.
5. Klein AW, Rish DC. Depilatory and shaving products. *Clin Dermatol* 1988;6(3):63–70.
6. Wickett RR, Walter LG. Beard length measurements by image analysis. *Cosmet Toiletr* 1990;105:71–74.
7. Scott MJ Jr, Scott MJ III, Scott AM. Epilation. *Cutis* 1990;46:216–217.
8. Duffy D. Causes of telangiectases. *Schoch Letter* 1993;43(3):10 (item 38).
9. Willis J. Some basics on hair removal products. *FDA Consumer* 1979; October: 25.
10. Cookson WOC, Harris ARC. Diphtheroid endocarditis after electrolysis. *Br Med J* 1981;282:1513–1514.
11. Hjorth N, Harring M, Hahn A. Epilation of upper lip hirsutism with a eutectic mixture of lidocaine and prilocaine used as a topical anesthetic. *J Am Acad Dermatol* 1991;25:809–811.
12. Bouman FG. Surgical depilation for treatment of pseudofolliculitis or local hirsutism of the face. *Plast Reconstr Surg* 1978;62:390–395.
13. Campbell DC. Thermoablation treatment for trichiasis using the argon laser. *Aust N Z J Ophthalmol* 1990;18:427–430.
14. Halder RM. Pseudofolliculitis barbae and related disorders. *Dermatol Clin* 1988;6(3):407–412.
15. Dunn JF Jr. Pseudofolliculitis barbae. *Am Fam Physician* 1988;38(3):169–174.

Subject Index